ESSENTIALS OF **HISTOLOGY**

Freeze-fracture preparation of an isolated β cell from islet of Langerhans of a rat. The nuclear envelope *(N)* with its pores is easily recognizable, and most of the globular profiles in the cytoplasm represent membrane faces of the secretory granules *(SG).* (×30,000.) (From Orci, L., and A. Perrelet. 1975. Freeze-etch histology, Springer-Verlag, New York.)

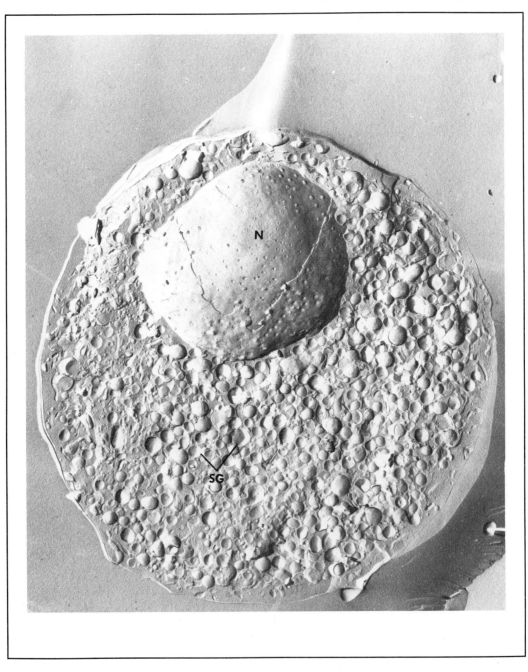

ESSENTIALS OF

HISTOLOGY

GERRIT BEVELANDER

Formerly the University of Texas, Dental Branch,
and the Graduate School of Biomedical Sciences,
Houston, Texas

JUDITH A. RAMALEY

University of Nebraska Medical Center,
Omaha, Nebraska

EIGHTH EDITION
with 446 figures and 6 color plates

THE C. V. MOSBY COMPANY

ST. LOUIS • TORONTO • LONDON   1979

EIGHTH EDITION

Copyright © 1979 by The C. V. Mosby Company

All rights reserved. No part of this book may be reproduced
in any manner without written permission of the publisher.

Previous editions copyrighted 1945, 1952, 1956, 1961, 1965, 1970, 1974

Printed in the United States of America

The C. V. Mosby Company
11830 Westline Industrial Drive, St. Louis, Missouri 63141

Library of Congress Cataloging in Publication Data

Bevelander, Gerrit, 1905-
    Essentials of histology.

    Includes index.
    1. Histology. I. Ramaley, Judith A., 1941-
joint author. II. Title. [DNLM: 1. Histology.
QS504.3 B571e]
QM551.B43   1979   611'.018   78-4847
ISBN 0-8016-0669-1

GW/CB/B 9 8 7 6 5 4 3 2 1

Preface

As in previous editions, our purpose in writing this book has been to provide a clear and concise introduction to the principles of histology, the microanatomy of tissues and organs. We have emphasized the relationship between structure and function to make the text more meaningful, more easily understood, and more relevant to other basic sciences. We have made the assumption that most of the people using this text intend to go into the health professions or biology, and we have attempted to lay the groundwork for the later study and recognition of differences that exist between normal and diseased or repaired tissue (pathology). Before one can understand the changes that occur during injury, healing, and disease, it is necessary to develop a clear idea of what normal tissues look like.

We have made a number of changes in this edition. In every instance our intent was to incorporate more structure-function correlations and to make clear the physiological implications of structure. Several chapters have been completely rewritten (the introduction, nervous tissue, lymphoid organs, male and female reproductive systems, and brain and special sense organs), and others have been substantially revised.

Our thanks go to the many colleagues whose micrographs appear in the text and to the many instructors and students who have given us help over the years in improving the presentation of the material. The text continues to evolve, and we are grateful for the support of our friends in this process.

Gerrit Bevelander
Judith A. Ramaley

Contents

COLOR PLATES

ESSENTIALS OF **HISTOLOGY**

1

Introduction

Histology (*histos*, Gr., web) is the science that deals with the detailed structure of animals and plants and the relationships between the structural organization of cells and tissues and the functions that they perform. The smallest functional unit of living material is the cell, an organized entity capable of maintaining its own integrity, its responsiveness to the environment outside its boundaries, and its unique chemical composition. A cell is fundamentally a container for a complex, chemical organization whose properties would be seriously disrupted if the environment had free access to the interior of the cell.

Tissues are communities of cells embedded in a structural framework or *matrix*. The arrangement of cells, their interconnections, the relationship of the cells to the extracellular matrix, and the properties of the matrix must be understood to develop a concept of how the tissue performs its characteristic functions. For convenience, cell communities are divided into four classes: *nervous tissue*, *muscle*, *connective tissue*, and *epithelial tissue*. As we shall see, each of these tissues has properties that differ considerably from those of the other tissue types.

Organs are composed of tissues arranged in characteristic ways. In this text we will begin with general considerations of cell structure and then go on to tissues and finally organ systems.

PREPARATION OF TISSUE FOR STUDY

Cell and tissue structure and cell products are made visible for study by treating the cells with chemicals that *preserve* the tissue from decay, *fix* the cellular and matrix components in place to prevent distortion, and *stain* the tissue to permit the visualization of cellular and matrix elements that otherwise would lack enough contrast to be easily visible using microscopic techniques.

Living systems are so heterogeneous in composition that no single fixative will work equally well for all constitutents of a cell, a tissue, or an organ. The method of fixation commonly used for routine laboratory work is chemical fixation. In dealing with a particular tissue, an investigator will select a method that meets certain criteria:

1. There should be a minimum of distortion.

2. The fixative should not dissolve tissue components, if possible.

3. The agent should prevent decay (that is, be bactericidal) and should halt the action of cellular enzymes that can cause autodigestion.

4. The agent should help hold cells and tissue in place so that the tissue can be sliced into thin enough sections to permit the visualization of detail. Most chemical fixatives are aqueous solutions containing reagents that work either by coagulating tissue components or by establishing cross-bridges between molecules so that the latter remain in place. An example of a coagulant is ethanol. Ethanol takes up water, thus permitting active groups of protein molecules to make new chemical bonds with each other. These bonds tend to hold the proteins in position. An example of a fixative that works in

a noncoagulating way is formaldehyde. Formaldehyde (HCHO) links to a nitrogen group on a protein to form a hydroxylamine $NH \cdot CH_2OH$, which then can link with another nitrogen group to form a carbon (methylene or CH_2) bridge. The result is that the proteins are linked together. Most fixatives are a mixture of coagulant and noncoagulant chemicals.

For rapid examination of tissue—during surgery, for instance—a tissue may be frozen to harden it and fix the tissue elements and then cut *(sectioned)* immediately.

Once a tissue is preserved and fixed, thin slices *(sections)* must be prepared. It is difficult to see the arrangement of cells in thick pieces of tissue, since the dimensions of individual cells are so small (an average of 7 to 20 micrometers [μm; formerly microns]; see Fig. 1-1). For routine microscopy thin sections of tissue not more than 8 μm thick are cut with an instrument called a *microtome*. Without further treatment, the tissue organization would not be easily visible, since cellular components are nearly uniform in optical density. Special optical systems such as *phase* or *interference microscopy* can be used to visualize tissue elements without staining. Although cell components are of similar optical density, their thickness and orientation within the cell are different, thus impeding to variable extent the light passing through them. If a specimen is illuminated with polarized light in which the light waves are in phase, the light passing through certain regions of a cell or tissue will be slowed down. If the light is split into two beams, one passing through the specimen and one not, the two beams will interfere with each other when they are recombined, since they will now be out of phase. The light waves will add to or cancel out each other, making a brighter or dimmer image that accentuates the contrast and permits visualization of cell components.

More commonly in routine histology, the problem of lack of contrast is solved by treating the tissue with chemicals (stains) producing a color reaction or a precipitate that will be visible under the light microscope. Various stains combine to different extents with particular cellular components and matrix elements, and the resulting color differences serve to highlight the composition of the tissue. To accomplish this, tissues are first stabilized by fixation and then embedded in a material to hold the tissue parts in a natural relationship to each other to prevent distortion during sectioning. Embedding media are chemicals that can be converted easily from a liquid that can penetrate a tissue into a solid that can hold the tissue in place during sectioning. The hardening process or solidification may involve covalent linkages between the embedding molecules, crystallization, or polymerization (that is, formation of long chain–like molecules from shorter ones). A frequently used embedding medium in routine histology is paraffin. It has the advantage of being a quick and simple agent to use; however, it also has the disadvantage of causing considerable shrinkage, since the tissue must be dehydrated before the liquid paraffin can penetrate it. For the much thinner sections that must be made for electron microscopy (see later), various plastics are used that polymerize to form a three-dimensional spongelike framework for the tissue. After a tissue is embedded in plastic, very thin sections can be cut with a minimum of distortion.

Color can be introduced onto a thin tissue slice by treating it with dyes. Often two or more dyes are used that have a selective affinity for tissue components to further heighten the contrast. The most commonly used combination in histology laboratories is hematoxylin and eosin (H and E). In a hematoxylin and eosin section the cytoplasm of cells stains red and the nucleus blue. The cytoplasm contains an abundant protein matrix, and at the pH normally used to stain tissue, many of these proteins have enough basic (positively charged) groups to combine with eosin, an acidic dye whose color is due to its negatively charged anions. The dye hematoxylin is not itself a basic dye but can be made to attach to negatively charged sites by the use of a *mordant,* an agent that has many positive charges, which can link hematoxylin to acidic groups. The nucleus contains nucleic acids whose acidic phosphate groups can combine with hematoxylin with the help of a mordant.

Several other dyes can be used to stain special tissue components such as glycogen or lipids (Table 1).

Color contrast can also be added to living cells by the use of agents that can be taken up by cells. These agents are called *supravital dyes* (Table 1, Janus green B).

Major advances in the understanding of cellular function and tissue organization have been made in the last few years as a result of the introduction of new ways to reveal the structure of cells and the location of constituents of these cells. These techniques have been used to examine the growth and repair processes of cells, the mechanisms by which cells manufacture materials for use outside the cell (such as matrix components or secretory granules), and the modulations of cell structure that occur during events such as cell division or the fertilization of an egg by a sperm. What has happened is that the old stop-action view of cells based on stained dead cells is being replaced by a dynamic view of cells caught in the midst of important functions. A description of these newer techniques will be given throughout the text where appropriate.

STUDY OF TISSUES AND ORGANS

One's view of the organization of cells and tissues is dependent on the degree of detail (smallest size visible) that can be seen through the microscope. The maximum magnification possible with a light microscope is about $1,000\times$, and the smallest detail visible with ordinary student microscopes is about $1\ \mu$m. The latter will vary according to the properties of the optical system and the wavelength used to illuminate the tissue specimen. The limit of resolution depends directly on the minimum contrast detectable by the human eye and the wavelength of the light used, and it varies inversely with the numerical aperture of the lens system. The term *numerical aperture* (NA) is a measure of the light-gathering properties of the lens system and depends on both the light-bending (refractive) properties of the medium used to embed the specimen and the angle at which light enters the field (controlled by

Table 1. Staining characteristics of cell components

	Cell constituent	Chemical constituent	Characteristics
Nucleus	Chromatin	DNA	Purple, blue, or black with hematoxylin—basophilia Blue with toluidine blue—orthochromasia Blue-green with methyl green—pyronin
	Nucleolus	RNA	Purple, blue, or black with hematoxylin—basophilia Red with toluidine blue—metachromasia Red with methyl green—pyronin
		Deoxyribose	Red-purple with Feulgen reaction
Cytoplasm			
	Ground substance	Protein	Pink-red with eosin—acidophilia, eosinophilia
	Mitochondria	Complex	Blue with Janus green B supravital, black with iron hematoxylin, red with acid fuchsin
Organoids	Centrioles	Protein	Rarely seen in hematoxylin and eosin, black with iron hematoxylin
	Chromophil substance	RNA	Same as nucleolus
	Fibrils	Protein	Special methods, argyrophil in nerve cells
	Lipids	Fats	Blackened by osmic acid—osmiophilia Negative image in hematoxylin and eosin removed by solvents
Inclusions	Zymogen	Protein	Red with eosin—acidophilia
	Mucigen glycogen	Carbohydrate	Removed by solvents in routine hematoxylin and eosin negative image; red to purple with PAS

the condensor). It follows, then, that the resolution of the field will depend on how well the slide was prepared and how well the microscope is adjusted, as well as on several other considerations.

The best theoretical numerical aperture obtainable with the light microscope is 1.4× for oil immersion and 1.0× for high dry (40× objective). This limits resolution to a theoretical maximum of about 0.2 μm using short wavelength (blue) light. The electron microscope employs beams of electrons having properties much like light but of ultrashort wavelength. However, since the electrons in the short wavelengths of the beam can be captured by air particles in their path, the beam and the specimen must be placed in a vacuum. The electron beam is focused by magnets that serve the same function as lenses in an optical system using visible light. The first electron microscope designs required that electrons pass through the specimen to generate an image. This technique is called *transmission electron microscopy.* Within the past few years, two new techniques have been developed in which whole specimens or thick sections rather than thin sections can be bombarded with an electron beam and a three-dimensional view of the tissue surface obtained by detecting the patterns of scattered electrons. These techniques are called *scanning electron microscopy* and *high-voltage transmission electron microscopy.*

Contrast in electron microscopy is ob-tained by treating the tissue with heavy metals that impede the passage of electrons (that is, electron-dense chemicals) or by forming precipitates that are electron dense using antigen-antibody reactions. A new field has arisen in which tissue compounds can be identified in this manner (*immunocytochemistry*). Heavy metal salts such as osmium are often used as combined fixative and "staining" agents. Osmium is taken up to a different degree by the various cellular components. To heighten contrast, other heavy metal salts of lead and uranium are applied to thin sections *after* they are cut. This process is called *shadowing* and can be employed to show the contours of cellular elements. A commonly used technique is *freeze-fracture etching.* In this technique a tissue is frozen quickly in liquid nitrogen and then shattered along natural lines of cleavage in the tissue. The surface is then etched with metals and an image obtained of the surface texture. Freeze-fracture etching permits visualization of the location of proteins within membranes, for example.

Fig. 1-1 gives an idea of the sizes of objects normally studied in anatomy. The usual range encountered in histology varies from the limit of resolution of most student microscopes (1.0 μm) to the limit of resolution of the unaided human eye (0.1 mm or 100 μm). Cells range in size from 8 μm (red blood cells) to 150 μm (ripe ova). The size of most cells falls between these two values. For approximating cell size in a tissue sec-

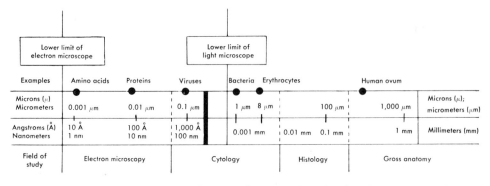

Fig. 1-1. Size of objects encountered in the study of anatomy. Note that there has been a terminology change in referring to the size of objects in histology. A micron (μ) is now a micrometer (μm), a millimicron (mμ) is now a nanometer (nm), and an Angstrom unit (Å) is now 0.1 nm. You are likely to encounter *both* sets of units, and so you should be familiar with both.

tion, the red blood cell is a useful standard. It measures approximately 8 μm in diameter and is usually present in the vasculature of most tissue. However, it must be remembered that processing tissues almost always causes some variation in the cell size.

One of the main objectives should be to develop an ability to visualize and construct a three-dimensional image of the cell or tissue from the flat, roughly two-dimensional object found on the microscope slide. To demonstrate how an object can apparently change in shape depending on how it is cut, one should consider the appearance of a simple spherical object such as an orange that has been cut in several planes (Fig. 1-2). The segments of the orange vary in shape depending on the *plane* of the section. The same kinds of variation will arise in connection with the study of cell and tissue structure.

Cellular detail visible with the light microscope is somewhat limited even when special stains are used, since most organelles are smaller than the resolution of the light microscope. For this reason it is essential to learn to recognize cells and tissues on the basis of several simple criteria. For example, one clue useful in identifying cell types is the appearance of the nucleus. In examining a slide of loose connective tissue (Fig. 3-7, for example), one can readily observe that the nuclei differ from each other in size, shape, staining intensity, presence or absence of nucleoli, degree of clumping of chromatin, and distinctness of the nuclear envelope (visible at the light microscope level only because of a rim of chromatin attached to it). Usually little if any cytoplasm is visible, and in addition the boundaries between cells may be indistinct. When cytoplasm *is* visible, the presence of variations in its staining properties (regions of basophilia, for instance) or the presence of visible inclusions (glycogen, pigment granules, vacuoles left by dissolved fats) should be noted. The identification of cells or tissues on the basis of color alone is not feasible because of

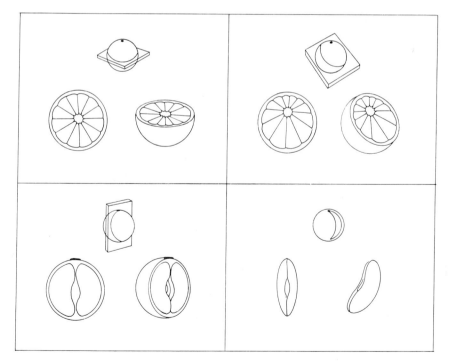

Fig. 1-2. Effects of plane of section on appearance of an object. Upper left, Orange cut perpendicular to long axis segments (cross section); lower left, orange cut parallel to long axis of segments (longitudinal section); upper right, orange cut obliquely to axis of segments (tangential); lower right, appearance of segments in space (three dimensional). (Drawing by Emily Craig.)

the diverse coloration that stained specimens may exhibit.

Another aspect of prepared specimens used in the study of histology both clinically and experimentally is the presence of *artifacts*. Poor tissue preservation or too long a delay before fixation results in autolysis (self-digestion) of the tissue and disruption and shrinkage or swelling of the cells. As slides age, the stain fades, reducing color contrast. Such distortions in the appearance of normal tissues may be present in the slides available for study.

THE CELL AND HOW ITS PROPERTIES CAN BE STUDIED

Most cells consist of a single *nucleus* embedded in *cytoplasm*. The entire unit is surrounded by a boundary called the *plasma* or *cell membrane* (Fig. 1-3). The membrane controls the movement of chemicals into and out of the cell and thus regulates the chemical environment in which cellular function takes place.

With the light microscope it is possible to see small areas of cytoplasm that differ from the rest. Early in the history of histology these regions were suspected of playing a role in cell function and were referred to as *organelles*. In the past 30 years the structure and function of these organelles, as well as other smaller cellular constituents not visible at light microscope level, have been elucidated by electron microscopy, by the study of cell fractions obtained from centrifugation, and by histochemical and autoradiographic techniques. Cellular components can be separated from each other in a centrifugal field because they differ in density, and it is possible to obtain *fractions* rich in membranes or organelles of different size and shape. The chemistry and ac-

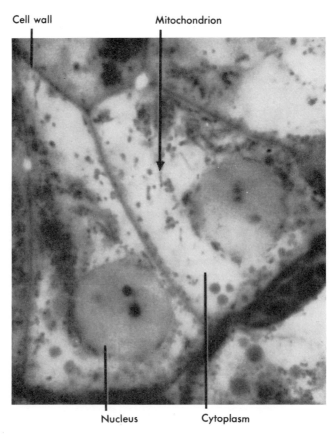

Fig. 1-3. Liver cells of turtle showing the nucleus, cytoplasm, mitochondria, and other cell features visible at a light microscope level. (Iron hematoxylin; ×1,000.)

tivities of these fractions can then be studied.

Autoradiographic techniques can be used to mark the position of cellular components. For example, a radioactively labeled amino acid can be used to indicate where cell protein synthesis is taking place. Also, once the amino acid has been incorporated into protein, the fate of the protein can be followed. *Histochemistry* consists of identifying products of enzyme activity in a cell by looking for accumulations of a marker substance such as a colored dye. In the ovary, for example, the enzyme steroid 3-beta-ol-dehydrogenase is necessary for progesterone synthesis, and its activity changes with age and with reproductive status. The location of the enzyme activity can be visualized by a series of chemical reactions in which the hydrogen ions released from a steroid nucleus as it is metabolized by the action of the enzyme are made to react with a dye called neotetrazolium. The resulting product is purple and easily seen in the tissue.

Within the past few years it has become possible to locate specific proteins within cells by means of the technique called *immunocytochemistry.* Proteins differ from each other on the basis of size, shape, and electrical charge, and they can be used as antigens (foreign chemicals) in an antigen-antibody reaction. As part of the immune defense system, animals are able to produce antibodies to specific antigens. Once an antibody reacts with a specific tissue protein, it can be visualized in various ways by tagging it with a chemical that will fluoresce or that will produce a colored product after suitable chemical conversions are performed. Such techniques have been used, for example, to locate which cells in the pituitary produce and store specific hormones.

Cellular membranes

The three types of cellular membranes that will be considered here are the cell membrane (plasmalemma), the endoplasmic reticulum, and the Golgi apparatus. The nuclear membrane will be considered later. All these membranes serve as partitions, separating one part of the cellular environment from another. Each compartment marked off by membranes has a unique chemistry and represents a miniature space in which particular cellular reactions take place. The plasmalemma forms the interface between the cell and the outside solution in which it resides. The other membranes form intracellular compartments intimately concerned with cellular *metabolism* (the sum of the chemical processes that take place in a cell).

The molecular architecture of cellular membranes has been studied primarily in the red blood cell, a source of readily available, easy-to-isolate membrane material. According to chemical analysis, the red blood cell membrane is about 50% protein and about 50% lipid. The lipid is made up of cholesterol (one third) and polar phospholipids (the remaining two thirds) whose primary property is that they have one end soluble in aqueous solutions and one end soluble in lipid. Lipids provide the matrix of membranes. Early electron micrographs of cell membranes stained with osmium showed two thin lines of electron-dense material separated by a narrow space. On the basis of this morphology and the chemical composition of membranes, Davson and Danielli and later Robertson developed a model of membrane structure, the unit membrane hypothesis, in which it was proposed that the phospholipids are arranged in a continuous bilayer (double layer) with the nonpolar ends of the lipids facing inward and the polar ends facing toward the surface of the membrane.* The heads of the phospholipids were thought to be embedded in a surface coating of protein running in continuous sheets. In recent years it has been possible to localize proteins within the membrane, and it is now clear that the older unit membrane hypothesis cannot adequately explain the properties of membranes. A new membrane model generally known as the *fluid mosaic model* was developed by Singer and Nicolson to take the

---

* For a review of membrane structure, see Singer, S. J., and G. L. Nicholson. 1972. The fluid mosaic model of the structure of cell membranes. Science **175**:720-731.

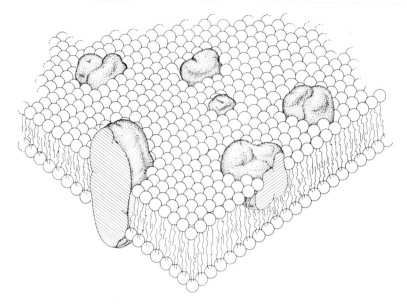

Fig. 1-4. Fluid mosaic model of cell membrane. Note lipid matrix consists of phospholipid bilayer with proteins floating in it, some passing through entire membrane, some projecting from one surface only. (From Singer, S. J., and G. L. Nicholson. 1972. Science **175:**720-731, Feb. 18; copyright 1972 by the American Association for the Advancement of Science.)

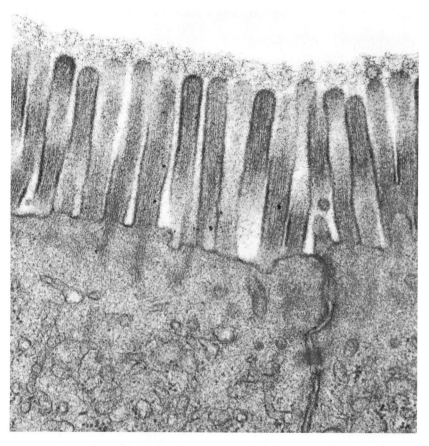

Fig. 1-5. Electron micrograph of microvilli forming striated border of small intestine of mouse and showing surface coat (glycocalyx) at periphery of microvilli. (×60,000.) (Courtesy Dr. Caramia, University of Rome.)

newer data into account. It is still suggested that the lipid forms a continuous bilayer, but it is now proposed that proteins float in this lipid, some proteins extending through the membrane and projecting onto both the intracellular and extracellular surfaces, others reaching only the inside or outside (Fig. 1-4). In this model the inner surface and the outer surface of the membrane have different properties.

Plasma (cell) membrane

The plasmalemma or cell membrane consists of two basic zones. Coating the surface of the cell membrane facing the outside world is a cell coat or glycocalyx (sweet husk) (Fig. 1-5) consisting of a fuzzy shell of carbohydrate-containing protein (glycoproteins) and lipid (glycolipids). The properties of the glycocalyx determine cell recognition, cell adhesiveness, movement, and maintenance of form. The inner zone consists of the basic fluid-mosaic membrane. Proteins projecting all the way through the membrane are probably involved in shuttle systems that move electrolytes and small metabolites such as amino acids and glucose into and out of the cell. Proteins that stud the inner surface of the membrane facing the cell cytoplasm are concerned with the regulation of cell metabolism and the initiation of cellular responses to chemical signals from outside, such as hormones.

Endoplasmic reticulum

The endoplasmic reticulum (ER) was originally named by early electron microscopists who found a series of intracellular membranes deep within the cell (the cell center was then called the endoplasm). Since that time it has become clear that the membranes are not confined to the deep parts of the cell. In all living cells, specific activities of great complexity are localized in different membrane types that channel the passage of macromolecules from one place to another within the cell. The ER consists of two basic components—granular (rough) and agranular (smooth). The rough ER consists of platelike flat channels (cisternae) stacked in piles.

Studding the surface of these plates are ribosomes, the cellular organelle on which protein synthesis takes place (Fig. 1-6). The rough ER is best developed in cells that elaborate a protein-rich secretory product. When subcellular fractions of the ER are obtained, they are referred to as *microsomes*. Other cells that make protein for internal use have many cytoplasmic ribosomes alone or in clusters (*polyribosomes*) but a poor membrane system.

Smooth ER consists of a latticelike arrangement of tubules. These membranes are involved in detoxification processes in the liver and in lipid and steroid metabolism in the testes and ovaries. In skeletal muscle the smooth ER plays a role in the coupling between surface stimulation of the cell and the initiation and cessation of muscular contraction (stimulation-contraction coupling). The membranes may serve as an intracellular transport system for nascent proteins and lipids and also a communication system be-

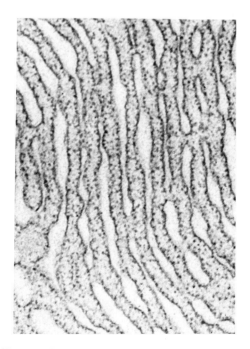

Fig. 1-6. Electron micrograph of portion of parotid gland showing profiles of the rough (granular) endoplasmic reticulum cisternae studded with ribosomes. (×50,000.) (Courtesy Dr. S. Luse.)

tween the surface and the interior of the skeletal cells, as in muscle cells.

Smooth and rough ER differ in chemical composition and enzyme content and clearly perform different functions. In the membranes from the enzyme-secreting part of the pancreas (acinar pancreas), for instance, the cholesterol-phospholipid ratio of the rough ER is about 0.02, whereas that of the smooth ER is 0.47. Differences in the lipid-protein ratio and the composition of individual lipids have also been found. The protein in rough ER is replaced every 5 days, on the average, with larger proteins being replaced more often than small proteins (an average of 4 and 28 days, respectively). The figures are dif-

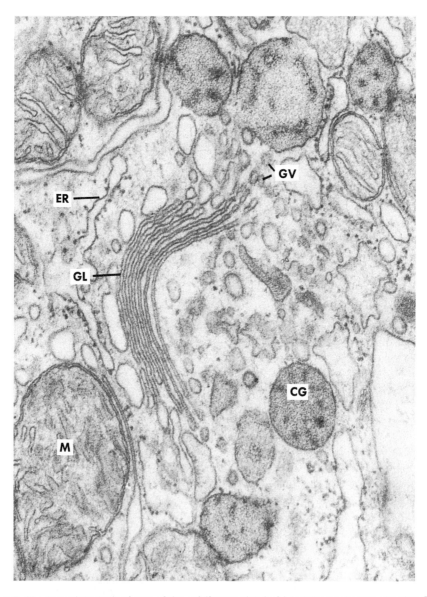

Fig. 1-7. Electron micrograph of part of the calciferous gland of *Lumbricus terrestris* showing Golgi apparatus. Note proximity of rough endoplasmic reticulum, *ER,* to stacks of Golgi lamellae, *GL,* which transmit and modify protein derived from *ER*. The material is then conveyed to the Golgi vesicles, *GV,* which undergo further changes in the cytoplasm, as represented by condensing vacuoles *(CG),* which are eventually extruded at the free surface of the cell. *M,* Mitochondria. (×77,000.)

ferent for smooth ER, being 3 and 13 days. The need for repair and replacement of membranes should be clear when it is considered that the pancreas produces 40 mg of protein in every secreting cycle (associated with a meal) for export. There is also a lot of intracellular traffic that requires a continual replacement of membranes (see discussion on Golgi apparatus). The enzymes detected so far in smooth ER are involved in glycogenolysis and steroid production, whereas those in the rough ER are concerned with energy transfer and release, which is required to provide the energy that drives protein synthesis.

Golgi apparatus

In light microscopy the Golgi apparatus or complex appears as a clear area in actively secreting cells such as the acinar cells of the pancreas or bone-forming cells (osteoblasts). It consists of a stack of more or less flat membranous vesicles called *saccules*, which resemble a pile of hotcakes (Figs. 1-7 and 1-8). The stack is curved so that the convex surface faces the ER. This face is referred to as the *immature* face, since it seems to be receiving a shower of small vesicles that are budded off the ER. The other face is called *mature* and appears to be discharging many small vesicles. The rough ER makes two sets of proteins, one for export and one for local use within the cell. As the newly synthesized protein is released from the ER, it can follow two not necessarily related routes. In secretory cells the protein becomes concentrated within *condensing vacuoles* that, in turn, mature into *secretory granules*. These granules eventually migrate to the cell surface, perhaps moved by contractile elements with-

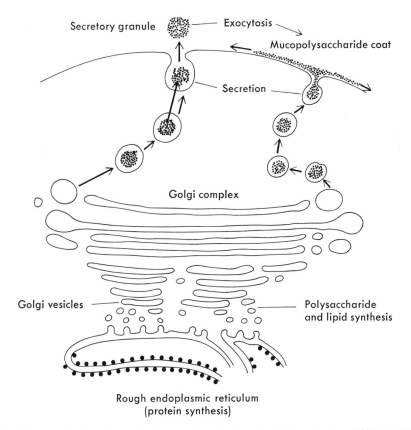

Fig. 1-8. Golgi complex showing origin from rough endoplasmic reticulum, fusion of Golgi vesicles to form stacks of smooth endoplasmic reticulum, and conveyance of product-containing secretory vesicles to cell exterior, liberating either secretory granules or extracellular coat. (From Berrill, N.J., and G. Karp. 1975. Development. McGraw-Hill Book Co., New York. Used with permission of McGraw-Hill Book Co.)

in the cell (microfilaments and microtubules, see later), and are discharged by a process called *exocytosis*. Other packets of newly manufactured protein arise from the Golgi apparatus or a complex meshwork of Golgi, ER, and enzyme-filled lysosomes (see later). This complex is referred to as GERL (an acronym formed from the words *Golgi, ER,* and *Lysosome*). The mature or forming face of the Golgi apparatus elaborates many *primary lysosomes* (see later).

The Golgi apparatus appears to act as a collecting system for large molecular weight (macromolecular) secretory products. Stacks of Golgi plates form clusters called *dictyosomes*, which may exist as a single large apparatus in some mammalian cells or as smaller membrane clusters scattered through the cell. Certain sugar-transferring enzymes (glycosyltransferases) are located exclusively in the Golgi membranes and serve as markers for biochemical studies of membranes. The Golgi apparatus appears to add terminal sugars to a number of glycoproteins (carbohydrate-containing proteins).

Lysosomes

A cell contains many round bubblelike vesicles sometimes with clear, homogeneous contents and sometimes with dense material or structured material within them. Some of these cell packets are concerned with intracellular functions, others with the packaging of materials for export.

The lysosome is a small, round membrane-bound organelle about 0.25 to 0.5 μm in diameter. It contains acid hydrolases, enzymes that break down proteins, nucleic acids, and carbohydrates at acidic pH. Lysosomes are found in almost all cells except red blood cells and fully keratinized skin cells. They seem to represent the "digestive system" of a cell. A freshly formed lysosome budded off the Golgi apparatus is called a *primary lysosome.* If the cell picks up foreign material (by a process called cell-eating or phagocytosis), the resulting food vacuole is called a *phagosome* (Fig. 1-9). The material in the phagosome is digested after a lysosome fuses with it and releases its digestive enzymes. The resulting packet of material, which represents a fused lysosome and phagosome, is called a *phagolysosome.* If the material inside the phagolysosome cannot be digested, usually due to a deficiency of a specific lysosomal hydrolase, lysosome storage diseases can occur. If the cell is situated along an excretory channel such as the bile

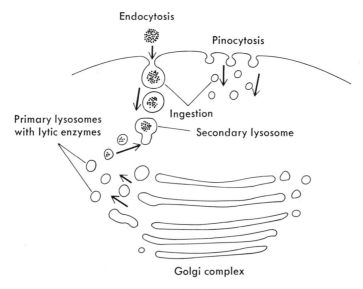

Fig. 1-9. Golgi–endoplasmic reticulum–lysosome (GERL) system is shown with primary lysosomes originating from Golgi complex and fusing with endocytic vesicles from cell surface (left) to form secondary lysosomes. (From Berrill, N.J., and G. Karp. 1975. Development. McGraw-Hill Book Co., New York. Used with permission of McGraw-Hill Book Co.)

canaliculi of the liver, the phagolysosome with its consumed material will eventually be extruded from the cell. If not, the packaged remnants will be retained within the cell to form an aging product often containing pigmented material called lipofuscin or lipochrome. In addition to assisting in the digestion of ingested materials, lysosomes take part in cellular growth and repair processes by removing damaged or excess cellular components. Cell breakdown during morphogenesis or cell death (autolysis) in many disease processes is due to the release of lysosomal enzymes. Self-destruction (autophagy) occurs when smooth ER envelops a structure to be consumed and an autophagic vacuole is formed. This vacuole is then inoculated with enzymes from a lysosome. Both phagocytic and autophagic vacuoles are called *secondary lysosomes* (Fig. 1-9). Gradually a cell fills up with these vacuoles, and as the contents of the vacuoles are processed and degraded, the vacuoles become residual or dense bodies.

Cell disruption can be activated by a variety of stimuli including starvation, ultraviolet irradiation, bacterial toxins, lack of adequate blood supply (ischemia), and the cell becoming filled up with autophagic vacuoles.

Some cells contain lysosomes with other materials in them in addition to acid hydrolases. Granular leukocytes, for instance, contain lysosomes with several basic proteins that destroy bacterial cell coats or attract other leukocytes to the scene of a bacterial invasion.

Microbodies (peroxisomes)

Microbodies are small membrane-lined vesicles 0.3 to 0.5 μm wide that resemble lysosomes except that they contain oxidative enzymes such as catalase and urate oxidase rather than acid hydrolases. They occur in abundance in liver and kidney cells and are primitive oxidative organelles that may serve to protect cells against hydrogen peroxide generated during oxidations.

Mitochondria

Mitochondria (Figs. 1-7 and 1-10) are the primary energy source for cells that are aerobic (that is, use oxygen in the process of energy production from glucose). Within mitochondria, molecular oxygen is used to oxidize metabolites to carbon dioxide and water. Much of the available energy liberated from the cleavage of pyruvate in the steplike sequence of oxidative phosphorylation is trapped by coupling the synthesis of adenosine triphosphate (ATP) to this process.

A mitochondrion is built of two membrane systems, an outer one about 7 nm (70 Å) in thickness and an inner one of about the same thickness, the two being separated by a narrow space 8 nm (80 Å) in width. The membranes form a continuous system like two sealed plastic bags, one inside the other. The inner membrane is folded into shelflike projections called *cristae*, which protrude into the center of the mitochondrion and greatly enhance the surface area available for energy production.

The outer membrane is selectively permeable to ions, thus controlling the internal environment of the organelle. It also contains monoamine oxidase, an enzyme required for oxidation of monoamines, chemicals that are important in neural transmission. The inner membrane is even more selective, allowing passage only of water, short-chain fatty acids, and a few small uncharged molecules like urea or glycerol. The compartment housed inside the inner membrane is thus different from the space between the two membranes.

The inner membrane contains the enzymes required for electron transport and phosphorylation and is studded with small knoblike projections (visible only after disruption of the membranes and special staining) that contain the enzyme complexes required for ATP formation. The space between the cristae is called the *matrix*. It is generally homogeneous and faintly granular and may contain occasional dense granules 30 to 50 nm in diameter. These granules can bind cations like calcium and are found in larger numbers in cells that accumulate calcium, such as osteoblasts. In the matrix are found the enzymes required for the tricarboxylic acid cycle (Krebs cycle), which provides the substrates for ATP formation,

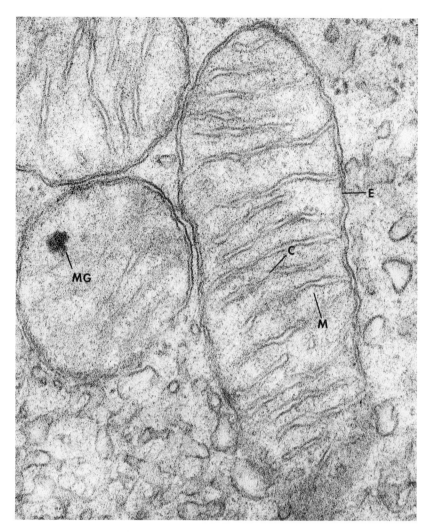

Fig. 1-10. Electron micrograph showing mitochondria from monkey kidney in longitudinal and transverse section. *C,* Cristae; *E,* external envelope; *M,* matrix; *MG,* matrix granule. (×70,000.) (Courtesy Dr. H. Nakahara.)

and some DNA, which codes for mitochondrial proteins.

Mitochondria are variable in size and shape and can be seen to be in constant movement within living cells. In section they may be caught at all angles and thus may appear to be even more variable than they really are. The number and shape of the cristae and the number and location of the mitochondria within the cell depend on the energy requirements and metabolic activity of cells. For example, cristae are usually platelike, but in steroid-producing or lipid-metabolizing cells the cristae are tubular.

Cells that have an active respiratory function have more mitochondria, with abundant cristae. In relatively inactive cells the mitochondria are few in number and are simple in structure. Cells involved in the active transport of materials across epithelial surfaces (as in the kidney or gut lining), synthesis of fat from carbohydrate (adipose cells), or conversion of chemical energy to mechanical work (muscle cells) have a larger number of mitochondria with a profusion of cristae. Many cells have mitochondria located in special cell sites. In cardiac muscle mitochondria exist in tight narrow rows between the con-

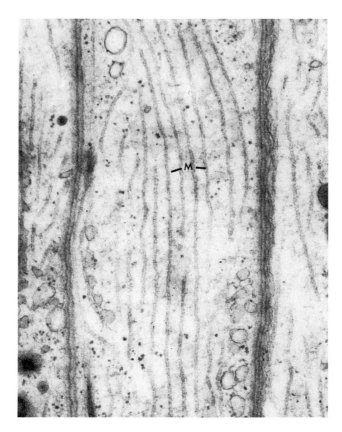

Fig. 1-11. Electron micrograph of longitudinal section of several microtubules, *M*, from marginal gland of *Littorina*. (×46,000.)

tractile elements. In the sperm tail the mitochondria are wrapped in a tight spiral around the upper end of the tail. In epithelial tissue that transports water or other materials from one side of the tissue sheet to the other, the mitochondria are in narrow compartments or interdigitations along the cell surface. In cells containing lipids, the mitochondria are often located along the edges of the lipid droplets.

Microtubules

Classical cytologists described a number of threadlike fibrils and filaments within cells, usually basing their classification on the cell or tissue type in which the fibrils were found. With the advent of the electron microscope, the fibrillar components of cells were resolved into two types, filaments and microtubules (Fig. 1-11). Under special conditions, microtubules can be seen in cells (in

tissue fixed in glutaraldehyde at room temperature) as hollow straight cylinders measuring 24 nm (240 Å) in diameter and of variable length. Each microtubule is composed of smaller spiralling filamentous structures about 4 to 5 nm in diameter, which themselves are made up of smaller globular subunits of a protein called *tubulin*. They are found in nearly all cell types; although they may play many roles, the functions most commonly ascribed to them are that they form part of a motile system (as in the central core of cilia and flagella, see later), an intracellular transport system (as in the axons of nerve cells, where they may serve as conveyor belts to move materials down the long cytoplasmic process), and a supportive or "skeletal" function (in red blood cells). Microtubules may play a role in the changes in cell shape that occur during cellular differentiation. They also are thought to be involved

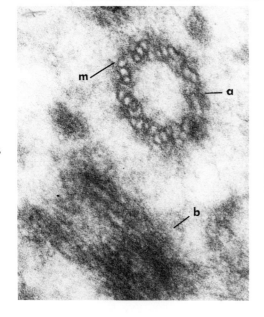

Fig. 1-12. A, Electron micrograph of rat eosinophil showing *C,* centrioles; *Cr,* crystalloid in specific granule; *G,* Golgi complex; *M,* mitochondrion. **B,** Electron micrograph of centrioles from rat nasal epithelium. *a,* Sectioned transversely; *b,* tangentially; *m,* triplets of fused microtubules. (**A** ×40,000; **B** ×140,000.) (Courtesy Dr. H. Nakahara.)

in the movement of chromosomes during cell division.

Microtubules exist either as single units or as groups in parallel array, fused sometimes into two's or three's, as in the core of cilia or the motile apparatus of the sperm tail (Fig. 18-1). They are constantly being dissolved and reformed from globular tubulin subunits, a process that can be blocked by the drugs colchicine or vinblastine. Only the tubules of cilia, centrioles, and basal bodies seem to resist these agents and hence are stable microtubule elements within the cell.

Basal bodies and centrioles

Near the nucleus is a specialized zone called the *centrosome,* which contains two small organelles called *centrioles* (Fig. 1-12). These two structures (together called the *diplosome*) are concerned with cell division and are the source of the mitotic spindle that forms during chromosome division. Basal bodies *(kinetosomes)* are similar structures associated with the motile processes of cells —the cilia and flagella (Figs. 1-13 and 1-14). Both organelles are hollow cylinders approximately 0.15 μm in diameter and 0.3 to 0.5

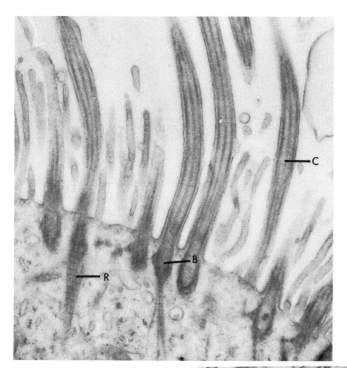

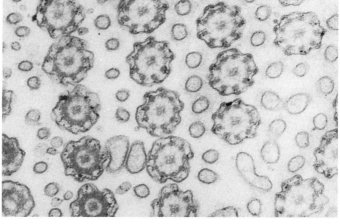

Fig. 1-13. Electron micrograph of longitudinal section of cilia, *C,* of epithelial lining of cat bronchiole; *R,* rootlet. Internal longitudinal filaments are continuous with basal bodies, *B.* ($\times$25,000.)

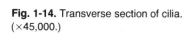

Fig. 1-14. Transverse section of cilia. ($\times$45,000.)

μm in length. The walls of these small barrellike organelles are composed of nine sets of three microtubules (triplets) arranged in an evenly spaced circle parallel to the long axis of the cylinder and embedded in a dense amorphous material, one end of which closes the cylinder. The two centrioles lie at right angles to each other in the nonmitotic cell and undergo replication as a cell prepares for mitotic division. After they replicate, the centrioles become associated with the microtubules of the mitotic spindle *(aster)* and are responsible for the movement of chromosomes during mitosis.

In cells that have motile processes, the centrioles replicate and the new centrioles migrate to the cell surface. Each centriole then becomes a basal body from which a cilium or flagellum arises.

Cilia and flagella

Cilia and flagella are composed of microtubules and are motile cellular processes. Ciliated cells are found in portions of the respiratory tract, in the female reproductive tract, and in the male reproductive tract. In all these channels the cilia serve to move along fluids and maintain a constant mixing action on the cell surface. In the respiratory tract they transport mucus. In the reproductive tracts, cilia move mucus and sperm and eggs along the tubes.

Each cilium or flagellum develops from a single basal body that is, as already indicated, a replicate of the cell centrioles. To form a cilium, microtubules of the ciliary shaft (called the *axoneme*) grow outward from the end of the basal body facing the cell surface and become the core of the cilium, which then pushes upward, taking a surface layer of cell membrane with it. As the axoneme grows, only two of the triplet microtubules elongate. As a result, the core of a cilium consists of a row of nine doublets instead of the triplets that make up the wall of the basal body. In addition, two single microtubules develop inside the ring of doublets.

Cilia beat at regular intervals to move fluids and mucus. The stroke consists of a stiff sweep forward, then a relaxation as the cilium is drawn back to its starting position. Mucus is swept forward in the active part of the stroke only, and then the cilium moves back through the mucus in a bent position. This permits a directional movement of mucus, since the limp backstroke does not move the mucus back in the opposite direction.

The only real differences between a cilium and a flagellum are that the latter is longer and cells generally possess only one or two flagella. In mammals the only flagellum-bearing cell is the sperm cell.

Fibers and filaments

Slender elongated threadlike structures occur in the cytoplasm of a wide variety of cells. They are of indeterminate length, vary from 3 to 15 nm in diameter, and are arranged as a meshwork of regularly oriented bundles. The terminology in reference to these structures is somewhat confusing but in general is related to size. A *filament* or microfilament is only visible with the electron microscope and has a diameter of 4 to 10 nm. A *fibril* consists of bundles or *fascicles* of filaments measuring 0.5 to 0.1 μm in diameter and is visible with the oil immersion lens. A *fiber* consists of a bundle of fibrils and is visible with low magnification. The term fiber is also used to designate some kinds of cells, for example, muscle (fiber) cells. The striated muscle cell illustrates all three subdivisions mentioned.

Microfilaments are closely related to microtubules. The larger filaments (10 nm) form cytoskeletal elements conferring rigidity to cytoplasm; the smaller filaments (3 to 7 nm) contain contractile protein (actinomyosin) and are associated with cell movement such as that occurring in a single-celled ameba or a muscle cell. Both large and small microfilaments are present in microvilli of epithelial cells as a *terminal web*, a supporting structure. Microfilaments are numerous in neurons and their processes where they serve as cytoskeletal structures; they may also be associated with transport of materials along the nerve fibers. In microvilli there are also contractile microfilaments.

Cytoplasmic inclusions

Inclusions are materials found in cells that may or may not be in organized organelles. A common inclusion is stored food, in the form of glycogen or fat. Glycogen is found primarily in liver and in skeletal muscle, usually in small clusters called rosettes or as individual particles 15 to 30 nm in diameter (Fig. 1-15). Glycogen is often found associated with smooth endoplasmic reticulum or within lysosomal particles. Fat is found as small globules within many cells but is most prominent in adipose cells where it is stored as triglycerides in a liquid form at body temperature.

Another type of inclusion is pigment. Some pigments are of exogenous origin, picked up from outside the body. Examples include dusts in the lung, minerals in bone, and lipochromes or carotenoids from food. There also are endogenous pigments such as hemoglobin or its pigmented metabolites hemosiderin (a golden brown pigmented deposit seen in phagosomes in liver and spleen) or bilirubin (a yellowish, noniron-containing breakdown product found in liver cells).

Cells in the skin and in the eye contain a brown-black pigment called melanin. As animals age, cells in the heart, liver, and central nervous system usually accumulate a brownish pigment called *lipofuscin.* This aging product may represent residual indigestible material in old lysosomes.

Finally, steroid-secreting cells may contain crystalline arrays of great complexity in the nucleus or the cytoplasm. The origin and function of these crystalline bodies are unknown.

Nucleus

The nucleus dominates the cellular architecture and forms at times the only identifiable characteristic of a cell at the light microscope level. At this level it is possible to identify a thin surrounding *nuclear envelope* or membrane, one or more darkly staining *nucleoli*, a series of finely granular or coarsely patchlike particles of *chromatin*, and regions of pale, amorphous material.

The nuclear envelope encloses a space in which are preserved most of the cellular deoxyribonucleic acid (DNA), the macromole-

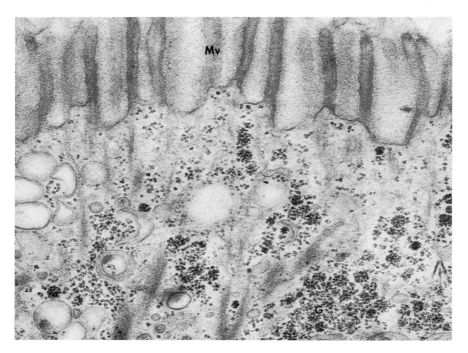

Fig. 1-15. Electron micrograph of part of epithelial cell showing clusters of dark granules, *G* (glycogen), arranged in form of rosettes. *Mv,* Microvilli. (×45,000.)

cules in which are stored the genetic information of the cell, along with associated basic proteins, especially *histones*. In procaryotic cells the genetic material is not segregated from the cytoplasm, whereas in eucaryotic cells it is enveloped in a membrane. The reasons for this segregation are only beginning to be understood. The properties of the nuclear membrane determine the chemical composition of the space surrounding the genetic material and govern the exchanges that take place between the contents of the nucleus and the cytoplasm (*nucleocytoplasmic interactions*). To understand the problems that must be solved by the nucleus, it is necessary to review briefly what we know about the process of copying information from the genetic material (*transcription*) and the means by which this information is used in protein sythesis (*translation*) for the regulation of cell function.

The process of genetic transcription requires an understanding of how information can be coded in the nucleic acids DNA and RNA. The primary information storage is in DNA. This information is read off onto a template that can be used for protein synthesis. The template is RNA. Nucleic acids consist of a sugar (pentose or deoxypentose), nitrogenous bases (purines and pyrimidines), and phosphoric acid. The long macromolecule of DNA or RNA is made up of a chain of linked units called *nucleotides*, each of which results from the combination of one molecule of phosphoric acid, one of pentose, and one of purine or pyrimidine. The phosphoric acid and pentose (ribose in RNA and deoxyribose in DNA) form a backbone joining the purines and pyrimidines together (Fig. 1-16). Attached to the sugar is a nitrogenous base (the purines adenine and guanine in both RNA and DNA and the pyrimidines cytosine and thymidine in DNA and cytosine and uracil in RNA). In DNA two chains of nucleotides wind around each other in a double helix, with the purines and pyrimidines projecting inward in complementary pairs. The varying sequence of the four nitrogenous bases along the DNA chain forms the basis for the coding of genetic information.

An incredibly large number of combinations of nitrogenous bases can be produced along a lengthy DNA chain. Information is stored in the form of "sentences" made up of three-base words (a sequence of three adjoining bases called a *codon*), which in turn are made from combinations of five "letters" (the nitrogenous bases). Since the only way that genetic information can ultimate-

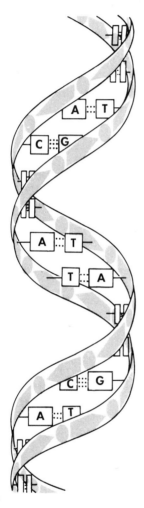

Fig. 1-16. DNA double helix. The two polynucleotide strands are said to be complementary to each other because sequence of bases in one chain determines sequence of bases in the other. Angles of bonds between backbone components cause double-stranded molecule to twist into double helix. Circles represent phosphate groups; pentagons, pentose sugar deoxyribose. (From Lane, T. R. 1976. Life, the individual, the species. The C. V. Mosby Co., St. Louis; modified from A. Cohen. 1975. Handbook of cellular chemistry. The C. V. Mosby Co., St. Louis.)

ly have an impact on cell function is by way of formation of proteins that become incorporated into the structure of cells or act to direct the metabolism of cells (as enzymes, for example), the nitrogenous base code within DNA specifies the positions of amino acids along a protein chain. Proteins are made up of 20 possible types of amino acids arranged in a sequence unique for that protein. The hormone calcitonin, which is a protein, has thirty-two such amino acids in a particular sequence. Other, more complicated proteins may have hundreds of amino acids whose sequence can be laboriously worked out using biochemical techniques. DNA is coded for each amino acid by a unique "word" consisting of a linkage of three bases. In addition to the basic code, the DNA contains "punctuation marks," that is, information needed to indicate where a particular sentence starts

and ends. At times there is some redundancy in the code. For example, the sequences TTT and TTG both code for the amino acid phenylalanine (T, thymidine; G, guanine).

Three types of RNA are required for the information carried in the DNA molecule to be copied (transcribed) and then used in protein synthesis (translated). These RNA species are messenger RNA (mRNA), transfer RNA (tRNA), and ribosomal RNA (rRNA) (Fig. 1-17). Gene transcription occurs when a strand of mRNA is synthesized alongside the exposed strand of a DNA molecule (Fig. 1-18). The bases on the DNA serve as the sites for the synthesis of complementary bases on the RNA molecule. rRNA is manufactured in the nucleus (see later) and is packaged into ribosomes that serve as the sites on which protein synthesis takes place using the mRNA as a template. tRNA con-

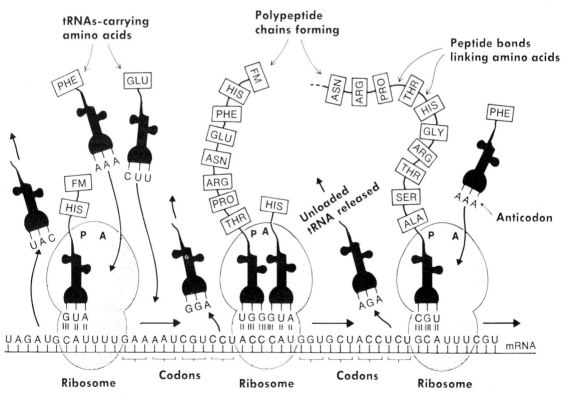

Fig. 1-17. Translation of mRNA on polyribosome. Horizontal arrows indicate direction of movement of ribosomes along strand of mRNA. Note growth of peptide chain. *FM,* Initiator amino acid formyl methionine. (From Lane, T. R. 1976. Life, the individual, the species. The C. V. Mosby Co., St. Louis; modified from A. Cohen. 1975. Handbook of cellular chemistry. The C. V. Mosby Co., St. Louis.)

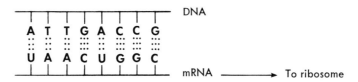

Fig. 1-18. Transcription of genetic message from DNA to mRNA. Mechanism of this process is identical to that of DNA replication, dependent on pairing of complementary bases, except that uracil is used in RNA in place of thymine, and product, mRNA, is single-standed. (From Lane, T. R. 1976. Life, the individual, the species. The C. V. Mosby Co., St. Louis.)

sists of RNA that contains a code for a single amino acid and picks up that amino acid for transfer onto a growing protein chain (Fig. 1-17). One section of the tRNA molecule recognizes the nitrogenous bases in the template mRNA; the other end recognizes and attaches to a particular amino acid. tRNA is thus able to translate the language of the nucleic acids into the language of another long-chain polymer, the proteins, and serves as an intermediary between them (hence the use of the term *translation* for the process of protein synthesis from a mRNA template).

The nucleus is a privileged microenvironment within the cell enclosed by a *nuclear envelope* consisting of two membranes. The outer membrane is broken at many points by small pores, producing an overall appearance of a whiffle ball. Information passes into and out of the nucleus through these pores. Each membrane is about 10 nm thick and is separated from the other by a space of variable thickness (10 to 15 nm) (Fig. 1-19). In most cells the outer nuclear envelope is continuous with the ER at many sites and resembles in structure the membranes of the endoplasmic reticulum. Except for the presence of DNA and RNA in the nuclear membrane fraction, the chemical composition of both membrane types is similar, with perhaps a slightly higher protein content in the nuclear envelope. It seems likely that the nuclear envelope performs some of the secretory and transport processes associated with the endoplasmic reticulum as well. The properties of the inner nuclear membrane may be different from those of the outer leaflet, but the arguments for this view are not well established.

The inner surface of the nuclear envelope maintains a stable relationship with the genetic material, which in interphase (not undergoing cell division) nuclei is found in condensed clumps called *heterochromatin.* Uncondensed chromatin is referred to as *euchromatin.* Many nuclei have a shell of chromatin attached to the nuclear envelope. Attachments to the nuclear membrane appear to be limited to preferential sites on distinct chromosomes. The most obvious example in mammalian cells is the extra X chromosome in female cells; it becomes condensed to form a Barr body, a visible large mass of chromatin in the nucleus, which attaches to the nuclear envelope. Chromatin attached to the nuclear envelope does not appear to be active in genetic transcription.

A distinguishing feature of the nuclear envelope is its pore structure. Only in special cases are pores lacking, as in the loop of nuclear membrane that folds down into the midpiece of a sperm. Pores are not unique to the nuclear membrane, since they also can be found in stacks of cisternae in the endoplasmic reticulum. Pores are sites of fusion of the two cisternal membranes, the inner and outer membranes of the nuclear envelope. The orifice itself is round or polygonal in outline, and there is some controversy about which shape is the "natural" shape in the living cell. The inner pore diameter is consistent within each nuclear type but may range in size from one nucleus to another 60 to 100 nm. Around the pore at its opening in both the inner and outer membrane is a ring or annulus of electron-dense material consisting of eight granular subunits that are radially symmetrical. The outer ring

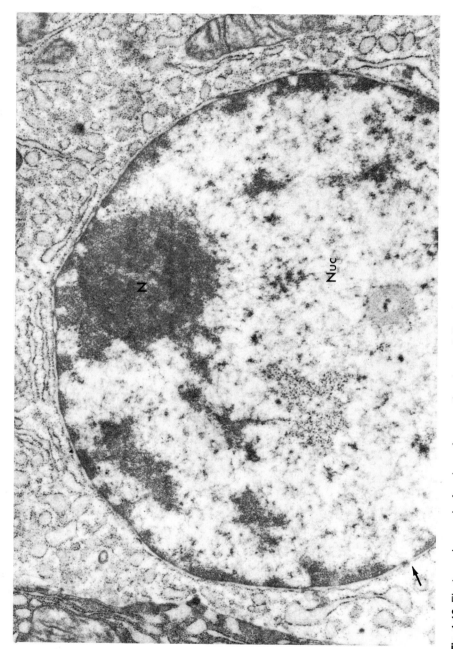

Fig. 1-19. Electron micrograph of nucleus of pancreatic acinar cell. Prominent nucleolus, *N*, is made up of granules arranged in irregular strands (nucleolonema). Nuclear envelope is made up of two membranes bonding narrow perinuclear cisterna. At frequent intervals nuclear membrane appears to be interrupted (arrow) by pores. Chromatin granules are scattered throughout nucleus, *Nuc*. (×18,000.)

is often associated with polyribosomes (clusters of ribosomes). Both the inner and outer rings frequently have small fibrillar material attached to the granular ring. The pores themselves are generally filled with clumps of densely staining material that may represent an occluding substance. The annuli appear to contain RNA.

Pores are considered gateways through which exchanges between the nucleus and the cytoplasm take place. Exchanges may also take place directly across the membranes by the formations of invaginations that traverse the nuclear envelope. Large particles such as RNA species seem to pass through the pores, but smaller materials may pass through the smooth parts of the envelope.

Chromatin was first defined as nuclear material that takes basic stains. It contains DNA and basic proteins, including histones. In electron microscopy sections treated with heavy metal salts, chromatin can be seen in several locations. Its structure is poorly defined in an interphase (nondividing) nucleus but occasionally fibrillar elements about 10 nm in diameter can be seen. The peripheral chromatin is found in dense clumps of irregular shape in close contact with the inner leaflet of the nuclear envelope, as already described.

Another mass of chromatin is associated with the *nucleolus*, an intensely staining concentration of RNA that may be found singly or multiply in cells. The nucleolus is known to produce most of the RNA found in cells, especially the rRNA that gives rise to ribosomes. The nucleolus is basophilic because of its overlying shell of chromatin, but its center is acidophilic due to the presence of ribosomal protein. Nucleoli vary in size and configuration according to the synthetic activity of the nucleus, shrinking in inactive cells. This can be seen in peripheral lymphocytes where rRNA synthesis is minimal. The nucleolus often appears solid at the light microscope level, but under electron microscopy it is seen to be heterogeneous, containing granular and fibrillar elements as well as amorphous spaces. The granular mate-

rial consists of RNA. The fibrillar elements (30 to 40 Å) serve as sites of synthesis of RNA. Some nucleoli in extremely active cells also contain a loose fibrillar network composed of 5 to 8 nm fibrils called a *nucleolonema*. In mature or nearly mature cells such as lymphocytes or smooth muscle the nucleolus may be ring shaped with RNA-containing material only at the periphery of the mass of the nucleolus. The central, lighter area represents a "resting" zone where little RNA synthesis is going on. Nucleoli do not contain much DNA, but in cells that are organizing for division, they are associated with specific regions on chromosomes called nucleolar organizing regions.

CELL CYCLES AND CELL DIVISION

Cells capable of division pass through a cell cycle consisting of an interphase condition and a mitotic stage. During interphase the cell passes through a period called G_1 or gap$_1$ when DNA is not being duplicated. This period lasts for variable lengths of time. At the end of this time, DNA is replicated during the S or synthesis phase, a process that takes about 7 hours to complete. During this interval the DNA molecules are copied so that a full DNA complement can be distributed to each of the two daughter cells that will result from cell division. There is then a short phase called G_2, lasting up to 2 hours, which precedes the onset of active cell division. As mitosis begins a dramatic change occurs in the chromatin; it coalesces into the identifiable bodies called chromosomes, which gradually shorten and thicken into characteristic shapes. The whole process of division of chromosomes and distribution into two newly organized nuclei takes about 2 hours and can be separated into four stages called *prophase, metaphase, anaphase,* and *telophase* (Fig. 1-20). Since the process is continuous, these stages tend to blur into each other. The most easily recognizable stage in tissue sections is anaphase, but it also is the shortest, lasting less than 4 minutes. Cells in the process of division are called *mitotic figures.* Even in tissues with active cell division, most of the cells will be

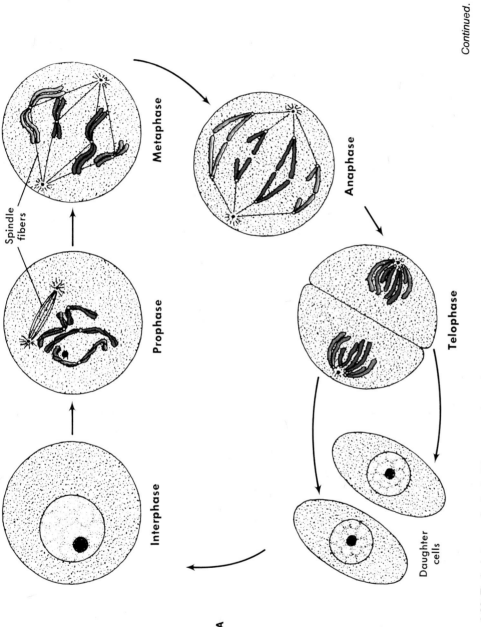

Spindle fibers

Prophase

Metaphase

Anaphase

Telophase

Interphase

Daughter cells

A

Fig. 1-20. Typical stages of mitosis. The process is continuous; each cell flows from one stage to next. **A,** Diagrammatic representation by a cell containing four chromosomes. **B,** Photomicrographs of mitosis in whitefish embryo. (**B** ×800.) (**B** courtesy V. B. Eichler, Wichita State University; from Lane, T. R. 1976. Life, the individual, the species. The C. V. Mosby Co., St. Louis.)

Continued.

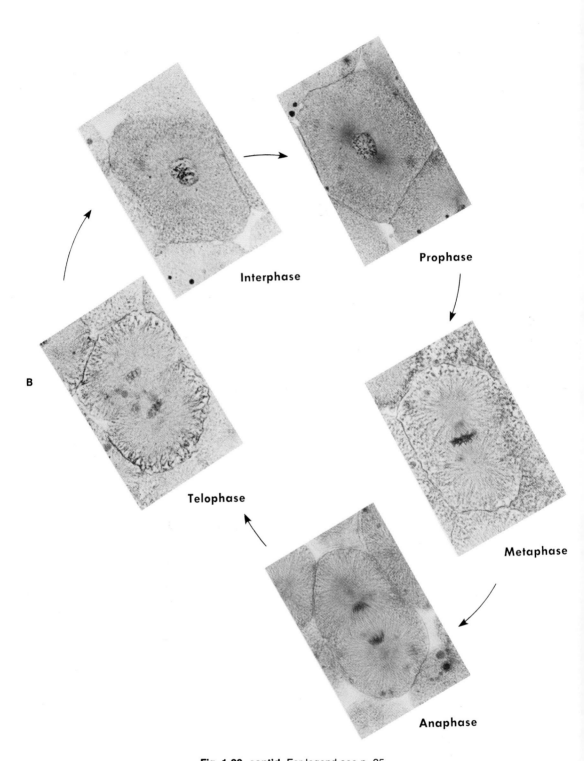

Interphase

Prophase

B

Telophase

Metaphase

Anaphase

Fig. 1-20, cont'd. For legend see p. 25.

seen in interphase, since it is by far the longest period of the cell cycle.

The longest mitotic phase is prophase. During this period the paired centrioles divide and take up an alignment at the opposite poles of the nucleus. As the centrioles come into position, microtubular arrays begin to form around them. In dividing sea urchin eggs a striking star-shaped basket of microtubules forms *(aster)*, but in dividing mammalian cells the display is less spectacular and is not visible at the light microscope level. The microtubules grow outward from the centrioles toward the opposite pair to form a *spindle apparatus.* As this occurs, the nuclear envelope melts away along with the nucleoli, and the chromosomes no longer lie in an enclosed space. The microtubules of the spindle contact the chromosomes at a coupling point called the *centromere.* Some microtubules do not become attached to chromosomes but pass to the opposite side to form the lattice of the apparatus itself.

During metaphase, which lasts less than 30 minutes, the chromosomes become aligned along the equator of the spindle. If a cell is treated with colchicine at this phase, the spindle apparatus will be "frozen," and the chromosomes can be seen clearly and analyzed. Analysis of metaphase figures is used in genetic analysis in humans, a process called *karyotyping.*

During the fleeting anaphase, which lasts less than 4 minutes, the bond holding the two sets of chromosomes (the original plus its exact replicate, called *chromatids*) splits so that the original and its duplicate become separated. Half of the chromosomes begin to move toward one pole of the spindle and half toward the other.

During telophase a new nucleus is organized around each cluster of chromosomes; and, in cells in which full cell division is going to occur, a cleavage furrow begins to develop between the two nuclear regions. The cytoplasm gradually divides in half (or sometimes unequally, as in the case of the formation of polar bodies during meiosis of female germ cells).

2

Epithelia

Epithelial tissues have two types of arrangement and two functions. First, they can be arranged in sheets, one or more layers in thickness, covering the surface or lining the cavities of the body to form a protective sheath or limiting membrane. Second, they are grouped in solid cords, tubules, or follicles, which have developed as outgrowths from an epithelial sheet and are specialized for secretion, absorption, or excretion. These organizations of cells are called glands (Chapter 11). The separation of function is not complete, however, since many lining epithelia have both a secretory and a protective function.

GENERAL FEATURES OF EPITHELIAL TISSUES

Covering and lining layers of epithelium, regardless of thickness or function, have several features in common.

1. The cells are somewhat regular in shape and lack extensive protoplasmic processes; most epithelial sheets fit tightly together and are held in this position by specialized portions of their cell surfaces known in general as *junctional complexes.*

2. Between the cells there is little structural framework (extracellular material or *matrix*). The matrix material present consists of *ground substance* composed of acid mucopolysaccharides (glycosaminoglycans) such as hyaluronic acid and the chondroitin sulfates. Calcium bound to the matrix is important in cell adhesion. Less is known about the composition of this matrix than is known about connective tissue matrices (Chapter 3).

3. Epithelial tissues lack a vascular supply and must be nourished by diffusion from underlying capillary beds.

4. Epithelial tissues are firmly bound to underlying connective tissue by a thin membrane called a *basal lamina* or *basement membrane* (Figs. 2-5, *B*, and 2-8).

5. Numerous mitotic figures may be observed in epithelia and, when present, are an indication of cell renewal. Estimates for the complete renewal of the cells of epithelial membranes range from a few days for the intestinal mucosa to a few weeks for parts of the lining of the respiratory tract.

SPECIAL FEATURES OF EPITHELIAL CELLS

Many epithelial tissues perform the function of maintaining a concentration difference between the fluid on one side of the cell sheet and that on the other. In this respect, epithelial sheets differ greatly from each other. Some boundaries such as the lining of the amphibian urinary bladder are very "tight" and can maintain extremely large concentration differences of fluid and electrolytes across their surface. Other epithelial membranes such as the lining of the gallbladder and the proximal convoluted tubule of the kidney are "leaky" barriers and allow large amounts of water and small solutes to pass from one face of the epithelium to the other. Some, such as the avian salt gland,

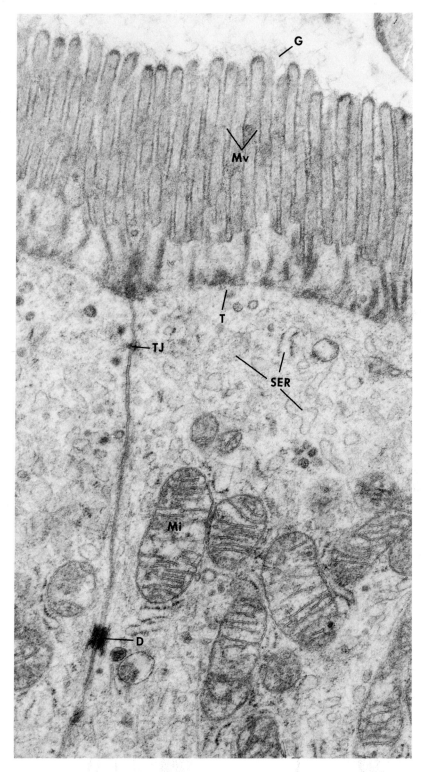

Fig. 2-1. Electron micrograph of portions of two epithelial cells from small intestine of monkey. *Tj,* Tight junction; *D,* desmosome; *Mi,* mitochondria; *Mv,* microvilli; *SER,* smooth endoplasmic reticulum; *T,* terminal web; *G,* glycocalyx. (×15,000.) (Courtesy Dr. H. Nakahara.)

transport hypertonic fluids. Others, such as the gallbladder, pass isotonic fluids. The cellular attachments, the cell bases, and the free cell surfaces of the cells making up an epithelial sheet are specialized for controlling fluid movement, absorption, or secretion, and many variations in cell morphology exist to support the different functional types of barrier.

Cell attachments. The plasma membranes of many epithelia are relatively impervious to fluids, and as a result, much of the fluid flux passes between the cells, governed by the properties of the membrane specializations that hold the membranes together. Some of these junctions encircle the cell completely; others are punctate regions somewhat similar to snap fasteners. Each type of junction has characteristic permeability properties.

1. The *zona occludens* or tight junction consists of a region where cell membranes are fused (Fig. 2-1). In tight junctions these zones of fusion are not continuous but are represented by several deep branching ridges of fusion on the cell surface (revealed by freeze-fracture techniques). More leaky epithelia have shallow zonae occludens containing one ridge. These zones form a tight seal between cells that extends all the way around the cell circumference. Large molecules injected onto the luminal surface of such an epithelial sheet will not pass through the region of cell fusion. Cells that have several zones of fusion within a zona occludens (represented by the ridges seen with freeze-fracture) have a tighter seal than do cells with only one such area of membrane fusion. When these regions of fusion are restricted to a small space on the cell surface, the junction is called a *macula* (L., spot) *occludens*.

2. Another type of cell attachment is the *adherens* type in which contiguous cell membranes are held together but do not fuse. At such sites an intercellular cell coat binds the two cells together. These points of attachment also serve as anchors for intracellular structural frameworks, the *tonofilaments*, that make up the cell web. These filaments may differ from ordinary contractile filaments in cells. *Cell webs* are accumulations of tonofilaments arranged in bundles large enough to be seen at light microscope level when properly stained. The cell web is especially prominent in cells lining the small intestine, where it is referred to as the *terminal web* (Fig. 2-1). The filaments of the terminal web extend up into the bases of the microvilli (numerous fingerlike projections of the cell surface) (Fig. 2-1). Together the terminal web and the microvilli appear at the light microscope level as a *striated border*. The microvilli alone appear as a *brush border* when the terminal web is not stained.

When the adherens region is continuous around the cell circumference it is called a *zonula adherens.* In epithelial linings such as the small intestine, a zonula adherens circles the cells in a ring just below the zonae occludens. Here the two cell membranes are separated by a 200 Å (20 nm) space filled with a lightly staining material. On the inner surfaces of the apposed cell membranes, there is a concentration of very electron-opaque material (a *plaque*) into which tonofilaments loop in and out.

When the adherens region is confined to a small area on the adjoining cell surfaces, it is called a *macula adherens* or *desmosome* (*desmos*, Gr., fastening) (Fig. 2-2). Cells anchored to underlying connective tissue have such membrane specializations without a corresponding partner on the facing surface. These single membrane specializations are called *hemidesmosomes.*

Some epithelia (best typified by the lining of the intestine) have a well-organized array of different cell junctions that together form a *junctional complex* (Fig. 2-1). Ringing the cells close to the luminal surface is a continuous zona occludens. Beneath this is a zonula adherens, below which are regions of desmosomal contact. The bases of the cells are tacked down to the underlying basal lamina by hemidesmosomal junctions.

VARIETIES OF EPITHELIA

The epithelia are divided into groups on the basis of cell shape and thickness, the number of cellular layers in the sheet, and whether the surface of the epithelium is wet or dry. Lining and covering membranes are

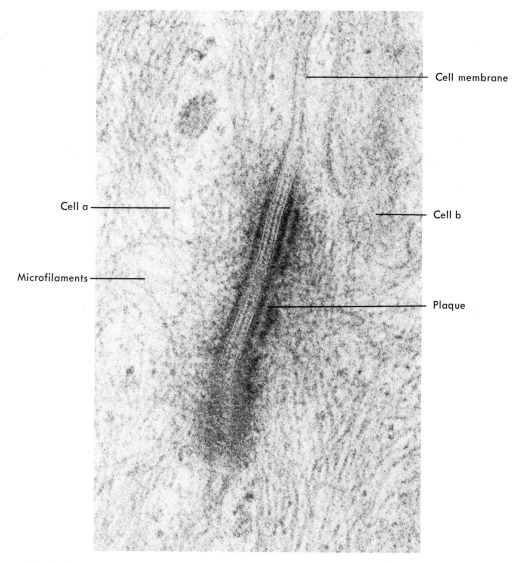

Fig. 2-2. Electron micrograph of a desmosome from nasal epithelium of mouse. (×130,000.) (Courtesy Dr. H. Nakahara.)

derived from ectoderm or mesoderm. The linings of the urogenital tracts, for example, are mesodermal in origin. For some reason, two types of epithelium are given different names. These are the *endothelium* lining blood vessels and lymphatic vessels (Fig. 2-3) and the *mesothelium* lining the body cavities and covering the viscera (Fig. 2-4).

Epithelial sheets one cell in thickness are referred to as *simple epithelia*, and multilayered sheets are called *stratified*. The two groups are further subdivided on the basis of the shapes of the cells that form them, as shown in the outline below.

Simple epithelia	Stratified epithelia
Squamous	Stratified squamous
Cuboidal	Stratified cuboidal
Columnar	Stratified columnar
Pseudostratified	Transitional

Simple epithelia

Squamous epithelium. The cells of simple squamous epithelium are extremely flattened and scalelike. Viewed from the sur-

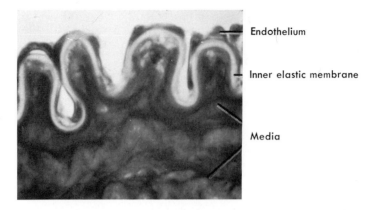

Endothelium

Inner elastic membrane

Media

Fig. 2-3. Endothelium lining lumen of medium-sized artery.

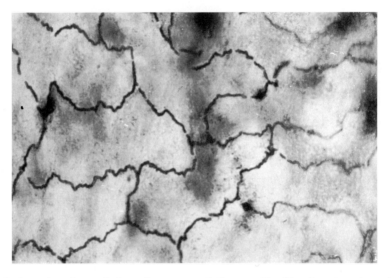

Fig. 2-4. Surface view of mesothelium of mesentery. Cells are outlined by silver deposits at their surfaces. (Silver nitrate preparation.) (×640.)

face, they appear as fairly large cells with clear cytoplasm. The nucleus of each cell is round or oval and eccentrically placed. Cell outlines are not ordinarily visible but may be demonstrated by the reaction of silver nitrate on intercellular substance. In such preparations the polygonal cell boundary may be somewhat wavy, serrated, or sometimes smooth (Fig. 2-4). In section, the cytoplasm is barely visible but may be seen in the region of the nucleus, where the cytoplasm appears to bulge (Fig. 2-3).

Simple squamous epithelium is not found in exposed regions or in sites where absorp-

tion and secretion are the primary activities. Generally it forms barriers in regions where diffusion or filtration rather than protection is the basic requirement. This is the case in Bowman's capsule of the kidney and in lung alveoli, which are used as examples of this tissue type in many histology courses. It forms the barriers of the blood–tissue fluid, tissue fluid–lymph, and tissue fluid–gas interfaces. *Endothelium* is the type of simple squamous epithelium found lining blood vessels, heart, lymphatic ducts, and bone marrow. It forms the entire thickness of the walls of blood and lymph capillaries. *Meso-*

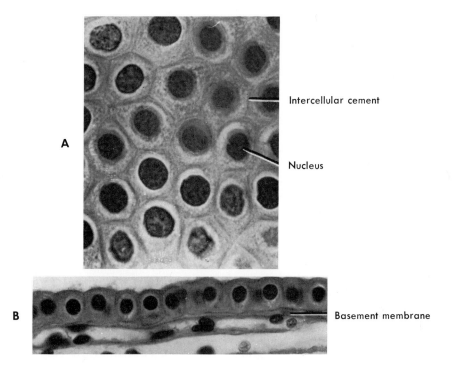

A

Intercellular cement

Nucleus

B

Basement membrane

Fig. 2-5. Cuboidal epithelium from kidney. **A,** Transverse section. **B,** Vertical section.

thelium is the same type of tissue found on the so-called *serous membranes* lining the peritoneal, pleural, and pericardial cavities of the body. Endothelium and mesothelium are not, however, morphologically distinguishable other than by location. They arise from mesoderm and mesenchyme and are said to be related to primitive connective tissue. In repair of mesothelial tissues, new cells are derived from cells of adjacent connective tissues; in repair of other types of epithelia, cells are replaced by mitosis of similar cells. For these and other reasons, mesothelium is often considered to be an epithelium with special properties or potencies. The mesothelium-like layer found lining the anterior chamber of the eye, the inner ear, and the cerebrospinal spaces is known as mesenchymal epithelium. The flattened cells lining joint cavities are said to be fibroblasts derived from the dense connective tissue in those regions and are not considered to be epithelial at all.

Cuboidal epithelium. In surface view the cells of cuboidal epithelium are smaller and more regular than simple squamous cells and appear roughly hexagonal in outline (Fig. 2-5, *A*). The cell boundaries are often clearly visible because of the presence of *terminal webs*. In vertical section (Fig. 2-5, *B*) the cell appears square with a rounded nucleus in the center of each, and in specially stained preparations the terminal bars are visible. The square shape is modified to that of a trapezoid when the cells are grouped around the lumen of a small duct. When they are closely packed around the lumen of some glands, the cells resemble a truncated pyramid and are accordingly called pyramidal cells. The cytoplasm of these cells may appear clear or granular, and in the latter case the cell boundaries are often indistinct in sectioned material. Simple cuboidal epithelium may be found in certain kidney tubules and as a covering over the ovary.

Columnar epithelium. In surface view, columnar epithelium fits the description given for cuboidal epithelium, including the same kind of junctional complexes of the occludens and adherens types. In sections, however, the cells are seen to be taller than they are broad, that is, they have the form of rectangles, with the long axis perpendicular to the free surface (Fig. 2-6). The nucleus is characteristically close to the base of the cell, except when the cells are extremely compressed. The free surface may be composed of a smooth plasma membrane covered by a thin or thick mucous secretion, or it may have microvilli or cilia. The cytoplasm may be clear or may contain granules, secretion droplets, or a large clump of secretion droplets in a vacuole near the surface of the cell (Fig. 2-7, *A*). (See discussion on goblet cells, Chapter 14.)

Mucous cells occur in varying numbers in the mucosa of the intestine and respiratory tract. They are modified columnar cells in which secretory droplets (mucinogen, the precursor of mucus) accumulate distally, resulting in a goblet-shaped cell. Eventually the cell surface ruptures, the secretion is discharged, and the cell repeats its secretory cycle.

The difference between cuboidal and columnar cells is not sharply marked. It depends on the height of the cells as seen in vertical section. An organ may be said by one author to be lined with *cuboidal epithelium,* whereas another will use the term *low columnar* in describing the tissue. An example of low columnar epithelium is shown in the illustration of the kidney (Fig. 2-5, *B*). Tall columnar epithelium is illustrated in Fig. 2-7.

In studying columnar epithelium, it is important to select a region in which the section passes through the tissue in a plane perpendicular to its surface. When a slanting (that is, tangential) section is studied, the appearance is that of two or more layers of cells, and the tissue may be erroneously classified as stratified or pseudostratified epithelium. Columnar cells are found in regions where the epithelial lining of an organ combines the function of secretion with that of a protective membrane (for example, digestive tract).

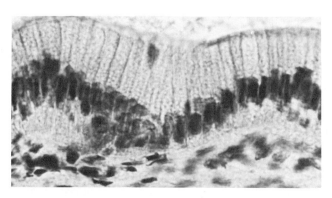

Fig. 2-6. Mucosa of human bile duct lined with tall columnar epithelium. (×600.)

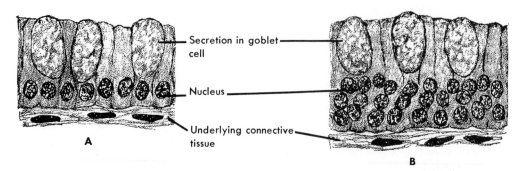

Secretion in goblet cell

Nucleus

Underlying connective tissue

A

B

Fig. 2-7. Tall columnar epithelium from intestine. **A,** Vertical section. **B,** Tangenital section.

Pseudostratified epithelium. Pseudostratified epithelium consists essentially of columnar cells, which are crowded very closely together (Fig. 2-8). Not all the cells reach the free surface of the epithelium. Those that do reach the surface have an upper part like a columnar cell and a much-constricted base, like the stem of a wine glass. Some have a wide base and an irregular spindle shape, and still others are short and rounded. The nucleus of each lies at its widest portion, and this gives the tissue the appearance of a stratified epithelium with nuclei at several levels. Only in the best preparations can it be demonstrated that, whereas approximately only one cell in three touches the free surface, all have a portion touching the basement membrane. In all preparations there seems, at the first glance, to be little difference between a vertical section of pseudostratified epithelium and a tangential section of simple columnar epithelium described. The nuclei of the two kinds of tissue offer the best means of distinguishing between the two. In pseudostratified epithelium these are of several types—theose at the base of the tissue being small and dark, those nearer the surface being larger and paler. In the tangential section of columnar epithelium, on the other hand, only one type of nucleus is present. The cytoplasm of the cells of pseudostratified epithelium is sometimes clear, sometimes granular. It may contain drops of secretions, and the surface cells are ciliated. The nuclei are round or oval according to the shape of the cells in which they lie. The usual appearance of this type of epithelium is illustrated in Fig. 2-8 (trachea). It is functionally adapted to serve as a fairly resistant yet flexible limiting membrane.

Stratified epithelia

Stratified epithelia serve a protective function and can withstand more wear and tear than simple epithelia can.

In all stratified epithelia a complete layer of small modified cuboidal or columnar cells lies next to the basement membrane. These cells are called *basal cells*. Above this, except with a two-layered epithelium, are one or more layers of polygonal cells. At the free surface lies a layer of cells that have a different shape in each subdivision of the group. The shape of the cells at the free surface of a stratified epithelium determines its classification into one of the four subdivisions.

Stratified squamous epithelium. These epithelial types are either wet (nonkeratinized) or dry (keratinized) and are the most protective linings in the body. The thickness and number of cells in each zone of stratified squamous epithelium vary from one place in the body to another but the basic arrangement is the same. The deepest or basal cells are polygonal in shape and are quite small. They frequently undergo mitosis and provide a stem line for the cells higher in the layers. As cells are pushed upward from the base,

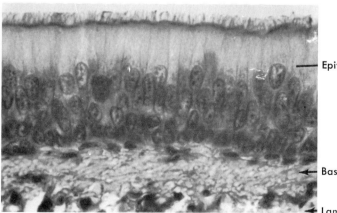

Epithelium

Basement membrane

Lamina propria

Fig. 2-8. Pseudostratified ciliated columnar epithelium from trachea of dog. (×640.)

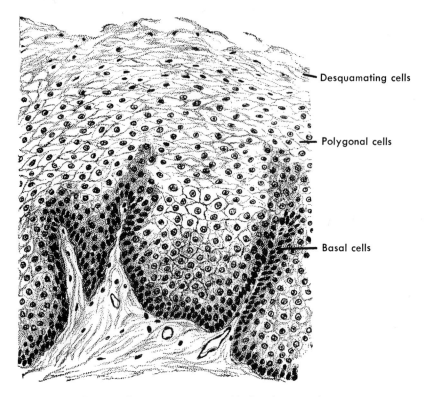

Desquamating cells

Polygonal cells

Basal cells

Fig. 2-9. Stratified squamous epithelium from esophagus.

they enlarge *(hypertrophy)* until they reach about the middle zone of the epithelium. Beyond this point, as they approach the surface they may become flattened, shriveled *(atrophic)*, and scalelike with small, darkened *(pyknotic)* nuclei, the situation seen in the mucous membranes of the oral cavity and esophagus (Fig. 2-9). In more exposed, dry surfaces such as the skin surface, the cells develop a tough resilient material (keratin) (Chapter 12). When this condition exists, the epithelium is said to be *cornified* or *keratinized.* This tissue is particularly well adapted to perform its protective function because of (1) its great thickness and keratinization, (2) its ability to slough off surface cells under the impetus of abrasion, and (3) the replacement of these cells from below.

The cells of stratified squamous epithelia are held together by desmosomal junctions. During ordinary fixation the cells shrink but cannot pull away from each other at the desmosome sites. The result is that the cells appear "prickly" (Fig. 12-3).

Stratified cuboidal epithelium. Stratified cuboidal epithelium is extremely rare, the best example occurring in the ducts of the sweat glands. A definite basement membrane is present, whereas the free surface bears a distinct border. Certain cell layers in the testis and ovary are also included in this group by some authors.

Stratified columnar epithelium. Stratified columnar epithelium differs from the pseudostratified type in having a continuous layer of small rounded cells next to the basement membrane. The columnar cells at the surface of the epithelium are thus entirely cut off from the basement membrane, and the epithelium is truly stratified. This type is of rare occurrence and is found only on a few moist surfaces where more protection is needed—in large exocrine ducts, for example.

Transitional epithelium. Transitional epithelium is a stratified epithelium whose surface cells do not fall into the truly squamous, cuboidal, or columnar categories. The basal cells are like those of stratified columnar

Pear-shaped
cell

Surface (dome-shaped)
cell

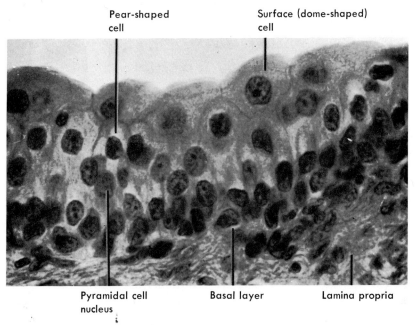

Pyramidal cell
nucleus

Basal layer

Lamina propria

Fig. 2-10. Section of mucosa of urinary bladder showing transitional epithelium. (×640.)

epithelium. Above them is a varying number of polygonal cells, of which those immediately below the surface layer tend to have an elongated, pearlike (*piriform*) shape. The layer at the surface is composed of large, somewhat flattened cells, generally described as dome shaped. One of these cells often covers three underlying pear-shaped cells, with indentations to receive the latter. The dome cells are so large that in sectioned material many of the nuclei are not visible because they are not in the plane of the section, although dome cells are known to have as many as two or three nuclei each. The cytoplasm just under the free surface of the dome cell appears to be more condensed and

deeply staining, which is an aid in the identification of this tissue at the optic level. Basement membrane, terminal bars, and cilia are not found in this nonsecretory tissue (Fig. 2-10).

Transitional epithelia are found in the urinary tract where they are adapted to permit considerable stretch as the tract fills with urine. The best place to examine this type of epithelium is in the urinary bladder. When it is not stretched, the surface cells appear round, but in the distended position the surface cells appear squamous. They can be pulled into a thin sheet because their membranes form pleated folds that provide extra membrane area in the distended condition.

3

Connective tissue proper

In the connecting and supporting tissues the arrangement of cells and intercellular substance is quite different from that seen in the epithelia. Rather than being closely applied to each other in the form of a sheet or a cord, the cells lie more or less scattered, sometimes not in contact, sometimes touching only at the ends of long protoplasmic processes. The intercellular substance is much more prominent than among the epithelia and becomes the most important part of the majority of the tissues in the group.

The type of cell most frequently found in these tissues is of an irregular branching form, sometimes called *stellate*. Its nucleus is vesicular and its cytoplasm is somewhat granular and prolonged in the form of processes. Cells of this type make up the mesenchyme (Fig. 3-1), the embryonic tissue from which the members of the group are derived. The original shape of the cell is retained in some of the connecting and supporting tissues after they have been fully differentiated. In others it is modified.

In loosely arranged connective tissue (tissue containing a soft, pliable matrix), these cells are called *fibroblasts*. In cartilage they are called *chondrocytes* and in bone, *osteocytes*.

The matrix or intercellular components of connective tissue consist of fibers, ground substance, and tissue fluid. All connective tissues contain these elements, but the various tissues can be differentiated from each other on the basis of (1) the arrangement of

fibers (ranging from loosely woven and highly pliable to tightly braided into bundles and extremely strong); (2) the chemical composition of the ground substance and its consistency (from a viscous sol to a semisolid gel); and (3) the arrangement and interrelationships of cells. Some connective tissue is designed as a type of excelsior or packing material, binding the skin surface down to underlying tissues or providing a coating or cushion for viscera. This form of connective tissue is called *loose* or *areolar connective tissue* because of its loosely woven consistency. Other connective tissue serves as a capsule for organs (*dense irregular connec-*

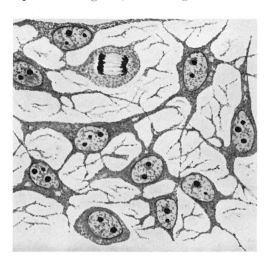

Fig. 3-1. Mesenchyme in 60 mm dog fetus. (Silver stain; ×1,200.) (From Nonidez, J., and W. Windle. 1953. Textbook of histology. McGraw-Hill Book Co., New York.)

tive tissue) or as the attachments of muscle (*dense regular connective tissue*).

In addition to the binding and packing functions, connective tissue has the role of providing a supportive framework for the body. The tissues involved in this function are stronger, more highly organized tissues, *cartilage* and *bone*. They constitute a separate class of connective tissue and will be considered in separate chapters. They do, however, contain the same basic elements as does connective tissue proper and should be considered as variants on the same theme.

In this discussion we will consider the matrix elements first and then the cellular inhabitants, both those that are fixed in place and those that can wander in and out.

FIBERS

The fibers are of three kinds (collagenous or white, reticular, and elastic) and are distinguishable by their appearance and chemical reactions.

Collagenous or white fibers. Collagenous or white fibers are the most common and occur in all types of connective tissue. They possess considerable tensile strength but little elasticity. They are dissolved by weak acids and yield gelatin on boiling. The fibers may be widely scattered, as in the loose areolar variety, or densely packed, as in a tendon.

Collagen fibers are often aggregated in bundles of varying thickness and indefinite length. Individual fibers observed in routine preparations are 1 to 10 μm in diameter. Following special treatment one may observe that collagen fibers are made up of smaller units, the *fibrils*. These are the fibrils of light microscopy and measure 0.2 to 0.5 μm in diameter. Many of the fibrils lie parallel to one another; this gives the impression that they are longitudinally striated. Fibrils are held together by a cementing substance that is removed by tryptic digestion.

Collagen fibers stain with acid dyes, pink with eosin and blue with Mallory's triple stain.

Electron microscopy has shown that the fibers which are visible with the optical microscope are made up of smaller fibrils known as *microfibrils*, having an average diameter of 100 nm. The microfibrils of mature collagen exhibit a periodic crossbanding of 64 nm (Figs. 3-2 and 3-3). Collagen microfibrils are composed of macromolecules 280 nm in length and 1.5 nm in diameter, known as tropocollagen (precursor of collagen). Tropocollagen consists of three polypeptide chains arranged in the form of a helix. Among the amino acids present in abundance are proline, glycine, hydroxyproline, and hydroxylysine, the latter being involved in the formation of cross-linkages between the macromolecules.

Tropocollagen macromolecules are polarized and have a characteristic intraband pattern. They are arranged in parallel rows, and all face in the same direction. The adjacent rows of macromolecules are arranged in a staggered or overlapping fashion, amounting to approximately one fourth the length of the 280 nm molecule, which gives rise to a periodic line at approximately 64 nm.

Reticular fibers. Reticular fibers are similar to collagenous fibers in that they exhibit the same 64 nm periodicity. They are finer in caliber, do not stain appreciably with eosin, but have an affinity for silver. Accordingly, they are not readily distinguished in sections prepared in the ordinary way. On boiling they yield reticulin, which differs slightly from gelatin obtained from collagenous fibers. Reticular fibers also resist peptic digestion longer than do the collagenous fibers.

Elastic fibers. Elastic fibers are highly refractile and occur singly or in the form of sheets. The fibers are usually thinner than collagen fibers except in some elastic ligaments such as the *ligamentum nuchae* where the fibers may reach a diameter of 10 μm. In ordinary preparations elastic fibers are barely distinguished from collagen fibers. With special stains such as resorcin, the elastic fibers are sharply differentiated, since this dye colors them deeply but leaves the collagen fibers pale. In such slides the elastic fibers appear as stout branching structures thicker than the individual collagen or reticu-

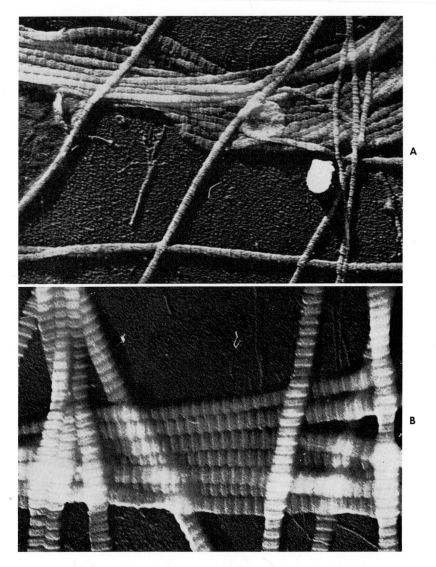

Fig. 3-2. Electron micrograph of connective tissue of skin. **A,** Reticular fibers (2 days). **B,** Collagenous fibers (90 days). Reticular fibers are smaller in diameter than are collagenous fibers but apparently have same periodicity. (×45,000.) (Courtesy Dr. J. Gross.)

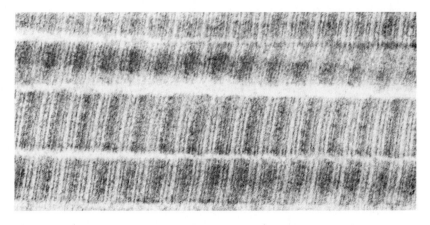

Fig. 3-3. Electron micrograph of rat tendon collagen showing major periodic bands at 64 nm and also smaller interperiodic bands. (×140,000.) (Courtesy Dr. H. Nakahara.)

lar fibers. (See the discussion of blood vessels in Chapter 9.)

Chemically, elastic fibers consist of a mucopolysaccharide moiety and a protein (elastin). Unlike collagen, an elastic fiber contains little hydroxyproline. It is extremely resistant to reagents but is digested by elastase, a pancreatic enzyme. These fibers have the property of elasticity. This is not apparent, however, in histological preparations.

At the electron microscope level (Fig. 3-4), it has been shown that elastic fibers are made up of two components—amorphous and fibrillar. The amorphous component consists of a homogeneous material of varying density in which the fibrils are embedded. The amorphous material also forms a coat surrounding the fibrils, which are composed of microfibrils. The microfibrils are relatively slender, measuring 30 to 150 μm in diameter. The amorphous material has the same amino acid composition as does elastin; the fibrils, however, are made up of a different protein that is rich in hydroxyproline.

Elastic fibers undergo age changes that are reflected in a decrease in the elasticity and resilience of the tissues in which they occur. For example, chemical changes in the elastic tissue in arteries give rise to sites that calcify. In the skin, changes associated with the polysaccharide moiety give rise to changes in resiliency. With aging the number of microfibrils also decreases.

GROUND SUBSTANCE

It has been said that the body is really an edifice of connective tissue in which cells are residents. The consistency of this edifice depends partly on its content of fibers and partly on the chemistry of the ground substance. The ground substance of connective tissue is a homogeneous semifluid material of a consistency varying from a viscous lubricant in joint cavities to a near-solid in vertebral disks. It is visible only after treatment with special stains. Ground substance consists primarily of acid mucopolysaccharides (glycosaminoglycans) arranged in a feathery

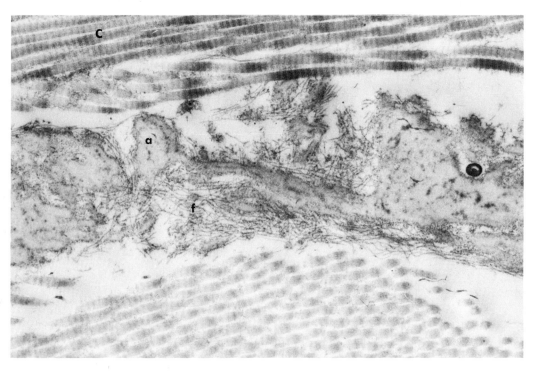

Fig. 3-4. Electron micrograph of section of elastic fiber enclosed by collagen fibers, *C*. Elastic fiber consists of two components: an amorphous portion, *a*, and a fibrillar portion, *f*. (×20,000.) (Courtesy Dr. R. Ross.)

mesh that is hydrophilic and therefore traps a large amount of tissue fluid. The predominant component is hyaluronic acid, a substance that acts as a water binder, lubricant, and shock absorber. The tissue fluids held by the hyaluronic acid serve as a medium through which nutrients and wastes pass back and forth between the cells and the capillary beds. The meshwork of polymerized hyaluronic acid serves also to obstruct the passage of larger particles such as dyes or bacteria through the matrix. Hyaluronidase produced by bacteria can depolymerize the ground substance and permit more rapid penetration.

The other main components in ground substance are the sulfated mucopolysaccharides, especially the chondroitin sulfates. The more hyaluronic acid a matrix contains, the more pliable it is and the more water it holds. As the proportion of sulfated mucopolysaccharides increases, the stiffness of the matrix also increases. Embryonic tissues have little chondroitin sulfate and are unusually soft and pliable.

Some tissues have unusual acid mucopolysaccharides that impart special properties to the site. For example, skin tendons and blood vessels have dermatan sulfate, a mucopolysaccharide associated with coarse collagen fibrils, which may contribute to the tensile strength of skin. This compound binds calcium, and its presence may help to explain why these sites are often places where calcification occurs.

The glycosaminoglycans in the ground substance can be visualized with special stains. In some connective tissue the matrix is clearly metachromatic, that is, it alters the color of the dyes that bind to the tissue. Toluidine blue, for instance, normally stains tissue blue, but it colors some connective tissues red, pink, or purple. Another dye that can be used is alcian blue, which becomes linked to the acidic groups on the glycosaminoglycans.

CELLS OF CONNECTIVE TISSUE

Some cells in connective tissue are permanent residents. They are responsible for the synthesis of both the fibers and the ground substance. Other cells wander into and out of connective tissue, removing debris after tissue injury or acting as a line of defense against invasion of the body by microorganisms. Not all the cells that will be described here can be found in every specimen of connective tissue, but various combinations of cells will be seen, depending on the history of that particular piece of tissue—its age, and whether it was involved in a process of growth, repair, or an inflammatory response to injury or invasion.

Fibroblasts. Primitive connective tissue develops from the mesoderm and rostrally from ectoderm. It is a soft, jellylike mass of ground substance with a few widely scattered cells that are thin and spidery in appearance (Fig. 3-1). This material penetrates almost everywhere in the developing embryo and gives rise to all the connective tissues. In connective tissue proper, the mesenchymal cells differentiate into *fibroblasts*, the matrix-forming cells of connective tissue. These cells have large oval nuclei with fine dust-like chromatin and widely dispersed, thin cytoplasmic processes that extend out into the matrix (Fig. 3-5). Young cells are more basophilic and have more cytoplasm. The appearance of the cells varies, depending on how much space they have. In tendons, for example, they become compressed between bundles of collagen, and the nuclei appear small and dark. When seen from the side, fibroblast nuclei are fusiform and somewhat easier to see. Fibroblasts are the most common cell type in connective tissue.

The fibroblast varies in appearance depending on its physiological state. In the resting cell the nucleus is small, the cytoplasm is pale, and the organelles are diminished in size and number. In an active state, when producing fibers or intercellular material, the cell enlarges, corresponding to an increase in the size of the nucleus and the number of organelles. The cytoplasm is more basophilic as a result of an increase in the rough endoplasmic reticulum.

An electron micrograph of an active fibroblast illustrated in Fig. 3-5 shows a cell with

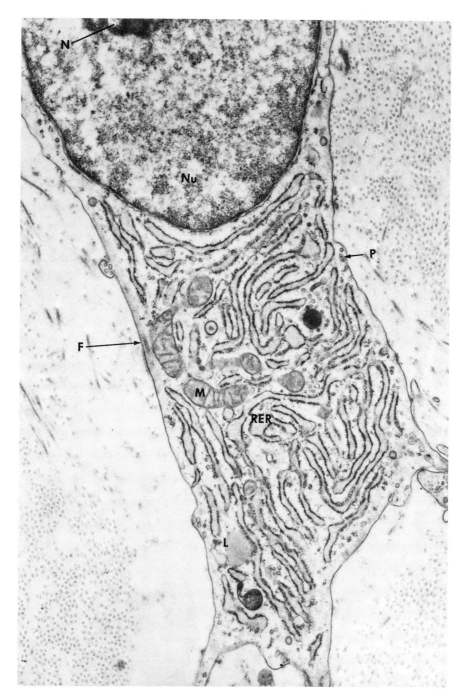

Fig. 3-5. Electron micrograph of an active fibroblast. *F,* Fibrillae; *L,* lipid droplet; *M,* mitochondrion; *N,* nucleolus; *Nu,* nucleus; *RER,* rough endoplasmic reticulum; *P,* pinocytotic vesicle. (×30,000.) (Courtesy Dr. R. Ross.)

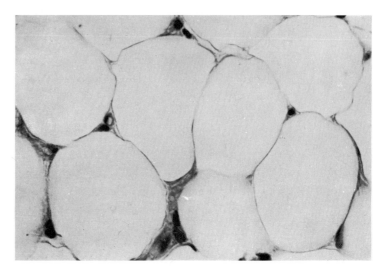

Fig. 3-6. Adipose tissue showing fibroblast nuclei between fat cells. (Hematoxylin and eosin stain; ×900.)

a large nucleus, extensive arrays of rough encoplasmic reticulum, cisternae, ribosomes, a Golgi complex, and mitochondria —a cell apparently actively synthesizing substances for the purposes of secretion.

The formation of collagen fibers takes place as follows: Amino acids are synthesized into polypeptide chains in association with ribosomes of the rough endoplasmic reticulum. From the cisternae of the endoplasmic reticulum the synthesized protein is transferred to the Golgi complex and further processed. It is then carried to the surface of the cell by way of vesicles derived from the Golgi complex. It is released as macromolecules of tropocollagen and then polymerized near the cell surface into fine threads or filaments exhibiting nodules at 64 nm intervals. The filaments serve as templates for additional polymerization of tropocollagen, and by aggregation give rise first to thin microfibrils that increase in length and size to thicker filaments exhibiting a periodicity of 64 nm. Microfibrils arranged in parallel arrays coalesce to form fibrils, the latter aggregate to form bundles.

When this process is followed using tritiated amino acids, it can be seen that collagen precursors are formed within about 30 minutes, are extruded from the cell by 4 hours, and are incorporated into the matrix within 35 hours.

The population of fibroblasts in connective tissue is not static or permanent. If injury occurs, new fibroblasts can be recruited from a population of undifferentiated mesenchymal cells that seems to persist in tissues after their embryonic development. These cells migrate into an injury site and further replenish their numbers by cell division. As they begin the process of wound repair, the fibroblasts secrete glycoproteins and mucopolysaccharides, the components of the ground substance. Later, the cells begin to manufacture collagen. As the collagen content of the injured site increases, so does its tensile strength until a scar is formed. This process demonstrates that some connective tissue proper has a considerable capacity for repair. This is especially evident in the skin.

Fat cells. Adipose or fat cells occur singly or in groups in loose connective tissue. A connective tissue is called adipose tissue when the fat cells are in abundance and organized into lobules (see later). Fat cells are easy to distinguish once they begin to store fat but resemble fibroblasts before that. Most cells have a few lipid droplets here and there, but fat cells specialize in this function and store large droplets of triglycerides that occupy much of the cell volume. Fat cells store nutrients, provide insulation, and act as cushions and crevice-filling tissue.

It appears that adipose cells (adipocytes)

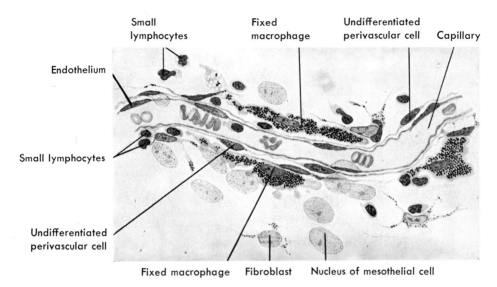

Small lymphocytes Fixed macrophage Undifferentiated perivascular cell Capillary

Endothelium

Small lymphocytes

Undifferentiated perivascular cell

Fixed macrophage   Fibroblast   Nucleus of mesothelial cell

Fig. 3-7. Stretch preparation of omentum of rabbit vitally stained with lithium carmine. (Hematoxylin stain; ×500.) (From Maximow, A., and W. Bloom. 1952. A textbook of histology. W. B. Saunders Co., Philadelphia.)

are a specialized connective tissue cell line and not simply a variant of the fibroblast. The fat stored in them is lost in the usual process of tissue preparation, and the cells appear as hollow vacuoles with a tiny rim of cytoplasm and a single fusiform nucleus (Fig. 3-6). At the electron microscopy level this cytoplasmic rim can be seen to contain a few free ribosomes, some rough and smooth endoplasmic reticulum, a Golgi apparatus, and mitochondria.

Mesothelial cells. The nuclei of mesothelial cells that occur in mesenteries and are frequently confused with the nuclei of fibroblasts. Mesothelial nuclei are much larger, somewhat lighter staining, and appear as elongated ovals, never fusiform in tissue spreads (Fig. 3-7). In addition, the mesothelial cytoplasm does not usually stain. These cells are not a regular feature of connective tissue but belong to the epithelium that forms the boundary of mesenteric and serous membranes.

• • •

The other cell types in connective tissue are transients. Only their morphological features will be considered here, since they will be considered in greater detail in later chapters. The cells we will discuss are plasma

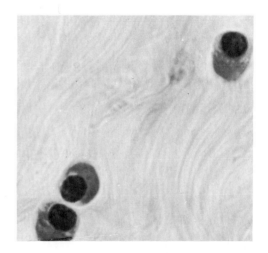

Fig. 3-8. Photomicrograph of plasma cells in connective tissue of mammary gland. Note eccentrically placed nucleus. (×1,600.)

cells, macrophages, mast cells, and various blood cells (lymphocytes, granular leukocytes).

Plasma cells (Fig. 3-8 and 3-9). Any invading organism enters the body by passing through the connective tissue. The matrix of connective tissue is thus the first line of defense against infection, and it should not be surprising that the cells concerned with defense against disease and with the maintenance of immunity are derived from con-

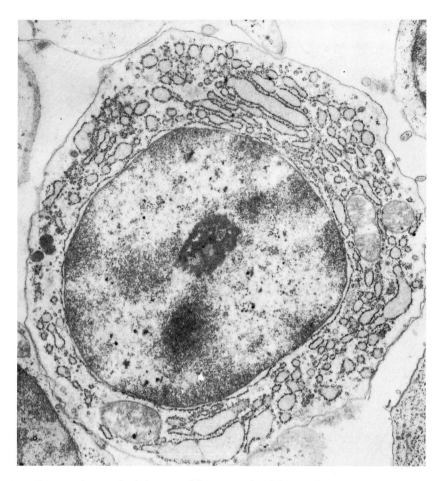

Fig. 3-9. Electron micrograph of plasma cell from a cat. In addition to the large nucleus, the characteristic feature of the cytoplasm is the extensive system of cisternae studded with ribosomes on which antibody synthesis occurs. (×17,000.)

nective tissue cell lines. Plasma cells can be found in abundance beneath moist epithelial membranes such as those of the intestinal and respiratory tracts—membranes across which invasion is especially likely. They are easy to see in standard hematoxylin and eosin sections. If they are lying free, they are rounded. If they are in crowded groups they may be more irregular in outline. The nucleus is rounded and placed eccentrically, with a trail of abundant, strongly basophilic cytoplasm extending out to one side in a wedge. The chromatin is mostly condensed, sometimes in flakes distributed like the spokes of a wheel, a so-called cartwheel nucleus.

These cells manufacture *antibodies* that are specific for foreign proteins (see discussion on *antigens* in Chapter 10). The cytoplasm of plasma cells is therefore filled with protein synthetic machinery and an abundant Golgi apparatus, since the cells are producing protein for export (Fig. 3-9).

Macrophages. These cells (also called histiocytes, "dust" cells, wandering cells) are specialized for phagocytosis. They are frequent residents of connective tissue, actively ingesting debris and bacteria. In some tissues, such as the hematopoietic tissues, phagocytic cells are attached next to the lining of the blood and lymph channels, where they are called reticular cells (Figs. 3-10 and 3-11).

The nucleus of macrophages tends to be

Connective tissue capsule   Peripheral sinus

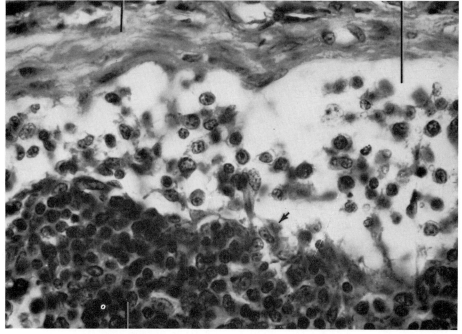

Lymphocytes

Fig. 3-10. Section of lymph node showing peripheral sinus. Arrow indicates reticulocyte. (×640.)

Medullary cord   Sinus   Lymphocyte

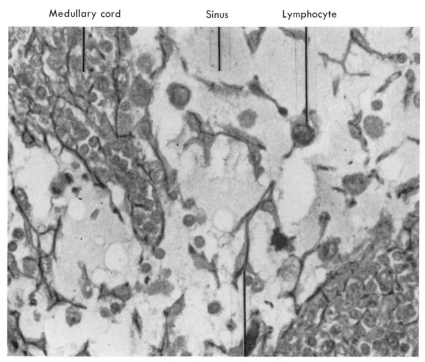

Reticulocyte and fiber

Fig. 3-11. Section of lymph node showing distribution of reticulocytes and reticular fibers in sinus. (Bielschowsky method; ×640.)

indented like a kidney bean and lies at one pole of the cell with its convex surface facing the rest of the cell. The nucleus is more condensed than that of a fibroblast and is slightly smaller. Macrophages are easier to see if the cytoplasm is filled with ingested debris or if the animal has been injected with a dye such as trypan blue or lithium carmine that will be taken up by phagocytosis (Fig. 3-7).

Macrophages are the representatives in connective tissue of a far-flung defense system called the *reticuloendothelial (RE) system*. This system is a collection of cells concerned with phagocytosis and defense against disease in widely scattered tissues of the body. The macrophages remove bacteria, dead cells, and debris and foreign particulate matter from body fluids and from the matrix of body tissues. Other elements of the reticuloendothelial system monitor tissue fluid, lymph, and blood; produce antibodies; and engage in blood cell formation. Tissue fluids are "cleaned" by fixed macrophages of connective tissue proper *(histiocytes)* and by wandering macrophages that enter the connective tissue from the blood. Other more organized communities of macrophages are formed around lymphatic channels and around vascular beds in bone marrow, liver,

and spleen. These macrophages will be discussed in subsequent chapters.

There is still some controversy on the origin and fate of tissue macrophages. Monocytes from blood (Chapter 6) transform into macrophages. According to one recent view, tissue macrophages are seeded in tissues during embryological development as cells migrate from hematopoietic tissue. Macrophages are replenished to some extent in adults as a result of monocyte transformations.

Mast cells. Mast cells exhibit basophilic and metachromatic cytoplasmic granules composed partly of polysaccharide. They are large round cells with pale nuclei frequently obscured by the abundant granules (Figs. 3-12 and 3-13). In hematoxylin and eosin preparations they are sometimes referred to as tissue basophils. They are frequently found in the vicinity of blood vessels and should not be confused with flattened cells known as undifferentiated perivascular cells. Mast cells contain heparin, an anticoagulant polysaccharide, and histamine. These cells may influence blood flow through capillary beds and are probably damaged during anaphylaxis. The properties of mast cells mimic

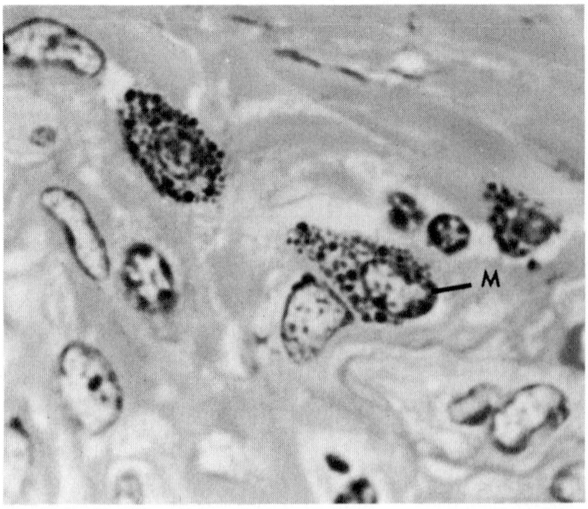

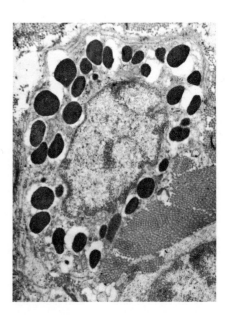

Fig. 3-12. Photomicrograph of mast cells, *M*, from gingival connective tissue. These cells contain metachromatic granules. (×1,200.)

Fig. 3-13. Electron micrograph of a mast cell from small intestine of mouse. Note numerous large electron-dense granules. (×10,000.)

those of the basophilic leukocytes (Chapter 6). Species that have large mast cell populations tend to have few basophils. It is presently thought that these two cell types, the mast cell and the blood basophil, supplement each other. During an infection, infiltration of a tissue by basophils may represent a quick response to foreign proteins (an antigenic stimulus), whereas in more long-lasting processes (chronic inflammation, parasite infestation, neoplasia) in which interaction between the host and foreign antigens is prolonged, basophils may gradually give way to new mast cells arising in the tissues.

Blood cells. Lymphocytes and leukocytes can migrate into connective tissue through blood vessel walls, and there is a steady traffic of such cells into and out of the connective tissue matrix, the volume of traffic depending on whether any injury has occurred. Lymphocytes in tissue appear as small round cells with darkly staining nuclei and little, if any, visible cytoplasm. A good place to look to get an idea of the appearance of lymphocytes is a nodule of a lymph node, where they will be found in great abundance (Fig. 3-10 and 3-11).

Scattered in loose connective tissue will be cells of the leukocyte series—neutrophils (polymorphs), eosinophils, and basophils. These cells migrate into tissues in great numbers whenever the tissue is injured and becomes inflamed. Eosinophils and basophils can be distinguished by their cytoplasmic content of granules that stain with acidic and basic dyes, respectively, and by their oddly shaped nuclei, which may be deeply indented or multilobular. Eosinophils are likely to be found in the lining of the intestine, in the lungs, and in the dermis of the skin. Basophils are rarely found there. Both cell types are involved in inflammatory and allergic responses.

Neutrophils (polymorphs) are highly mobile and phagocytic and are attracted to sites of injury. The granules contained within the cytoplasm are not readily visible in tissue sections. The nuclei are distinguishable because they are multilobed (see Chapter 6 for further details).

TYPES OF CONNECTIVE TISSUE PROPER

Connective tissues are classified primarily according to the arrangement of fibers in the matrix. In the looser tissues there are relatively few fibers (irregularly arranged), a large amount of tissue fluid, and many cells. In denser tissues, there is an increase in the number of fibers (more regularly arranged) and a corresponding decrease in ground substance and cells.

Mucous connective tissue

Mucous connective tissue is found in the embryo (where it is called mesenchyme), but it is retained in a few places in the adult. The cells are spindle shaped or branching, and the matrix is the dominant feature of the tissue. In the adult it is found in the vitreous humor of the eye. In histology laboratories it is usually studied in sections of the umbilical cord (Wharton's jelly), and it is of interest primarily because the relationships of cells and collagen are clearer here as there are so few fibers.

The vitreous consists of approximately 99% water and 0.1% macromolecules, the remainder being low molecular weight solutes. The protein that makes up the ground substance is dispersed in a thin, three-dimensional fibrillar network made up of a collagen-like protein called vitrosin and hyaluronic acid. Occasional cells are trapped in the matrix.

Fibrous connective tissue
Areolar or loose connective tissue (Fig. 3-7)

In this tissue, the collagenous fibers predominate, although some elastic fibers are found. This type of tissue is found in mesenteries, in the omenta of the alimentary canal, in the subcutaneous tissue of the skin (beneath the dermis), and immediately below the mucosal epithelium of the alimentary canal. The predominating collagenous fiber bundles branch and are of variable thickness. They also intertwine to form a network. In sections they are cut in all possible planes, and since they twist and interlace, bundles can be traced for only short distances. Elastic fibers are usually nearer the surface of the tissue and, when stretched, form a network of straight fibers that give rise to Y-shaped branches, often curling at the free ends. In hematoxylin and eosin–stained sections, elastic fibers are not generally distinguishable from the white fibers. Sectioned materials stained with orcein (dark brown), resorcin-fuchsin (dark blue), or Verhoeff–van Gieson (dark purplish brown) show elastic fibers as scattered short single pieces cut obliquely. Together the fibrous elements, collagen and elastin, produced and maintained by fibroblasts, form the major structural support of the matrix and are woven into a mat of considerable flexibility. The intercellular fluid fills in the spaces between fibers and cells and provides the medium for movement of nutrients and metabolic wastes between the cells and the capillary beds.

Loose connective tissue is usually studied in spreads of mesenteries. The reader is cautioned to distinguish between cells that are properly a part of the connective tissue itself and epithelial cell types that lie over the connective tissue—the mesothelial cells.

Dense fibrous tissue

Irregular. In irregular dense fibrous tissue the number of collagenous fibers is increased tremendously, whereas intercellular fluid and number of cells are definitely decreased. The result is a tough, resilient tissue of great strength and flexibility. The thick collagenous bundles are arranged in an intertwining network (Fig. 3-14). In routine hematoxylin and eosin–stained sections the whole mass stains a bright yellowish pink or red; widely scattered fusiform fibroblast nuclei are also a feature of this tissue. In some dense connective tissue such as the dermis of the skin, there are a large number of elastic fibers, especially in the scalp and on the face. They form a loose lattice to support sweat glands, hair follicles, and the capillary bed of the dermis and to anchor the epidermis to the dermis.

This tissue can occur in the form of sheets in the perichondrium, periosteum, dermis, and capsules of many organs. In certain encapsulated organs, pillars of dense irregular connective tissue known as *trabeculae* penetrate and subdivide the structure. The trabeculae usually contain blood vessels,

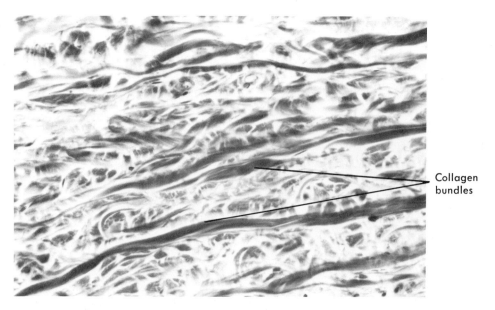

Collagen bundles

Fig. 3-14. Section of irregular dense connective tissue from skin. (×800.)

nerves, and sometimes the ducts of glands. The trabeculae are composed almost entirely of collagenous fibers but, in some instances, may include elastic and reticular fibers and even smooth muscle.

Regular. Regular dense fibrous tissue occurs in cords or bands and is typified by tendons, ligaments, and aponeuroses. In the tendon the fibers are densely packed in thick, parallel, unbranching bundles. These bundles are so closely crowded that the cells between them are flattened to a platelike form (Fig. 3-15). The cells lie in rows parallel to the fibers. In profile the nuclei are extremely long and thin, whereas in surface view the individual nuclei are elongated ovals. In cross section the cells are so compressed that they appear as winglike projections between adjacent bundles. Tendons are composed almost entirely of collagenous fibers.

Collagen fibers

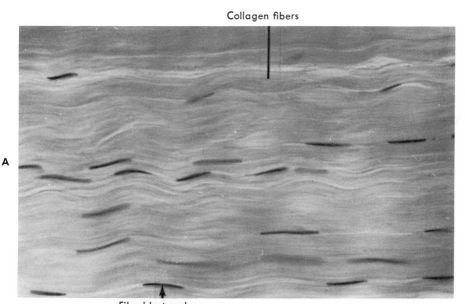

Fibroblast nucleus

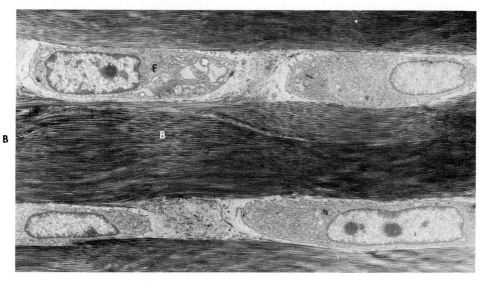

Fig. 3-15. Longitudinal section of tendon. *B*, Collagen fibers; *F*, fibroblast. (**A**×640; **B**×2,500.)

Elastic tissue

Elastic fibers are of rather general occurrence in connective tissue, but they are not considered elastic tissues. In certain situations the elastic fibers predominate, whereas the collagenous fibers are sparse. In the walls of arteries elastic fibers have developed and fused to such an extent that they form an incomplete (fenestrated) membrane, enclosing cells and a few collagenous fibers. As such, this arrangement might be termed dense irregular elastic tissue. A form of dense regular elastic tissue is found in the neck ligament of the ox (ligamentum nuchae) and in the smaller ligaments between the vertebrae (ligamentum flavis). In this type, thick, long, branching elastic fibers lie in nearly parallel arrangement in association with very few cells and an extremely small number of fine collagenous fibers. In such a dense arrangement the fibers, especially in older animals, appear yellow in color, hence the new obsolete term *yellow fibers.*

ADIPOSE TISSUE

Adipose tissue is commonly included in the groups of connective and supporting tissues, although it differs from the other members of the group in several respects. The cells composing it do not form intercellular fibers or matrix but are specialized for the storing of fat. They thus form a reserve of foodstuffs as well as supporting pads of tissue. The cells are mesenchymal in origin, like those of connective tissue. They lose their protoplasmic processes early in the course of their transformation and become round, with abundant cytoplasm and central nuclei. The fat is deposited in the cytoplasm in minute droplets that gradually increase and unite in one large drop, which pushes the nucleus to one side of the cell. As still more fat accumulates, the nucleus becomes flattened and the cytoplasm is reduced to a mere film enclosing the fat globule. In tissues that have been treated with ordinary fixatives followed by alcohol, the fat is dissolved out, leaving the cytoplasm of the cells in the form of large irregular rings, each having a dark flat nucleus at one side. In preparations made with osmic acid the fat is retained and appears as a darkly stained black or brown occupying the center of each cell. There is no intercellular substance elaborated by adipose tissue cells. They lie embedded in reticular or areolar tissue, the fibers among them being the product of reticular cells or fibroblasts. Adipose tissue is illustrated in Fig. 3-6.

Fat is made up of glycerol esters and fatty acids. They are synthesized from carbohydrates and may be stored or called on as a reserve source of food in time of body need. Adipose tissue serves as a padding for organs, mechanically protecting them from shock; as a reserve food supply; and lastly as an agent in thermoregulation by aiding in the conservation of body heat, particularly in the newborn.

SEROUS MEMBRANES

Serous membranes—the pleura, peritoneum, and pericardium—consist of a thin layer of loosely arranged connective tissues covered by a layer of relatively flat mesothelial cells (Fig. 3-7). The membrane is made up of loosely arranged collagenous fibers, scattered elastic fibers, fibroblasts, macrophages, mast cells, adipose cells, and a varying number of other cells. The amount of fluid exudate and the variety and number of cells suspended in it increase greatly in adverse physiological or pathological conditions.

4

Cartilage

In the connective tissue proper described in Chapter 3 the elements present consist of cells and fibers embedded in a viscid ground substance and tissue fluid. The noncellular elements are collectively known as the matrix. In the supporting tissues such as cartilage and bone, the character of the matrix varies. In cartilage the ground substance is semirigid and contains a protein-carbohydrate complex known as chondromucoid. On partial hydrolysis the latter yields chondroitin sulfuric acid. Chondromucoid is PAS positive and basophilic and stains metachromatically with toluidine blue because it contains chondroitin sulfate as the predominant proteoglycan in the ground substance. Cations, for example, calcium and strontium, are bound strongly to chondroitin sulfuric acid, and the cartilage in these regions stains orthochromatically with toluidine blue and appears intensely basophilic with hematoxylin and eosin. The presence of condroitin sulfate makes the matrix pliable, a bendable supportive framework. In older individuals, mineralization of cartilage, for example, in the larynx, may occur and is usually accompanied by degenerative changes of the cells. As a result, the cartilage becomes brittle and can shatter under strain.

DEVELOPMENT OF CARTILAGE

Cartilage forms the skeleton of the embryo and is exemplified in the adult by the tracheal rings. Throughout the matrix collagenous fibers interlace much as they do in the fluid matrix of areolar tissue. The cells lie in minute spaces in the matrix called the lacunae (Fig. 4-1). These vary in shape according to their position in the plate of cartilage. They are thin and oval shaped near the edges of a cartilage plate and larger and rounder near the center of a plate. The cells, originally stellate like other mesenchyme cells, have lost their protoplasmic processes and have assumed the shape of the lacunae in which they lie. Unlike other connective tissue, cartilage contains no blood vessels so that nourishment must reach the cells by seepage through the matrix.

Cartilage develops from mesenchyme, as do the other supporting tissues. Mesenchyme cells first elaborate the fibers and later lay down the solid matrix on them. Each cell forms a circumferential layer of matrix, thus enclosing itself in a lacuna. As growth and development proceed, the amount of matrix between cells increases, pushing them farther apart, so that ultimately the condition is reached in which the cells lie in lacunae scattered through a relatively large amount of intercellular substance. For a time, at least, after the embryonic period, growth may be effected interstitially by the division of cartilage cells and the laying down of matrix around each daughter cell (interstitial growth). Later, however, the increasing solidity of the matrix renders this type of growth more difficult, and increase in the size of the cartilage plate is caused by the addition of new layers at the periphery by the

Collagen fibers   Chondrocytes

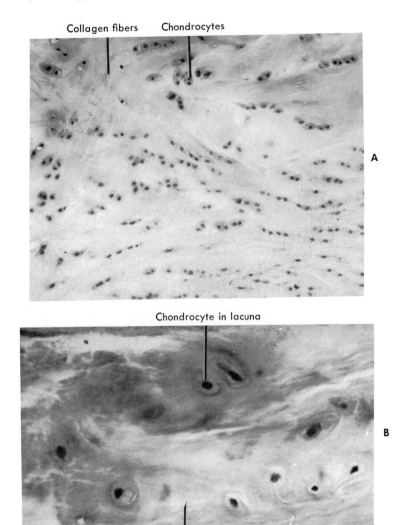

Chondrocyte in lacuna

Collagen fibers

Fig. 4-1. Fibrocartilage from symphysis of rabbit. (**A,** ×160; **B,** ×640.)

cells of the surrounding connective tissue capsule, called the *perichondrium*. This process is referred to as appositional growth. In adult cartilage one may, as previously stated, find two or four lacunae close together separated by very thin walls of matrix. These and the lacunae that contain two cells indicate that interstitial growth is proceeding by mitosis but that matrix formation is slow.

TYPES OF CARTILAGE

Cartilage occurs in three forms—fibrous, hyaline, and elastic; these are distinguished by the character of their fibers, the relative proportions of fiber types, and the consistency of matrix, which varies from resilient and pliable (as in fibrocartilage) to elastic and deformable (elastic cartilage) to tough and weight-bearing (hyaline cartilage).

Fibrocartilage

Of the three cartilage types, fibrocartilage most nearly resembles connective tissue proper (Fig. 4-1). In the intervertebral disks, fibrocartilage forms a layer between the connective tissue capsule of the disks and the hyaline cartilage overlying the bony surface of the vertebrae. Here it blends on one side with connective tissue and on the other with hyaline cartilage, and, as will be explained, it is intermediate between the two kinds of tissue in qualities as well as in position. It consists of a network of coarse collagen fibers, which take the usual red color when stained with eosin. These fibers are embedded in a solid matrix, which fills the interstices between them. The extent of the matrix varies somewhat in different specimens. In some cases it replaces the fluid matrix only partially and appears merely as fine purplish lines between the red fibers and as thin capsules surrounding the cells. In others its amount is greater and it forms darker lines among the fibers and definite branching islands containing lacunae. In the former condition it is not easily distinguished from dense connective tissue, but one characteristic feature is always to be seen: the round or oval lacunae that contain the cells called chondrocytes, which manufacture fibers and ground substance. In connective tissue the cells are flattened by the pressure of the surrounding fibers; in cartilage, they are protected by the capsules of matrix in which they lie.

Hyaline cartilage

The collagenous fibers of hyaline cartilage are not gathered in bundles but are dispersed throughout the tissue in a fine, close network completely filled in by the substance of the matrix. The union is so close as to form a mass that, though pliable, is very firm and able to bear weight. The fibers and matrix have, moreover, the same staining capacity and refractive index so that in ordinary preparations they are not morphologically distinguishable. Hyaline cartilage is so named because the matrix appears clear (*hyalos*, Gr., glasslike), and special techniques are required to demonstrate that the intercellular substance consists of fibers and matrix.

Hyaline cartilage occurs in the form of definite plates, in each of which the cells and matrix exhibit a definite plan of organization. If one studies a cartilage plate from the tra-

chea, for instance, certain regions may be distinguished, and the plan found will be typical of all cartilage plates. At the periphery of the plate is a fibrous layer, the perichondrium. This is, on the outside, similar to the surrounding areolar tissue with which it blends. It is well supplied with blood vessels. Toward the cartilage the perichondrium becomes denser; that is, the fibers become heavier and more closely crowded, and the interfibrillar spaces containing the cells become smaller. The outer layer of the perichondrium is called the fibrous layer; the inner, the chondrogenic layer. At the inner border of the chondrogenic layer a condition is reached in which individual fibers are no longer distinguishable, their identity being obscured by the solid matrix in which they are embedded. Both fibers and matrix are pink in this region in well-stained hematoxylin-eosin preparations. The cells, known as chondroblasts, are no longer free as in the fluid matrix of the perichondrium but are enclosed in spindle-shaped lacunae (Fig. 4-2).

Cartilage is unique in that it has no blood supply except at the edges of each plate. As a result, the cells in the center receive all their nutrients by diffusion. Since cartilage is a weight-bearing connective tissue, any blood supply would be occluded by pressure. This problem is prevented in bone, another form of specialized dense connective tissue: the calcified matrix provides for blood vessels a protective series of passageways that cannot be collapsed by pressure. One consequence of the absence of a blood supply is that cartilage can be transplanted without fear of immune rejection because foreign proteins in the cells and matrix cannot escape into the host circulation to initiate a graft rejection response.

Toward the center of the plate, which is the farthest from the blood supply, changes occur in cells and matrix. The latter becomes chemically basic and accordingly stains blue rather than pink in the region of the chondrocytes (territorial matrix). The region between the cell groups, known as interterritorial matrix, becomes increasingly nonbasophilic with age because of loss of chondroitin

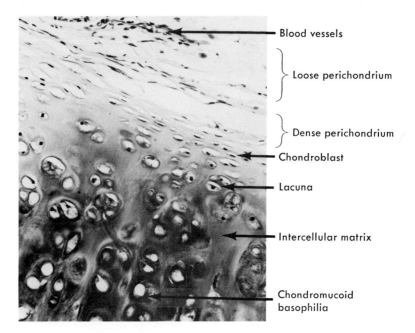

Blood vessels

Loose perichondrium

Dense perichondrium

Chondroblast

Lacuna

Intercellular matrix

Chondromucoid
basophilia

Fig. 4-2. Hyaline cartilage from trachea. (×400.)

sulfate and increase in albuminoid substances chemically related to keratin. The color is pale except immediately around the lacunae, where it is often very dark blue. The shape of the lacunae also changes toward the middle of the plate; they become round rather than flattened. Often they are found in pairs or groups of four, with the facing sides flattened. The cells *(chondrocytes)* occupying these central lacunae are spherical and in the living tissue fill the entire space. They are separated from the matrix by a fine capsule, which rarely may be distinguished. In fixed preparations the cytoplasm is usually shrunken, and the only prominent feature is the nucleus. This is surrounded by an irregular cytoplasm. The shrinkage occurs because the fixatives penetrate slowly through the matrix and do not reach its center until after postmortem changes have taken place there and because the cartilage cells contain large amounts of glycogen and some fat that are lost in processing. When cartilage cells are well preserved, they are roughly spherical and have a prominent, centrally placed nucleus. The cytoplasm is granular and basophilic. Large mitochondria, varying amounts of glycogen, numerous vacuoles, and lipid

droplets are present. At the electron microscope level the surface of the cell is irregular, and the rough endoplasmic reticulum occupies the greater part of the cytoplasm. The appearance of hyaline cartilage is illustrated in Figs. 4-2 and 4-3.

Elastic cartilage

Elastic cartilage is similar to hyaline cartilage in the arrangement of perichondrium, matrix, cells, and lacunae. The difference is that elastic cartilage contains, besides the invisible collagenous fibers, a network of elastic fibers, which may be readily demonstrated by the use of the appropriate stain. This type of cartilage occurs in the epiglottis and is present also in the external ear (Fig. 4-4). The areas in which elastic cartilage will be found in the embryo exhibit connective tissue fibers and fibroblasts. The fibers are wavy and do not react characteristically for either collagen or elastin. These peculiar fibers apparently transform into elastic fibers and then chondrocytes develop. A perichondrium located on the periphery of the growing cartilage subsequently initiates appositional growth during the ensuing embryonic period.

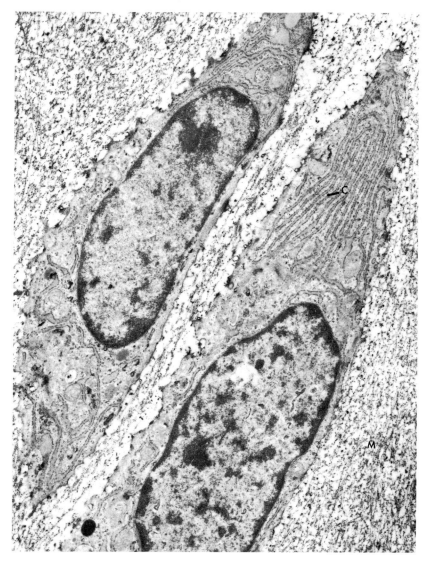

Fig. 4-3. Electron micrograph of young cartilage cells and surrounding cartilage matrix. The most characteristic features of these cells are prominent arrays of cisternae, *C,* studded with ribosomes. The matrix, *M,* surrounding the cells shows delicate reticular fibers and dark granules, which are probably acid mucopolysaccharide. (×12,000.)

Connective tissue

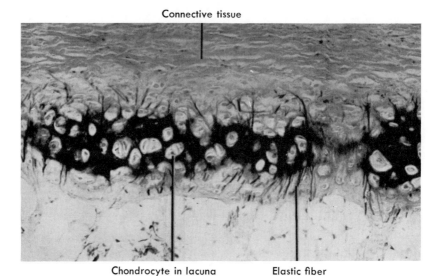

Chondrocyte in lacuna   Elastic fiber

Fig. 4-4. Elastic cartilage from external ear. (Verhoeff's method; ×160.)

FUNCTIONS OF CARTILAGE

The function of cartilage varies and serves the organism in many ways. Hyaline cartilage forms a large part of the temporary skeleton of the embryo. This variety of cartilage makes up the articulating surface of movable joints: in this capacity it exhibits properties of unusual strength for support and also allows the bones to move freely. In the respiratory system the cartilage prevents the collapse of passageways. Hyaline cartilage participates in and contributes to the growth and calcification of long bones. Nutritional and vitamin deficiencies and hormonal imbalance modify the normal participation of cartilage in bone development and result in the production of abnormalities of the skeletal system.

Elastic cartilage forms a more flexible support in movable nonweight-bearing structures such as the epiglottis and the external ear. Fibrocartilage is essentially an unusually tough binding tissue similar to the dense connective tissue of organ capsules.

5

Bone

bone - sheath - periosteum;
cartilage - sheath - perichondrium } vascular .

COMPARISON BETWEEN BONE AND CARTILAGE AS TISSUES

Both bone and cartilage are specialized forms of dense connective tissue whose matrix is especially resilient and pliable. Both tissues perform structural and weight-bearing *skeletal functions* in the body. Bone is designed architecturally to be a light-weight, extremely strong weight-bearing tissue whose lines of strength follow the lines of strain induced by weight-bearing. To accomplish this, the matrix is mineralized along highly organized fiber arrangements.

In both tissues the cells that form and maintain the matrix become trapped within shells of matrix called *lacunae*, but the shape and distribution of these lacunae are characteristic for each tissue type. Both tissues are covered by a sheath of dense irregular connective tissue (the *perichondrium* and *periosteum*) containing an abundant blood supply and a population of stem cells that continuously give rise to new matrix-forming cells, chondrogenic and osteogenic cells, respectively, for cartilage and bone. Both tissues can grow by layering on from the edges (appositional growth). In cartilage the stem cells proliferate and form chondrocytes that rapidly surround themselves with matrix. In bone the stem cells (called *osteoprogenitor cells*) first develop into *osteoblasts*, extremely active matrix-forming cells that gradually wall themselves off in a lacuna and become *osteocytes*. These cells, unlike cartilage cells, remain in contact with each other through channels in the matrix and do not die as the matrix around them becomes calcified. Unlike cartilage, bone retains an abundant blood supply running through the matrix. This is possible because the mineralization of the matrix provides protective channels through which the vessels can run without risk of being occluded by outside pressure on the tissue when it is bearing weight.

Adult cartilage can also continue to grow by interstitial growth, the proliferation of chondrocytes inside the cartilage plate. Adult bone cannot add to its mass in this manner. Instead, the internal areas of bone are continuously subject to a process of erosion (*resorption*) to remove old bone, which is then followed by remodeling to replace the removed bone. This continual remodeling process is required for the physiological role of the skeleton in mineral balance (regulation of blood calcium levels) and provides a mechanism for adjusting the organization of bone in response to changes in stress and strain lines. To accomplish this remodeling, cells called *osteoclasts* actively remove matrix, leaving a space for new bone formation.

Another difference between the two tissues is that the matrix of cartilage only calcifies under special conditions, such as during aging. In bone, mineralization is a normal process required for the structural organization of the matrix. In cartilage, mineralization is a pathological condition and seals off the chondrocytes from nutrients that cartilage must obtain by diffusion from the vascular bed in the perichondrium.

The matrix of bone contains the same elements as do other connective tissues—fibers and ground substance. The laying down of this matrix by osteoblasts is called *ossification*. The deposition of calcium salts in this matrix is called *calcification*, a process that occurs normally in bone but can occur pathologically in other connective tissues such as cartilage or the walls of blood vessels. If calcification has not yet occurred in the bone matrix, the area is referred to as *osteoid*. There is always a rim of this material around osteoblasts and osteocytes.

The fibers that form the framework of the matrix are highly organized, and their arrangement imparts considerable resilience and strength to the bone. Bone can be classified according to its fiber arrangement as *woven* or *lamellar*. Woven bone is found in

adults in tooth sockets, in sutures between the skull bones, and in regions of tendon-bone attachment. In these areas the fibers are woven together into a dense mat. In the embryo most bone contains the woven arrangement of fibers. Elsewhere in mature bone the fiber arrangement is uniform and regular and appears laminated. It is called lamellar bone.

Bone can also be classified as spongy *(cancellous)* or compact. Bone is porous because it is built up around the vascular spaces, and, when the spaces are visible, this honeycomb appearance is called *cancellous*. In *compact* bone the porous spaces are small, 10 to 20 μm in diameter, whereas in *spongy* or cancellous bone the spaces are larger and visible to the naked eye (Fig. 5-1). The fiber arrangements tend to be different in these two bone types.

The lamellar arrangements of fibers can be

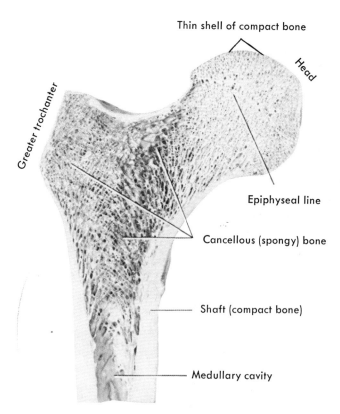

Thin shell of compact bone

Head

Greater trochanter

Epiphyseal line

Cancellous (spongy) bone

Shaft (compact bone)

Medullary cavity

Fig. 5-1. Longitudinal section through upper end of femur of adult male. (From Copenhaver, W. M., (ed.) 1964. Bailey's textbook of histology, 15th ed. Copyrighted 1964, The Williams & Wilkins Co., Baltimore.)

seen in three configurations in compact bone.

1. The concentric *Haversian system,* consist of rings of bone deposition around a central vascular channel (Fig. 5-2). These systems are actually solid cylinders extending for considerably distances along the long axis of the bone. By being organized this way, the long bones acquire extensive strength without having to sacrifice lightness. To imagine this, think of the advantage of holding many small straws, each bearing weight, rather than one large heavy cylinder.

2. Between the cylindrical Haversian systems are remnants of old, remodeled systems that have been partially removed by the process of resorption, called *interstitial lamellae* (Fig. 5-2).

3. Along the outer edges of the bone surface where growth occurs by apposition are found *circumferential lamellae:* layers added on, from the periosteal surface, that conform to the outer contour of the bone.

Not all adult lamellar bone has fully developed Haversian systems. In long bones, for example, only the regions of compact bone show this arrangement. The smaller spicules of spongy bone that form the core of the head of the femur, for example, contain coarse cancellous bone made up of an irregular, haphazard arrangement of fragmented lamellae similar to the interstitial lamellae of compact bone. Only the thicker trabeculae of spongy bone have fully developed Haversian systems.

With this introduction to the cell types and fiber arrangements of bone as a background, the discussion can now proceed to a consideration of how bone is formed and remodeled. Bone is an unusual tissue in that it is constantly remodeling and being reorganized in the process of performing its functions of support and of calcium regulation. It is necessary from the very beginning to view bone as an extremely dynamic tissue whose structure is being continuously altered.

DEVELOPMENT

Bone always forms within a preexisting framework of connective tissues. Differences in development occur because in the embryo some of the bones are laid down in undifferentiated mesenchyme (*intramembranous bone formation*), whereas in other parts of

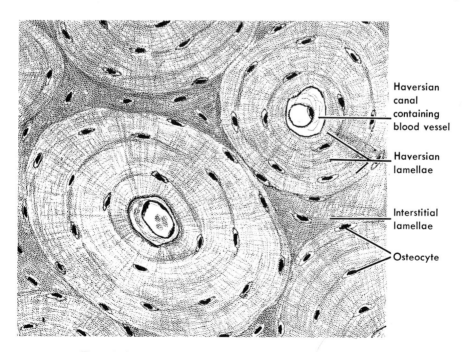

Fig. 5-2. Compact bone decalcified, showing organic constituents.

Haversian canal containing blood vessel

Haversian lamellae

Interstitial lamellae

Osteocyte

the body a temporary supporting system of cartilage precedes bone formation (*endochondral bone formation*). The essential process by which bone matrix is formed and ossified is the same in both cases. Membranous ossification occurs principally in the flat skull bones and clavicle while endochondral ossification is characteristic of most of the rest of the skeleton. The difference between these two kinds of bone formation lies in the tissue that precedes each in the place where it develops. The immediate result is also the same in both cases: the formation of a mass of irregular trabeculae of bone penetrated by blood vessels and connective tissue. Such bone is called woven bone, because the fibers of the matrix form a dense, irregular mat.

In whatever manner it has been formed, the newly developed bone undergoes secondary changes. These consist of (1) erosion or resorption and (2) rebuilding. Differences in the manner and extent of rebuilding in different parts of the bone result in the development of two types of adult structure. In some regions the bone is eroded and rebuilt in its original form (spongy). In others, rebuilding follows a new pattern and is more extensive so that the tissue develops organized Haversian systems and becomes compact bone. Compact and spongy bone are alike in their essential elements—each is made up of lamellae. They differ, however, in the arrangement and relative amounts of matrix, blood vessels, and marrow spaces.

In the following outline the development of bone has been divided, for convenience, into four steps: spicule formation, confluence of spicules, erosion, and rebuilding.

A. Formation of spicules of matrix
 1. Intramembranous—spicules laid down directly in mesenchyme
 2. Cartilage replacement
  a. Bone formed around the outside of the cartilage (perichondral)
  b. Erosion of the center of the cartilage and penetration of blood vessels
  c. Bone laid down on fragments of disintegrating cartilage (endochondral)
B. Confluence of spicules to form woven bone
C. Secondary erosion

D. Rebuilding
 1. In the form of new spongy bone
 2. In the form of compact bone

The division is arbitrary, and it should be remembered that different parts of the same bone may be in different stages of development at any one time and that the steps merge gradually into each other. Although all the processes involved are most active during fetal and early postnatal life, they continue slowly until old age is reached, and any one of them may be accelerated by metabolic or traumatic changes. Longitudinal growth of the long bones of the skeleton (such as the femur) occurs by endochondral bone formation, but transverse growth of the shaft takes place by intramembranous bone formation resulting from periosteal activity. This latter process allows for a slow but progressive increase in the diameter of the bones in adults even after the body has reached its full height.

Intramembranous bone

The regions in which the process of intramembranous bone formation occurs are determined by the proximity of blood vessels. In an area where bone will develop, mesenchymal cells differentiate to form osteoprogenitor cells and osteoblasts (Fig. 5-3). The osteoprogenitor cells are irregular in shape and somewhat elongated. They have pale-staining cytoplasm and nuclei. They are similar in appearance to mesenchyme cells and are identified by their association with osteoblasts. The cells are connected with one another by their processes and are surrounded by delicate bundles of reticular fibers. The cells and fibers are loosely arranged in a jellylike ground substance.

The initiation of bone formation consists in the production of an increased amount of ground substance between the cells, often trapping some of the cells within it. At the same time, the cells increase in size, assume a polyhedral form, and maintain, meanwhile, the numerous processes by which they are connected with adjacent cells. At this stage they are known as osteoblasts (Figs. 5-3 and 5-4).

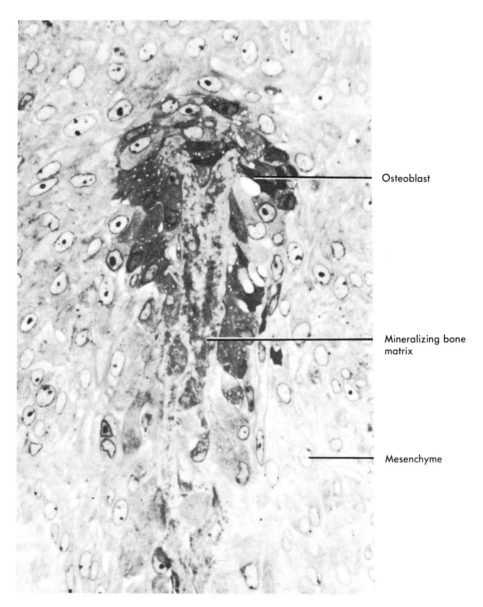

Osteoblast

Mineralizing bone matrix

Mesenchyme

Fig. 5-3. Developing bone spicule. (×800.) (From Bevelander, G. 1971. Outline of histology, 7th ed. The C. V. Mosby Co., St. Louis.)

Osteoblasts, as their name implies, are associated with bone formation and are invariably found on the margin of growing bones (Fig. 5-5). During the period of growth they are arranged in a closely packed layer of cuboidal or low columnar cells joined together by slender processes. The nucleus, usually located in the basal region, exhibits a prominent nucleolus. By appropriate staining methods a diplosome and well-developed Golgi apparatus can be observed adjacent to

the nucleus. Mitochondria are numerous and usually elongated. The cytoplasm of the active cell is intensely basophilic and also contains PAS-staining granules, as well as considerable amounts of alkaline phosphatase. At the electron microscope level (Fig. 5-4) the osteoblast exhibits an extensive, rough endoplasmic reticulum; numerous free ribosomes; well-developed Golgi membranes and vesicles; lysosomes; and other inclusions. The general appearance of the cell is

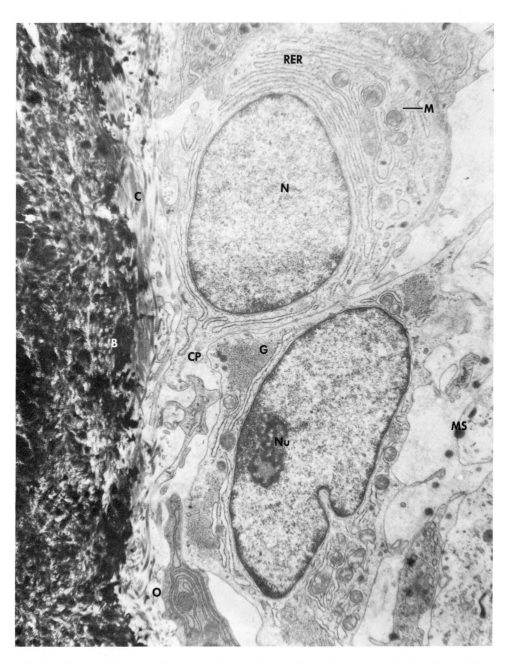

Fig. 5-4. Electron micrograph of two osteoblasts and adjacent bone. *B,* bone crystals; *C,* collagen; *CP,* cell process; *G,* glycogen; *M,* mitochondria; *MS,* marrow space; *N,* nucleus; *Nu,* nucleolus; *O,* osteoid; *RER,* rough endoplasmic reticulum. (×10,000.) (Courtesy Drs. J. H. Martin and J. L. Matthews.)

Osteocytes

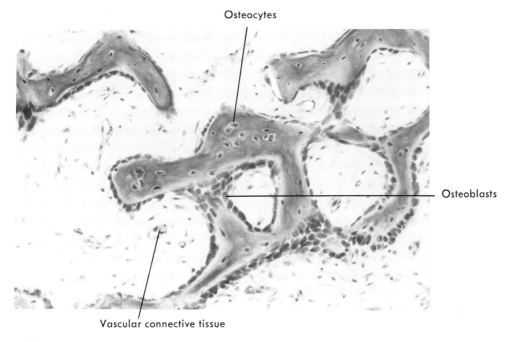

Osteoblasts

Vascular connective tissue

Fig. 5-5. Section of developing bone. Trabecula containing osteocytes and lined by osteoblasts. (×200.)

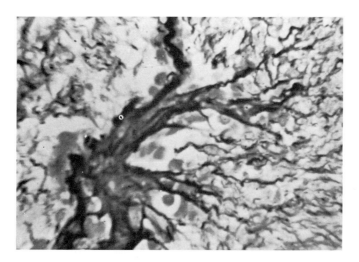

Fig. 5-6. Developing spicule of membrane bone showing origin and incorporation of fibers before mineralization occurs. (Reticulum stain.)

similar to other cells known to be engaged in protein synthesis.

When certain conditions are attained in the elaboration of cells and matrix, the tissue undergoes calcification; that is, mineral is deposited in the matrix in the form of hydroxyapatite $(Ca_3[PO_4]_2)_3\text{-}Ca(OH)_2$. In addition, bone mineral may contain other cations such as sodium, magnesium, carbonate, and citrate. The mineral or inorganic part of a bone may vary from 35% dry weight in young bones to 65% in adult bones.

The organic or interstitial component of bone contains numerous reticular fibers (Fig. 5-6), which are surrounded by an amorphous ground substance. In the embryonic state this substance is PAS positive and metachromatic, the latter property being correlated with the presence of a sulfated polysaccharide.

The mechanism for the deposition of bone salts is unknown, although many theories have been developed to explain the process. One crucial factor seems to be the ratio between calcium and phosphate. Bone mineralization becomes defective whenever the blood calcium level falls or when the ratio of calcium to phosphate falls. One theory holds that mineralization occurs when the local ion concentration exceeds the limit of solubility of these ions in tissue fluid, but there are a number of difficulties with this theory. It seems likely that both cellular and physiochemical factors are involved. Mineralization may occur around collagen chains or proteoglycans in the matrix that act to precipitate bone salts from a supersaturated solution in extracellular fluid. The chief difficulty in explaining how bone and other structures mineralize is due in part, at least, to the fact that the exact manner in which minerals are transported from tissue fluids to the matrix that undergoes mineralization has as yet not been elucidated. In any case, bone is formed under the influence of osteoblastic activity in two successive stages: (1) matrix formation and (2) mineralization. Matrix formation involves the biosynthesis of collagens and of the proteoglycans (glycoproteins) of the ground substance. Mineralization involves the initial deposition of an amophorous tricalcium phosphate that is slowly converted to crystalline hydroxyapatite in two stages. In the first stage (primary mineralization) about 75% of the mineral content of the matrix is deposited within a few days under the control of osteoblasts. The remainder of the mineralization process takes place slowly over a period of several months and is apparently not under the control of bone cells.

Following the initial stages of bone formation just described, other changes occur: the osteoprogenitor cells divide by mitosis and give rise to osteoblasts by a process known as modulation and then arrange themselves on the surface of the developing bone in a continuous layer. The osteoblasts appear to form a barrier between the surface of developing bone on one side and the connective tissue and blood vessels of marrow on the other. The cells are probably joined by tight junctions, but since the cells are not sealed together over their entire surface, there are many small channels between them. Adjacent to the osteoblasts is a layer of unmineralized matrix (the *osteoid seam*), which is separated from mineralized bone by an intermediate zone 3 to 4 μm wide, known as the *mineralization front*. Reticular fibers are added to the matrix from the surrounding mesenchyme to give rise to the so-called osteogenic fibers on which calcification subsequently takes place. As mineralization occurs, these fibers become collagenous. The bone increases in thickness by adding successive layers of matrix resulting from osteoblastic activity. During this phase of development, some of the osteoblasts with their processes become entrapped in the matrix, and when calcification occurs, they occupy a space in the matrix known as a lacuna. These are the true bone cells or osteocytes (Figs. 5-4 and 5-5), and approximately one osteoblast in ten will become trapped in the developing spicule in this manner.

An osteoblast, after it is surrounded by bone matrix, remains in the tissue as a bone cell or osteocyte. The spicule thus formed contains all the essential elements of the bone: fibers, a calcified matrix, and cells situated in lacunae. It differs from cartilage in two respects: the chemical composition of the matrix and the shape of the lacunae. In cartilage the lacunae are round or oval and are entirely separate from each other, whereas in bone the spindle-shaped lacunae are connected by tiny channels in the matrix, through which cellular processes of the osteocytes maintain contact with each other. The fibers of a new spicule are arranged in a woven pattern (woven bone), whereas the fibers of adult bone are usually arranged in layers (lamellar bone).

Osteocytes, or bone cells, occur in lacunae within the calcified matrix. The main portion of the cell is flattened, conforming to the shape of the lacuna that it occupies. Numerous slender processes extend from the cell body into canaliculi at right angles to the surrounding matrix. Although the extent of these processes is controversial, it is generally believed that they are linked to adjoining cells by gap junctions. The osteocyte is a less active cell than the osteoblast; accordingly, the organelles are not as prominent as those occurring in the osteoblast (Fig. 5-7). The osteocyte is not concerned with bone formation but rather with metabolic activities necessary for the maintenance and modification of the bone matrix and with mineral balance. The thin layer of bone against which osteocyte processes lie (the perilacunar bone) differs from other kinds of bone. It has fewer collagen fibers and crystals, contains more

amorphous bone salt, and differs in permeability and staining properties. This region of low density bone contains more labile minerals than do other parts of bones and is of special importance, since the osteocytes contribute to the regulation of body calcium balance (calcium homeostasis) by a process known as osteolysis. Osteocytes also play a role in the detection and repair of fatigue microfractures (tiny fractures in bone matrix due to pressure and tension), and help to prevent major damage to the bones.

Other osteocytes line the 70% or so of bone surface where neither formation nor resorption is taking place. These cells, sometimes called surface osteocytes to distinguish

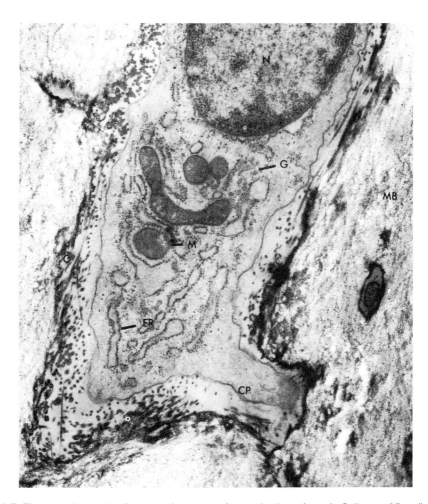

Fig. 5-7. Electron micrograph of portion of osteocyte from calvarium of rat. *C,* Collagen; *CP,* cell process; *ER,* endoplasmic reticulum; *G,* Golgi vesicles; *M,* mitochondrion; *MB,* bone matrix; *N,* nucleus. (×23,000.)

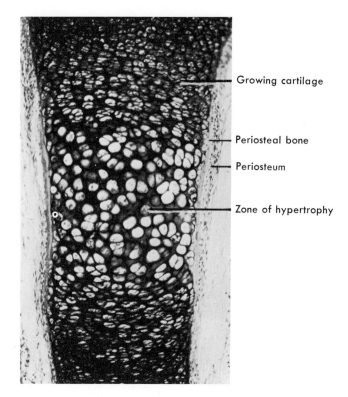

Growing cartilage

Periosteal bone

Periosteum

Zone of hypertrophy

Fig. 5-8. Central part of shaft of developing long bone.

them from the "deep osteocytes" trapped in lacunae, form a layer of thin flattened cells that provide an incomplete film of tissue covering the bone surface. These same cells also form the outer lining of bone marrow and extend through the channels in bone as well as over the endosteal and trabecular surfaces.

Cartilage replacement (endochondral) bone

In many parts of the embryo a model of the skeleton is laid down in cartilage first. This must be replaced by bone in a gradual manner so that the embryo will not be left unsupported at any time. The process is well illustrated in the femur, a typical long bone. The process of endochondral bone formation and remodeling allows the femur to bear weight continuously all through the growth period of childhood while it changes progressively in length (Figs. 5-15 and 5-16).

The first indication of mineralization in the cartilage model appears in the center of the future shaft. The cartilage cells in this region

undergo proliferation and hypertrophy (Fig. 5-8). This results in an increase in the number and size of the lacunae and a decrease in the amount of matrix (partitions). The partitions become infiltrated with mineral salts and stain intensely with basic dye (Fig. 5-9). This region is known as the primary ossification center. At the same time that the above events are taking place, cells in the perichondrium assume an osteogenic function and lay down a collar of membrane bone around the ossification center. This bone is closely adherent to the underlying cartilage and aids in the support of the bone. The *periosteal collar* is thin walled and short, but becomes progressively thicker and longer. The perichondrium covering the cartilage has now assumed a bone-forming function and is accordingly known as the periosteum.

When the periosteal collar has been established, vascular connective tissue sprouts derived from the periosteum, known as *periosteal buds* (Fig. 5-10), pierce the bone collar and enter the cartilage matrix. These buds

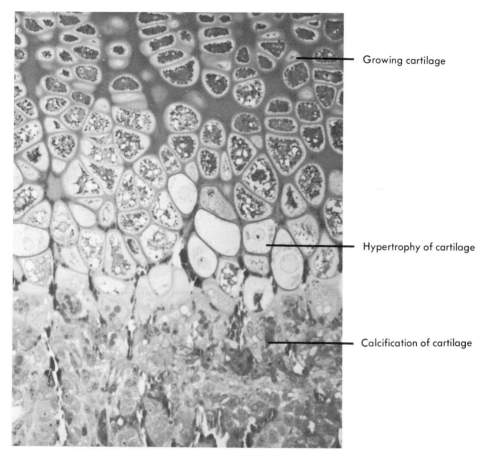

Growing cartilage

Hypertrophy of cartilage

Calcification of cartilage

Fig. 5-9. Part of epiphyseal region of 4-day-old rat femur showing cellular differences during growth. (Plastic section; ×250.)

consist of blood vessels and osteogenic cells. They penetrate the cartilage and form cavities, the *primary marrow spaces.* The osteogenic cells brought in by the periosteal buds give rise to osteoblasts that align themselves on the margins of the calcified cartilage remnants. Osteoblastic activity results in the deposition of bone matrix (osteoid), which subsequently becomes mineralized. By means of the processes just described, a series of interconnecting spicules and trabeculae with a central core of calcified cartilage matrix are formed. The primary bone deposited on the surface of the calcified spicules, together with the calcified cartilage, is then resorbed by osteoclastic activity that results in the formation of the *primary bone marrow cavity* (Fig. 5-11). Hemopoietic ele-

ments brought in by the periosteal bud give rise to vascular elements and a primary bone marrow. The resorption of the bone trabeculae is a gradual process, and there are always some trabeculae retained for purposes of temporary support during growth of the bone.

The essential process of endochondral bone formation is similar to that occurring in intramembranous bone. The difference between the two processes is that in endochondral ossification each spicule is deposited around a fragment of calcified cartilage matrix, whereas in intramembranous bone spicules no such framework is present.

The calcification of the cartilage matrix and bone formation that is first observed in the center of the *diaphysis* (that is, the shaft of

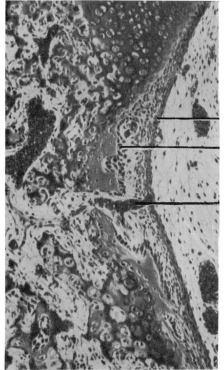

Periosteum

Osteoblasts

Periosteal bud

Fig. 5-10. Section through center of shaft of developing long bone showing periosteal bud and associated structures.

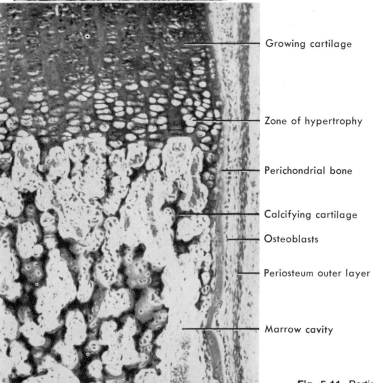

Growing cartilage

Zone of hypertrophy

Perichondrial bone

Calcifying cartilage

Osteoblasts

Periosteum outer layer

Marrow cavity

Fig. 5-11. Portion of shaft of developing long bone showing calcification of cartilage.

the bone) subsequently extends in two directions toward each end *(epiphysis)* of the developing bone (Fig. 5-12). The extension of the zones of ossification takes place by means of an orderly sequence of changes in the cartilage similar to those occurring during the formation of the primary ossification center. These changes, however, occur in distinct zones (Figs. 5-11 and 5-12), each of which exhibit different activities.

1. The *zone of resting (reserve) cartilage* is the most distal and is relatively long. It consists of small randomly distributed chondrocytes.

2. Next is the *growth zone (zone of cell multiplication)*, composed of cells that are arranged in rows parallel to the long axis of the cartilage model. There is a considerable amount of matrix formed between the chondrocytes. The cellular activity results in lengthening the bone.

3. Nearer the diaphysis is the *zone of cell*

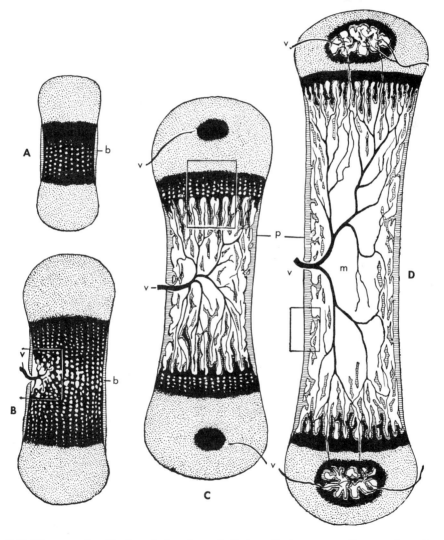

Fig. 5-12. Diagrams of ossification of a long bone. **A,** Early cartilaginous stage; **B,** stage of eruption of periosteal bone collar by osteogenic bud of vessels; **C,** older stage with primary marrow cavity and early centers of calcification in epiphyseal cartilages; **D,** condition shortly after birth with epiphyseal centers of ossification. Calcified cartilage in all diagrams is black. *b,* Periosteal bone collar; *m,* marrow cavity; *p,* periosteal bone; *v,* blood vessels entering centers of ossification. (From Nonidez, J., and W. Windle. 1953. Textbook of histology. McGraw-Hill Book Co., New York.)

hypertrophy and lacunar enlargement. In this zone the cells enlarge, which results in a further increase in the length of the cartilage. The cytoplasm of the cells accumulate glycogen, lipid droplets, and alkaline phosphatase. The nuclei enlarge and then become pyknotic prior to degeneration and death of the cells.

4. The *zone of calcification* is narrow and variable. The matrix between adjacent lacunae dissolves, leaving the matrix between the rows as jagged spicules of calcified cartilage matrix.

5. The previous zone is gradually transformed into a *zone of cartilage removal and bone deposition.* As was the case in the formation of bone in the primary ossification center, vascular sprouts arising from the primary bone marrow cavity grow into the lacunae between the jagged trabeculae, carrying with them osteoprogenitor cells and osteoclasts (Figs. 5-13 and 5-14). Osteoblasts lay down bone on the calcified cartilage spicules, and increased vascularization occurs; then osteoclastic resorption of the calcified cartilage matrix and bone follows, which results in further enlargement of the bone marrow cavity. The region where the diaphysis and epiphysis meet, that is, the zone where cartilage is resorbed and in which bone is being formed, is known as the *metaphysis*, the region connecting the shaft with the articular ends of the bone.

At the same time that changes noted above are taking place within the cartilage model, the periosteal collar increases in length and thickness. The marrow cavity also enlarges by means of longitudinal extension and increase in diameter, the latter being due to resorption on the inner surface of the bone collar. The zone of reserve cartilage is maintained during growth of the bone. It becomes reduced in length as ossification proceeds.

Later, new and independent centers develop in the ends of the cartilage model without the preliminary formation of perichondrial bone. These new centers in the epiphyses represent secondary centers of ossification that spread radially. The growth zone of cartilage, on which the increase in length of the bone as a whole depends, thus comes to lie between two centers of ossification that encroach on it from opposite directions. The growth zone persists during the early years of life, and as long as it remains, the individual continues to grow in height. Ultimately, at

Trabecula   Osteoclasts

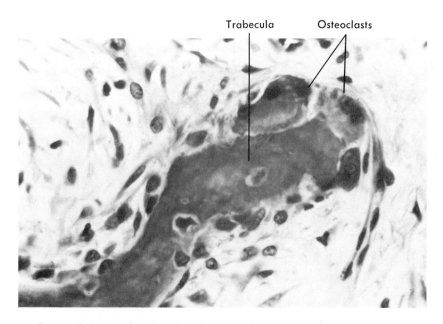

Fig. 5-13. Portion of a bone trabecula undergoing resorption by means of osteoclastic activity. (×600.)

about the twentieth year of life, ossification outruns cartilage growth and the epiphyses and diaphysis unite. The time at which the epiphyses fuse differs for each bone, and analysis of the degree of ossification in various sites can give a rough idea of the developmental age of an individual (a gauge of *bone age*, often used to evaluate disorders of growth and development). After fusion has occurred, the bone ceases to grow in length, but additions in thickness may be made by osteoblasts in the surrounding periosteum. The importance of this layer, as well as its

structure, will be discussed in connection with the histology of the adult bone.

The process of erosion of bone actually begins soon after the first trabecula of spongy bone has been laid down and continues actively throughout life even after the bones stop growing. Initially, it starts at the point where bone formation began: at the borders of the primary marrow cavity. Thus as mineralization of the diaphysis of a long bone moves toward the ends of the cartilage model, it is followed by a secondary breaking down and resorption of part of the newly

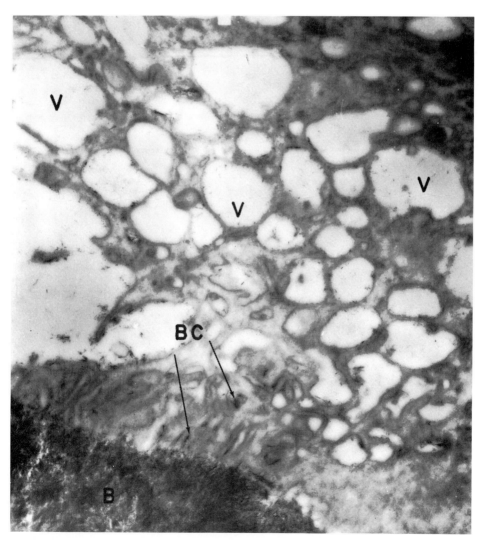

Fig. 5-14. Electron photomicrograph of an osteoclast showing crystals. *B,* Bone; *BC,* bone crystals; *V,* vacuole. (×20,000.) (Courtesy Dr. F. Gonzales.)

formed tissue so that the bone is maintained in a proper shape, rather than becoming progressively thicker at the ends. The result is an enlargement of the marrow cavity and a resculpturing of the ends, which prevents the bone from becoming too heavy and solid. During the internal reconstruction of the bone, the tips of the trabeculae at either end of the marrow cavity are constantly being resorbed. Resorption is necessary for the overall growth of the bone. This process tends to maintain a metaphysis of a constant length, whereas the overall length of the bone shaft increases.

Osteoclast

Large multinucleated cells, the osteoclasts, are associated with bone resorption and are often located in concavities of the bone surface (Howship's lacunae) (Fig. 5-13). The cytoplasm is only slightly basophilic and exhibits a vacuolated appearance. The nuclei are similar in appearance to those of the osteoblasts. At the electron microscope level it has been shown that the surface of the cell adjacent to the bone appears to be characterized by numerous infoldings of the cell membrane, giving rise to clefts (Fig. 5-14). Evidence suggests that bone salt crystals are loosened from the bone matrix by enzymatic activity and taken up by the folds in the surface, then by vesicles in the cytoplasm where they undergo demineralization. The mechanism whereby the collagen fibers and matrix are degraded is accomplished, according to suggestive evidence, by proteolytic enzymes elaborated by the osteoclasts.

The area of the osteoclast in contact with bone surface has a ruffled appearance in active erosion. This ruffled border consists of many cytoplasmic extensions infiltrating the disentegrating bone surface. In adult bone approximately 0.5% of the free bone surface is being remodeled continuously.

Erosion is not confined to the central portion of the bones where its effect is a progressive enlargement of the marrow cavity. It occurs throughout the mass of all bony tissue, but in all places except the marrow cavities it is followed by rebuilding. In the ends of the long bones and in the central portions of other bones the rebuilding keeps pace with erosion and follows the pattern of the original formation of the tissue, resulting in a renewal of spongy bone. In the peripheral parts of all bones, however, rebuilding is more rapid than erosion, and a compact layer of bone is established.

Formation of Haversian systems. Compact bone is more regular in its arrangement than spongy bone. Its development may be described as follows. The marrow spaces, containing reticular tissue and blood-forming cells, are penetrated throughout by a rich vascular network. The vessels at the periphery of the bone follow a more or less regular pathway parallel to the surface. In long bones, they run mainly in the long axis of the bone. In places where compact bone is to be formed, an area of bony matrix is first removed by osteoclasts. This erosion follows a definite plan, rounding out the matrix so that cylindrical cavities are formed around the blood vessels (Fig. 5-17). After the matrix has been reshaped in this manner, the cavity is lined by successive concentric layers (lamellae) of new bone. The process continues until the space is almost filled with lamellae, and the channel eventually persists as a central canal containing blood vessels, nerves, and connective tissue. Such a grouping of concentric layers of bone, with its central canal, is called a Haversian system (Fig. 5-2).

When a new remodeling process begins in an area of compact bone, it is first necessary to clear a space (resorption) for new bone. This is followed by a period of bone deposition by osteoblasts. Normally, refilling follows immediately behind excavation in a line advancing through the cortex either alongside or parallel to an existing Haversian system. This wave of cellular activity can be called a cortical remodeling unit that passes through a cycle. Although mesenchymal cell proliferation, osteoclastic resorption, and osteoblastic deposition follow one another in unvarying succession, little is known about these processes. Normally a conelike front of resorption cuts through the cortex at the rate

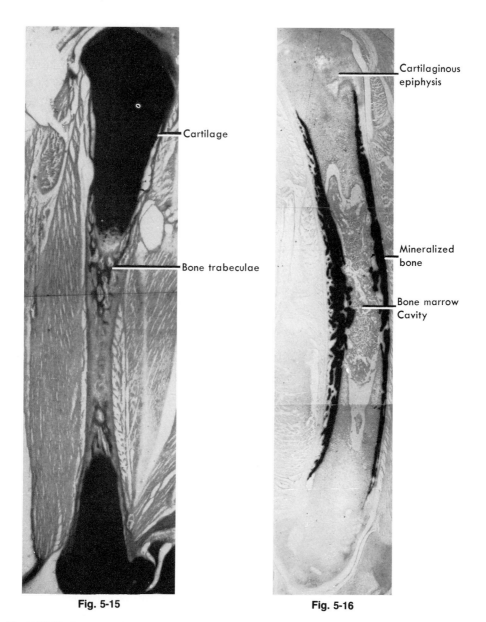

Cartilaginous
epiphysis

Cartilage

Mineralized
bone

Bone trabeculae

Bone marrow
Cavity

Fig. 5-15   **Fig. 5-16**

Fig. 5-15. Radioautograph of femur of 14-day-old chick injected on thirteenth day with ^{35}S. Note uptake in cartilage matrix and to lesser degree in bone matrix. Black areas are metachromatic. Compare with Fig. 5-16.

Fig. 5-16. Radioautograph of longitudinal section of femur of 14-day-old chick injected with ^{45}Ca on thirteenth day. Black areas show regions of ^{45}Ca uptake. Practically no endochondral ossification is present in chick bone at this time.

of about 20 μm/day longitudinally and 5 μm/day wide. The time required for the entire sequence of resorption and refilling to take place is conventionally referred to as sigma (σ) and is at least 100 days, about 20 days of which are spent in resorption and the rest in bone deposition. Variations in this rate can occur in response to age, stress, metabolic status, and other factors.

Although cortical bone occupies about 80%

of the total adult skeleton by volume, it only provides 20% of the surface available for remodeling. The remainder of remodeling takes place on the trabeculae, apparently by a similar succession of cellular events. In general, bone remodeling occurs continuously both during development and in the adult in spatially discrete locations. Within each site of remodeling there occurs an unvarying sequence of cellular events, each lasting

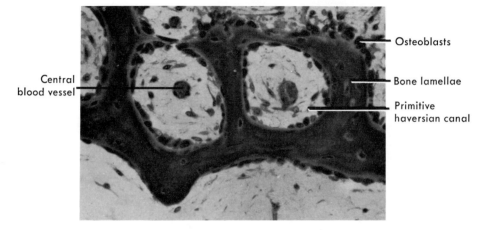

Central blood vessel ⎯ Osteoblasts

Bone lamellae

Primitive haversian canal

Fig. 5-17. Remodeling of bone to form Haversian systems.

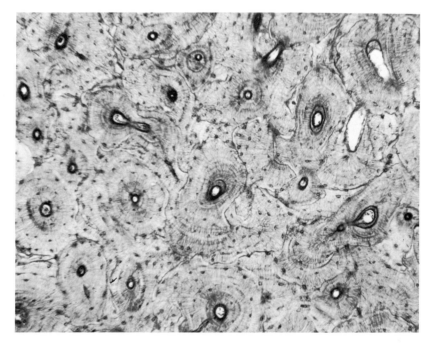

Fig. 5-18. Ground section of compact bone showing arrangement of Haversian systems. ($\times$100.)

about the same time and replacing about the same volume of bone that was present before the remodeling began.

The remodeling of bone does not end when the primary Haversian systems are laid down, but continues into adult life. The primary systems are partially destroyed to provide space for new ones in response to changes in mechanical stress. The final result is a mass of bone composed of secondary and tertiary Haversian systems embedded in the remains of earlier systems. The lamellae that form the background for the Haversian systems, holding them together in a solid mass, are called interstitial lamellae. The surface of the bone is formed by circumferential lamellae that have been laid down by the osteoblasts of the periosteal tissue. This region contains no Haversian systems. Endosteal lamellae of the same character line the shaft where it borders the marrow cavity.

ADULT BONE

Gross examination of adult bone that has been sawed in half will show that it is composed of both spongy and compact tissue. In the long bones the spongy arrangement is confined to the epiphyses and inner part of the shaft, and there is a central marrow cavity entirely devoid of bone matrix. In flat bones the spongy tissue forms trabeculae crossing from one side to the other so that there is no large marrow cavity but several small irregular marrow spaces. Either form of bone has an outer layer, or cortex, of compact tissue that is, in turn, covered by the periosteum, a tough fibrous coating.

Microscopically the most characteristic feature of bone is its lamellar structure. Sections of decalcified spongy bone present a picture much like that of developing intramembranous bone except for the greater extent of the trabeculae and bone marrow. Osteoblasts and osteoclasts are less common but may be found in portions of the tissue that are undergoing changes in arrangement. The matrix stains red with eosin and is lamellated; the cells are dark in color and disposed, one in each lacuna, between adjacent lamellae. With special techniques one may demonstrate the canaliculi and the fibers on which the matrix was deposited, but these are not ordinarily visible in hematoxylin-eosin preparations.

Ground sections of bone do not show the cellular elements of the tissue, since these are destroyed in the making of the preparation. Such sections are useful in studying the architecture of compact bone. In transverse ground sections the following features are to be noted (Figs. 5-18 to 5-21). The Haversian canals appear as empty circular spaces, each

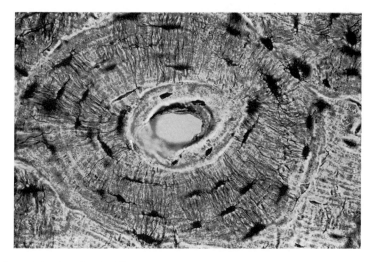

Fig. 5-19. Ground section showing Haversian system (osteone) with concentrically arranged lamellae and centrally located Haversian canal.

of which is surrounded by six to fifteen concentric lamellae. The lacunae and the canaliculi radiating from them are readily visible. The concentric lamellae, the cells, and the central canal constitute a *Haversian system* or *osteone*. Between Haversian systems is the packing of interstitial lamellae, and a section taken from the periphery of the bone will contain periosteal lamellae. Canals running diagonally or at right angles to those of the Haversian systems are the canals of Volkmann. They provide for transverse connections and anastomosis between the blood vessels and are distinguished from Haversian canals by their direction through the tissue and by the fact that they are not surrounded

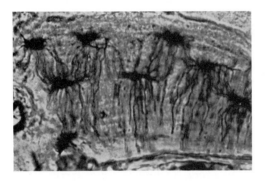

Fig. 5-20. Higher magnification of portion of Fig. 5-19 to show detail of lacunae and canaliculi in bone matrix.

by concentric lamellae. The vascular pattern of bone is best seen in longitudinal sections in which, however, the concentric arrangement of lamellae is not to be observed. The appearance of decalcified bone is shown in Fig. 5-2.

Despite its physical rigidity, bone is a tissue that retains considerable ability to respond to environmental changes. The most obvious of these are traumatic changes such as fractures, which are repaired by the osteoblasts in the periosteum and at the border of the marrow cavity. Some disturbances of the endocrine glands (acromegaly, for example) provide a stimulus to the osteoblasts of the periosteum that results in the laying down of additional cortical layers of bone. Also, the skeleton serves as a storehouse for calcium, and the rates of erosion and rebuilding respond to variations in the mineral metabolism of the body. It is essential to life that a certain amount of calcium be present in the body fluids. When this amount is not supplied by the diet, it may be withdrawn from the bones, or, conversely, excess calcium may be stored in them.

The skeletal system is under the influence of several hormones. Parathyroid hormone, calcitonin, and vitamin D are responsible for the maintenance of normal levels of calcium

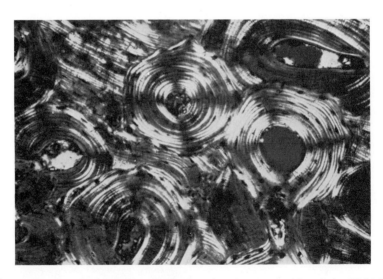

Fig. 5-21. Cross section of compact bone; ground section photographed in polarized light. Note high degree of orientation of fibers and crystals of bone.

in the blood. The activity of the parathyroid gland appears to depend on calcium levels in the circulation. When blood calcium is low, secretion of the gland is stimulated. In hyperparathyroidism, bone is resorbed to an unusual degree and is replaced by fibrous tissue; this condition is known as osteitis fibrosa or von Recklinghausen's disease. Calcitonin is a hormone that is derived from the parafollicular cells of the thyroid gland (Chapter 20). It has an action antagonistic to that of parathyroid hormone, lowering blood calcium and inhibiting bone resorption. In addition to the two hormones mentioned, it has been shown that growth hormone elaborated by the hypophysis maintains the cartilage plates of the long bones and is necessary for normal bone growth. Gonadal hormones play a role in the rate of skeletal maturation by affecting the rate of closure of the epiphyseal growth plates due to depletion of the reserve cartilage.

It is obvious that normal bone growth and maturation are dependent on several nutritional factors. This is especially true of the adequate supply and availability of minerals such as calcium and phosphorus, which are the main inorganic components of bone. It has been shown that a dietary insufficiency of either calcium or phosphorus leads to a rarefaction and brittleness of bones. In situations where dietary calcium and phosphorus are adequate but vitamin D is deficient, interference with mineral absorption occurs and mineralization of the growing epiphysis is inhibited, giving rise to a condition known as rickets. When subjected to stress, bone in this state becomes deformed.

Adult rickets (osteomalacia) is a condition in which bone exhibits considerable amounts of osteoid tissue. The situation is caused by a long-term deficiency of dietary minerals and vitamin D. Deficiency in vitamin A results in an inhibition of the rate of growth of the skeleton by interfering with the ratio of osteoblasts and osteoclasts responsible for growth and resorption, respectively.

Retardation of growth and of healing of fractures is correlated with a deficiency of vitamin C. In this case, there is insufficient production of the elements needed to form the bone matrix.

PERIOSTEUM

The periosteum is a connective tissue layer covering the bone except at the articular surfaces. It is divisible into two layers. The outer of these is a network of densely packed collagenous fibers with blood vessels. The inner layer provides the penetration fibers (of Sharpey), which are inserted into the bone and attach the periosteum to it. In the inner layer of the periosteum, one may also find fine elastic fibers loosely arranged. Osteoblasts occur here also whenever appositional growth of the bone is taking place. The endosteum is a thin layer of connective tissue lining the marrow cavity and the smaller cavities within the bone. In addition to the more obvious function that the periosteum performs, such as anchorage for tendons and ligaments, it is also concerned with repair and regeneration of bone.

BLOOD SUPPLY AND NERVES

The blood supply of bone comes by two routes. Near the middle of the shaft is a medullary or nutrient canal that pierces the bone and leads to the marrow cavity. The nutrient artery passes through this canal, giving off branches to the Haversian canals on the way. In the marrow cavity it divides into an ascending and a descending branch, both of which supply the marrow.

The other supply of blood for the bone tissue comes by way of the numerous arteries of the periosteum. These enter the substance of the bone through Volkmann's canals, which, in turn, lead to Haversian canals.

Veins leave the bone through the nutrient canal, and it is here also that the myelinated and nonmyelinated nerves enter. The nerves accompany the blood vessels into the Haversian canals.

The circulation of blood occupies a central role in the physiology of bone. In humans approximately 25% of the cardiac output goes to bone, a volume comparable to the amount of blood flowing to the kidneys. Little is known about the control of skeletal blood flow.

Cartilaginous callus

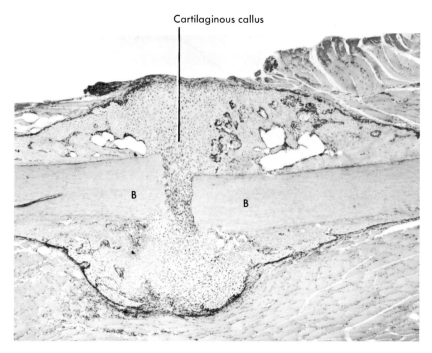

Fig. 5-22. Partial repair of bone fracture (rabbit rib). Space between fractured ends of bone, *B*, is filled in with fibrous tissue. On the periphery a cartilaginous callus, later replaced by bone, has developed. (×40.)

Most pain sensitivity in bone is localized in the periosteum, but patients also often complain of discomfort when bone marrow is aspirated during biopsy, suggesting that the blood vessels of the marrow are also innervated.

Lymphatic channels exist in the periosteum but not within the cortex or medulla of bones.

MARROW

Although marrow is not actually a part of bone as a tissue, it is included in sections of decalcified bone and should be mentioned here. It is of two kinds, named red and yellow marrow according to their color in the fresh state. Both kinds have a framework of reticular tissue. Red marrow is the chief site of the formation of certain types of blood cells, including the red corpuscles and contains a great number of blood vessels. The details of its structure will be considered in the following chapters. In yellow marrow the blood-forming elements have been replaced by adipose tissue, and the amount of reticular tissue is reduced. Red marrow is present in the cavities of all bones during fetal life and early childhood. It is gradually replaced by yellow marrow, and red marrow remains in the adult chiefly in the epiphyses of long bones and in the ribs, vertebrae, cranial bones, and sternum.

BONE REPAIR

After bone fracture the following events occur in connection with the repair of the injured bone. First, a hemorrhage is caused by the rupture of blood vessels, which is soon followed by the formation of a clot. Subsequently fibroblasts and capillaries migrate into the area formed by the clot, which results in the formation of granulation tissue. The granulation tissue then becomes infiltrated with dense fibrous tissue, giving rise to a fibrous union *(procallus)*. The fibrous tissue soon is transformed to cartilage, which constitutes a temporary union or *callus* (Fig. 5-22). The cartilaginous callus is gradually replaced by bone because of the stem cell activity of the cells in the periosteum. Finally, excess bone present in the callus is partially or completely resorbed. The repair of bone

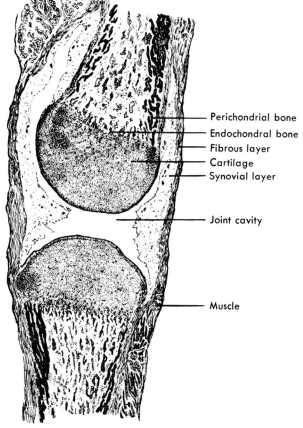

Fig. 5-23. Joint from finger of newborn child. Process of cartilage replacement is still going on, and one may distinguish between endochondral and perichondrial bone.

Perichondrial bone
Endochondral bone
Fibrous layer
Cartilage
Synovial layer

Joint cavity

Muscle

as described here is dependent on an adequate blood supply, on the activity of the bone-forming cells in the periosteum, and also on adequate vitamin and mineral supplies.

JOINTS

The bones are joined together to form the skeleton by a series of articulations, the structure of each varying with the degree of movability of the joint. Articulations that are immovable or nearly so are called synarthroses. In the skull, for instance, the bones are held together by ligaments composed of short fibers, of which some are elastic and others are continuations of the fibers of Sharpey. The vertebrae are less closely joined, allowing a limited amount of movement, and the spaces between them are occupied by intervertebral disks of fibrocartilage.

The movable joints or diarthroses are characterized by a space between the bones, which is the articular cleft. Each bone bordering on this space has at its end a cap of articular cartilage, which is the remainder of the embryonic cartilage model of the bone. This cartilage is of the hyaline type but has no perichondrial fibrous layer (Fig. 5-23).

The capsule that encloses the articular car-

tilages and the space between them has two layers. The outer part is the stratum fibrosum, composed of dense fibrous tissue continuous with the outer layer of the periosteum of the bones. The stratum fibrosum is blended with the tendons and ligaments of the muscles attached at this point. The inner or synovial layer is of looser and more vascular connective tissue. Where it borders on the articular cavity, it is lined with a layer of dense connective tissue. This consists of fibers and fibroblasts arranged around the border of the cavity. The synovial layer sometimes forms projections into the joint cavity, which may contain fibrocartilage. The synovial fluid, or synovia, is believed to be secreted, at least in part, by cells of the synovial membrane. It is a yellow viscid fluid containing mucoproteins and cellular debris. It serves to lubricate and thus facilitate the smooth movement of the articulating surfaces.

6

Blood and blood formation

Mesenchyme, an embryonic connective tissue derived from the mesoderm, contains characteristic cells that are stellate in shape and connected one to the other by their cellular processes. These cells undergo many changes, which result in the elaboration of blood, lymph, blood vessels, connective tissue proper, cartilage, and bone. In blood and lymph the intercellular substance is fluid; in connective tissues, fibers occur; in cartilage the intercellular substance is semirigid and contains fibers; whereas in bone the fibers present are impregnated with mineral salts.

Blood may be considered a specialized form of connective tissue consisting of free cells and a fluid matrix (plasma). Blood cells develop in reticular connective tissue of blood-forming organs and enter the bloodstream as fully formed cells.

The structural elements of the blood consist of red cells (*erythrocytes*), white cells (*leukocytes*), and platelets. Together they are about equal in bulk to the plasma. Red cells are more numerous than white; the number of red cells in human males is 5 to 5.5 million/mm³; in females, 4.5 to 5 million/mm³. These values are subject, however, to wide variation. White cells are present in the amount of 8,000 to 10,000/mm³. The total volume of blood in an average individual of 60 kg (150 pounds) amounts to 5 to 6 liters, or roughly 8% of the body weight.

BLOOD
Red blood corpuscles (erythrocytes)

When a drop of freshly drawn blood is examined under the microscope, red corpuscles are seen as biconcave disks having a diameter of approximately 8 μm (Fig. 6-1). In the fresh state they appear greenish in color rather than red. The depression in the center of each corpuscle makes a light spot that might at first sight be mistaken for a nucleus. Adult red cells are, however, nonnucleated in mammalian blood. Often they stick together in rows, or rouleaux. As a drop of blood dries at its edges the red cells lose fluid and change their shape. Some are cup shaped, others are irregular in outline. In sections of organs and tissues stained with hematoxylin and eosin, the red blood cells have a bright orange or red color. The disk shape is the most common in such preparations, but, especially in small vessels, the cells are sometimes cup shaped, sometimes compressed into angular forms. The usual method of preparing blood for microscopic study is to spread a drop on a slide so that it forms a thin smear and then to stain it with a special stain. Wright's stain is commonly used. The red corpuscles when so treated lose volume without changing shape. Those at the center of the smear, when there have been no changes caused by rapid drying, have the form of biconcave disks (Fig. 6-1), which average about 7.5 μm in diameter. The cells are nongranular and colored pale brown or pink by the stain.

About 1% of the erythrocytes examined in a smear, although having lost their nuclei, have a diffuse bluish stain and are somewhat larger than the red-staining cells. When stained with cresyl blue, a network of reticulum appears in the cytoplasm; they are ac-

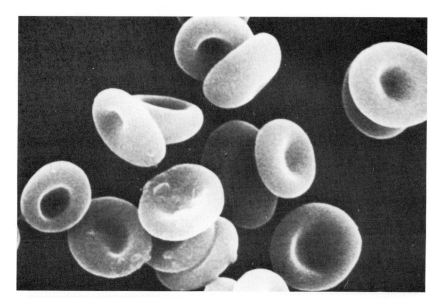

Fig. 6-1. Scanning electron micrograph of erythrocytes. (×3000.) (Courtesy Dr. H. Nakahara.)

cordingly known as *reticulocytes*. They are immature erythrocytes.

Because the red blood cells are nonnucleated, it is sometimes said that they should not be called cells. The name erythroplastid may be used, but erythrocyte is the more common term. The cytoplasm of the red corpuscles contains a protein called hemoglobin, which combines with oxygen and is transformed to oxyhemoglobin. In the body tissues, where the oxygen concentration is less than in the lungs, the oxyhemoglobin is released and the oxygen is utilized in metabolic processes of the cells. Hemoglobin is also important in the transport of carbon dioxide from the tissues to the lungs.

Hemoglobin imparts a reddish tint to cells containing it if the latter are stained with Wright's stain. This fact is important in recognition of early stages of development of red blood cells. (See discussion on bone marrow later in the chapter.)

White blood corpuscles (leukocytes)

The leukocytes as a group respond differently from the red cells to the treatment involved in making a smear. Erythrocytes lose a slight amount of volume and are therefore smaller in the smear than in the fresh state. Leukocytes, on the contrary, are flattened by the treatment and acquire a greater diameter.

The leukocytes contain a nucleus and cell organelles. They exhibit a limited degree of ameboid movement and, for convenience, may be divided into two main groups: the granular variety and the nongranular or lymphoid types. In sections stained with hematoxylin and eosin the leukocytes stand out among the erythrocytes because of their darkly stained nuclei. It is sometimes possible to identify lymphocytes, granulocytes, and monocytes in such preparations, but for critical examination of white cells one must use preparations made with special stains, such as Wright's or Giemsa.

Granular (polymorphonuclear) leukocytes

An outstanding feature of the granulocytes is the presence of granules in the cytoplasm. Each variety of granulocyte has a different kind of granule readily identified at both the optical and the electron microscope levels. A second characteristic feature of these cells is the nucleus, which is multilobed. Although several criteria may be used to distinguish and classify the granulocytes, the two most commonly employed are based on the morphological characteristics of the nucleus and the size, shape, and tinctorial properties of the granules. The granulocytes make up from 60% to 70% of the white cells. In a blood smear or bone marrow smear treated with Wright's stain, the types of cells illustrated in Plates 1 to 4 may be distinguished.

Neutrophilic (heterophilic) leukocytes. The nucleus of neutrophilic leukocytes consists of from three to five irregular oval lobes connected by thin chromatin strands. In dry smear preparations from females an appendage appears on one of the lobes in about 3% of the cells. This chromatin appendage, known as a "drumstick" (not to be confused with irregularities on the margin of the nu-

clei), represents the chromatin material in which one female (X) chromosome is located. The cytoplasm (except for a clear homogeneous peripheral zone) is slightly acidophilic and contains numerous fine granules, which appear purple or lavender. These cells measure about 8 μm in the fresh state and attain a size of 12 μm in a dry smear preparation. At the electron microscope level the granules appear diverse in size and shape (Fig. 6-2). They can be divided into three morphological and biochemical varieties: (1) Relatively large, electron-dense, *azurophilic* or *primary granules* that contain peroxidases and hydro-

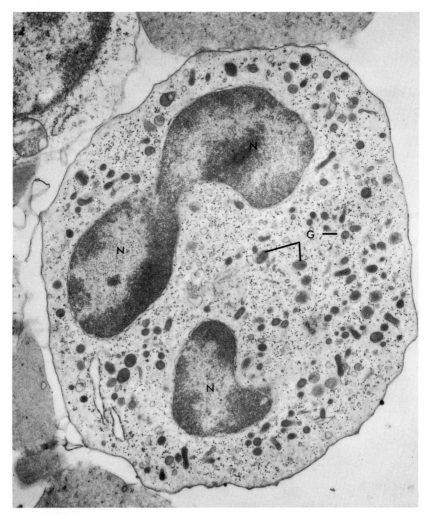

Fig. 6-2. Electron micrograph of neutrophilic leukocyte from bone marrow of cat. Granules are bounded by membrane and vary in density. They contain hydrolytic enzymes. Ribosomes are scattered throughout cytoplasm. *G,* Specific granules; *N,* lobes of nucleus. (×19,000.)

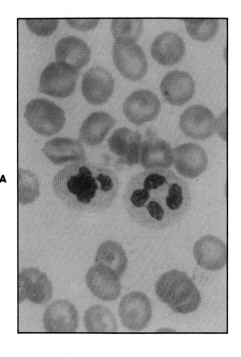

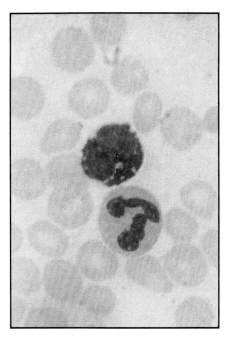

A

B

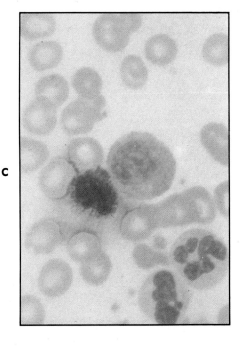

C

Plate 1. A, Segmented neutrophil, which shows at least one filament. The strict criterion for a filament is that it represents a bilayer of nuclear membrane with no chromatin in between. The cell to the left shows a little thicker filament than this but is still acceptable. **B,** A typical basophil (above) and a band neutrophil. A typical basophil in normal blood is characterized by an abundance of blue-black granules that vary in size and usually obscure the nucleus. **C,** The difference between a basophil and an eosinophil is shown here. Note that although the eosinophil granules are not a pure orange-red, they are uniform in size and have pale centers. (From Miale, J. B. 1977. Laboratory medicine: hematology. 5th ed. The C. V. Mosby Co., St. Louis.)

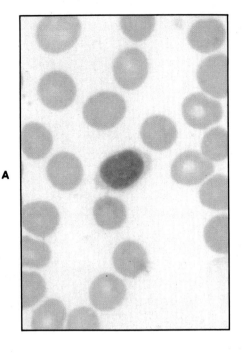

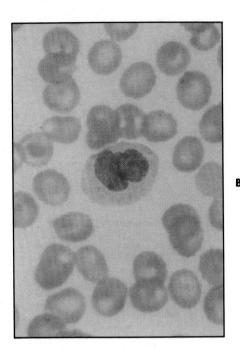

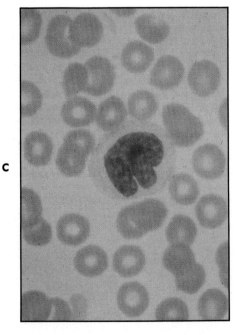

Plate 2. A, This cell is the typical small lymphocyte found in normal blood. Note the dense, pachychromatic nucleus and the smudged chromatin-parachromatin junction. The cytoplasm is clear, but normal lymphocytes may have small cytoplasmic granules. These are, however, peroxidase negative. **B** and **C,** These monocytes are from normal blood and are considered typical. Note the monocytoid nucleus and the very fine, dustlike, pink, cytoplasmic granules. These characteristics can be obscured by overstaining or if the stain is not good. The most common error is to call a poorly stained monocyte a neutrophilic metamyelocyte. (From Miale, J. B. 1977. Laboratory medicine: hematology. 5th ed. The C. V. Mosby Co., St. Louis.)

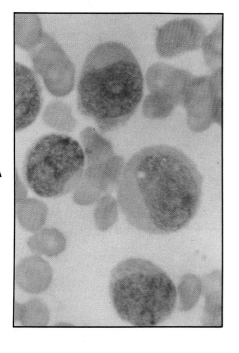

A

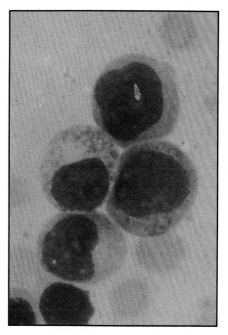

B

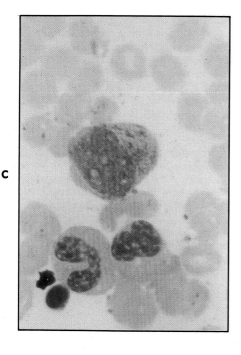

C

Plate 3. A, Myeloblast, which is usually about three times the diameter of a red blood cell but may be only two times the diameter in some acute leukemias. The high nucleus-cytoplasm ratio, the leptochromatic and delicately structured nucleus, and the nucleoli indicate the blast nature of these cells. As shown, the nucleoli may be multiple or single and are usually more numerous than in the lymphoblast, but this is not a reliable differential feature. **B,** Progranulocyte. The two cells on the right have immature nuclei with faintly visible nucleoli and a few cytoplasmic granules. The cell on the left above is a late myelocyte, and the cell below is a metamyelocyte. **C,** Myelocyte, which shows a still immature nucleus with several nucleoli and prominent, nonspecific, coarse granulation of the cytoplasm (center). The typical myelocyte seldom shows more than one nucleolus, and this is usually obscured by overlying granules. (From Miale, J. B. 1977. Laboratory medicine: hematology. 5th ed. The C. V. Mosby Co., St. Louis.)

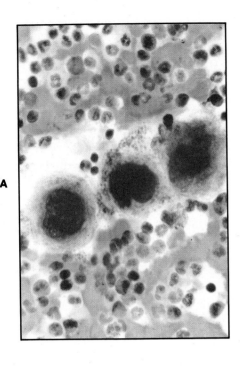

A

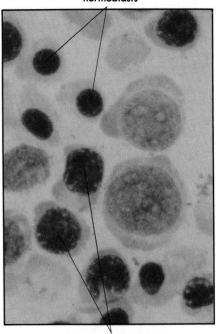

B

Orthochromic
normoblasts

Polychromatophilic
normoblasts

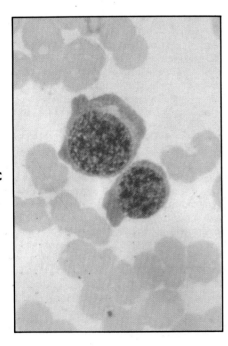

C

Plate 4. A, Megakaryocyte, which is a very large cell. There is good platelet formation shown here. **B,** Pronormoblast, which is sometimes difficult to distinguish from other blasts, but characteristically the nucleus tends to be round rather than oval and the cytoplasm more abundant than in the myeloblast. Some of its features, especially the blue nucleoli, are similar to what is assumed to characterize hemopoietic stem cells. **C,** Basophilic normoblast, which is distinguished from the pronormoblast by the coarser nuclear structure and the intense basophilia of the cytoplasm. The intense basophilia reflects the greater content of RNA preceding the synthesis of hemoglobin. At this stage of erythroid maturation, roundness of the nucleus is seen, which is characteristic of this and more mature erythroid cells. (From Miale, J. B. 1977 Laboratory medicine: hematology. 5th ed. The C. V. Mosby Co., St. Louis.)

lases; (2) smaller, less electron-dense *specific granules* that contain alkaline phosphatase and some antibacterial substances; and (3) a heterogeneous group smaller than specific granules that contain acid hydrolase. These and the primary granules are considered to be lysosomes.

Acidophilic (eosinophilic) leukocytes. The acidophilic leukocytes, which are approximately spherical, measure 9 μm in diameter in the fresh condition and in dry smears may attain a diameter of nearly 12 μm. They make up from 2% to 5% of the total leukocytes in the peripheral blood. In contrast with the nuclei of the neutrophils, the nuclei of the acidophils usually consist of two oval lobes connected by chromatin strands. Except for a centrally located area occupied by the cytocentrum, the cytoplasm contains numerous coarse granules, which in humans are spherical. When stained with acid dyes, the granules vary in appearance from pink to bright red. When observed with the electron microscope, the granules exhibit dense crystalline bodies that vary in appearance in different species (Figs. 6-3 and 6-4). Eosinophils increase in number during allergic conditions and certain parasitic infections. They apparently phagocytize antibody-antigen complexes that are then acted on by enzymes present in the granules.

Basophilic leukocytes. The basophils are the least numerous of the leukocytes and comprise less than 0.5% of the total count. They are approximately the same size as the neutrophils. The nucleus often appears S-shaped, is constricted in two or more regions, and stains less intensely than the other varieties. The granules are extremely coarse and with Wright's stain appear a dull blue. They are metachromatic and contain histamine, heparin, and serotonin. These granules also give the impression of being partially extruded from the cell surface because the

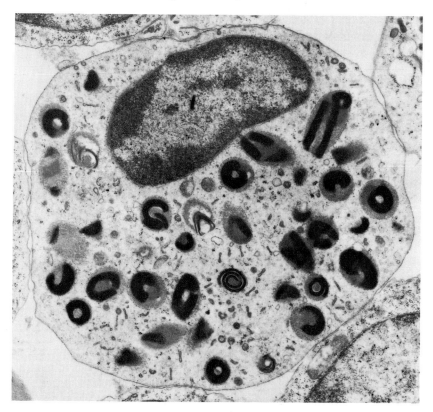

Fig. 6-3. Electron micrograph of eosinophilic leukocyte from bone marrow of cat. Note that granules are dense and contain dark organic crystals of varying shapes and sizes. (×17,000.)

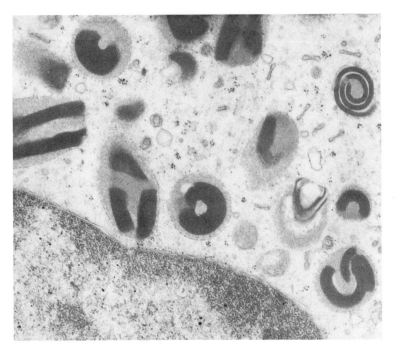

Fig. 6-4. Electron micrograph of part of eosinophilic leukocyte from bone marrow of cat showing detail of organic crystals in membrane-bound (specific) granules. (×33,000.)

cells are easily fragmented. They often partially obscure the nucleus. Viewed with the electron microscope, the granules appear membrane bound; the material enclosed by the membrane varies in appearance in diverse species. Scattered mitochondria and Golgi vesicles are usually present (Fig. 6-5).

Nongranular leukocytes

Lymphocytes. In the human the lymphocytes make up from 20% to 25% of the total number of white cells of the blood. They are spherical and measure from 6 to 8 μm in diameter, although some of them may be slightly larger. The most characteristic morphological feature of these cells is the presence of a large, dense nucleus with a distinct indentation on one side, which is not, however, observed in dry smear preparations. Prominent nucleoli may be observed in well-prepared sections at both the optical and the electron microscope levels. The cytoplasm appears as a thin rim surrounding the nucleus. It is homogeneous and basophilic, which is referable to numerous ribosomes observed at the electron microscope level. Occasionally, purple azurophilic granules may be ob-

served in the cytoplasm but these are inconstant features that represent early stages in granule development.

The larger lymphocytes are relatively few in number, and their increase in size results from the presence of a greater amount of cytoplasm. The cytoplasm usually contains a few scattered mitochondria and granules.

Monocytes. Monocytes resemble the lymphocytes, especially in forms that appear to be transitional. A typical monocyte measures from 9 to 12 μm in diameter. In dry smear preparations, however, they may appear to be 20 μm or larger. The mature monocyte exhibits considerably more cytoplasm than does the lymphocyte and often, though not invariably, has an eccentrically placed nucleus that is oval or kidney shaped. It stains less intensely than the lymphocytes. Organelles such as mitochondria and a Golgi apparatus are usually observed. The monocytes comprise from 3% to 8% of the leukocytes of the circulating blood.

Monocytes migrate from the bloodstream and become phagocytic. They are indistinguishable from macrophages that are normally present in connective tissue.

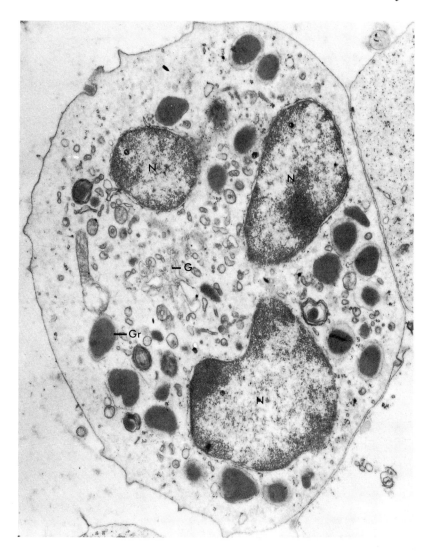

Fig. 6-5. Electron micrograph of basophilic leukocyte from bone marrow of cat. This cell contains three nuclear lobes, *N,* but does not show connecting strands of chromatin. Also shown are Golgi apparatus, *G,* and large dense membrane-enclosed granules, *Gr.* (×17,000.)

Functions of leukocytes

The leukocytes in the bloodstream appear to be inactive, and their function is not well understood. Outside the bloodstream, they exhibit ameboid movement. Leukocytes constantly migrate from the vessels to the tissues. This is particularly noticeable at the site of local injury or infection, where the granulocytes migrate in response to chemotactic stimulation. Later, monocytes also accumulate in these areas. Among the granulocytes only the neutrophils exhibit phagocytosis. Many types of bacteria are ingested by this process. After phagocytosis, the specific granules of the cell break down and disappear, meanwhile liberating hydrolytic enzymes, which are responsible for the destruction of bacteria. The neutrophils also release enzymes in surrounding tissues. This results in the intercellular destruction of bacteria. The neutrophils meanwhile die and form pus cells. Various other enzymes are present in leukocytes, but their function is not known at present.

In recent years the function of lymphocytes has received considerable attention.

This is especially true of the small lymphocytes, which are believed to play a significant role in the initiation of immune responses. Small lymphocytes are made up of two types of populations. This differentiation is based on the region in which they arise, the duration of life span, and reaction to certain drugs. The precursors of *T-lymphocytes* (CFU cells) arise in bone marrow and migrate to the thymus where they multiply and differentiate into T cells. Following this they may return to either the bone marrow or lymph organs, where they are retained for long periods. *B-lymphocytes* migrate by way of the blood stream to the generalized lymphoid tissues. This variety survives only a few days. When B-lymphocytes are exposed to antigens in the body, they produce antibodies. They inactivate or destroy such material or facilitate phagocytosis by macrophages. T-lymphocytes also act against foreign materials and give rise to a delayed hypersensitive reaction. For more information on lymphocytes, see Chapter 10.

Platelets

In addition to the cells just described, blood contains groups of minute cytoplasmic fragments that are called platelets or thrombocytes and are not generally included under corpuscles. The individual platelet, about 2 μm in diameter, is composed of a cytoplasm, which stains blue with Wright's stain. It has a dark granular center, the chromomere, and a light peripheral area, the hyalomere.

Thrombocytes or platelets are believed to liberate the enzyme *thromboplastin* involved in the clotting of blood (Fig. 6-6). Thromboplastin transforms prothrombin to thrombin, which, in turn, transforms fibrinogen to fibrin. Thromboplastin also has been identified in blood plasma. Platelets are formed by the budding off of cellular fragments from megakaryocytes in bone marrow.

Plasma

The fluid part of blood containing dissolved electrolytes and proteins is called *plasma*. One liter of plasma contains 940 ml of water; the rest of the volume is occupied by 60 gm of protein. Plasma makes up about 55% of the blood volume and cells make up the remainder. The relative amounts of blood cells and plasma (the hematocrit) vary under different physiologic conditions. In addition to electrolytes and

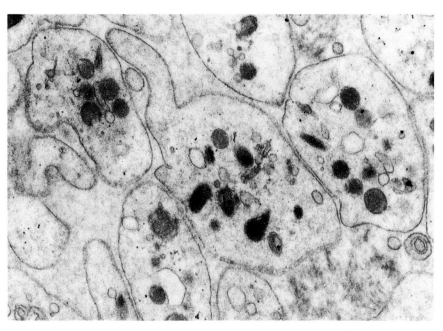

Fig. 6-6. Electron micrograph showing several blood platelets (thrombocytes). (×29,000.)

proteins, plasma contains a number of dissolved substances such as nutrients, gases, hormones, and clotting factors. One of the constituents of plasma, *fibrinogen,* is converted on standing to a fibrous clot in which erythrocytes and platelets become enmeshed. Clots help to control blood loss during hemorrhage. The clear, straw-colored fluid from which cells and clotting factors have been removed is called *serum.* Plasma transports the nutritive substances derived from food, the waste products of various tissues, and secretions of the endocrine glands.

LIFE SPAN AND DISPOSAL OF BLOOD CELLS

In comparison with many cells, red and white cells are relatively short lived. Isotope tracer studies have shown that red cells live for approximately 120 days. White cells are believed to remain in the circulating blood for about 24 hours. They may return to the circulating blood or remain in the tissue spaces.

Most red cells are removed by the reticuloendothelial cells in the liver and spleen. After destruction of the red cells by the phagocytes, the hemoglobin is converted to hematin and globin. The hematin is further reduced to iron, which is stored and reutilized.

Platelets survive 4 to 5 days and are removed from circulating blood by phagocytes in the liver and spleen.

LYMPH

Lymph consists of a fluid plasma that is somewhat different chemically from blood plasma. In it are floating leukocytes, principally lymphocytes and large mononuclear leukocytes. In sections of lymph vessels one sees only a fine granular coagulum with occasional lymphocytes.

BLOOD FORMATION

In the adult body, blood cells are normally formed in two organs that are alike in having a framework of reticular tissue but different in the kinds of corpuscles that they produce. Bone marrow is the normal source of the red blood cells and the granulocytes, and probably also the monocytes, and lymph nodules are the source of the lymphocytes.

Bone marrow

It will be remembered that, in the formation of a bone, a space is left at the center by the resorption, first, of the cartilage and, later, of endosteal bone. This space is invaded by mesenchyme, which develops into an organ having no part in the supportive function of the bone itself. This is the red bone marrow, which in the adult is the source of the majority of the blood corpuscles. The primitive mesenchyme of the embryo develops in this location into three main types of cells: (1) framework of reticular tissue, (2) adipose tissue, and (3) hematopoietic or blood-forming cells (Fig. 6-7). In early life all three kinds of cells are present in the marrow of any bone (Fig. 6-8). Later the hematopoietic cells disappear from the marrow of some of the bones, leaving only reticular tissue and fat cells, which make up the yellow marrow. In other bones the marrow continues to form blood cells throughout life, and their presence makes the tissue red.

Marrow may be studied in smear preparations or in sections. For critical examination a blood stain must be used.

Reticular tissue cells. In sections reticular tissue cells are somewhat obscured by the hematopoietic cells, but may be distinguished in smears or thin sections.

Adipose tissue cells. Adipose tissue cells are generally scattered in red marrow and appear under the low power of the microscope as holes in the marrow because of the loss of lipid during fixation. About half of normal bone marrow is occupied by fat cells (Fig. 6-7).

Hematocytoblasts (stem cells). Hematocytoblasts are from 10 to 12 μm in diameter and have a basophilic, usually nongranular, cytoplasm. The form of the cell is pear shaped or polygonal, without cytoplasmic processes. The nucleus is large and is situated at the widest part of the cell. As the name implies, these were once regarded as the cells from which the blood cells are de-

Erythrocytes

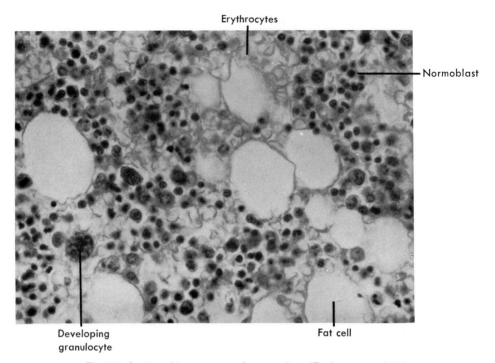

Normoblast

Developing
granulocyte

Fat cell

Fig. 6-7. Section of bone marrow from monkey. (Eosin-azure; ×640.)

rived. On the basis of cell culture and genetic marker studies, it has been established that all blood cells derive from a free stem cell called a *colony-forming unit (CFU)*, a much smaller cell than the hematocytoblast. As befits a stem cell (that is, an undifferentiated cell involved in active cell division), this cell contains only a bare minimum of organelles, including mitochondria, free ribosomes (to produce the new proteins required for cell division), and a small Golgi complex for manufacturing cell membrane and surface coats. In cell culture this single cell type gives rise to two cell lines, one committed to differentiating into the granulocyte series and monocytes and another that is destined to produce erythrocytes. This latter cell is sensitive to a growth-promoting hormone called *erythropoietin*, the precursor of which is produced by the kidneys. The precursor stimulates red blood cell production in conditions in which oxygen supplies are limited (anoxia).

Promyelocytes, myelocytes, metamyelocytes. There are three intermediate stages between the stem cell (CFU) and the gran-

ular leukocyte. They are characterized in general by the development of cytoplasmic granules, which are neutrophilic, eosinophilic, or basophilic, according to the kind of leukocyte destined to develop from each. It is possible, with sufficient care, to recognize three main types or stages of this group.

1. The youngest (promyelocyte) is a spherical cell with a basophilic cytoplasm much like that of the hematocytoblast except that it contains a few granules. The nucleus of the promyelocyte is large and pale.

2. The second stage (myelocyte–marrow cell) is the most common of the group and is the most easily distinguished. The myelocytes divide rapidly, giving rise to successive generations of cells in which one may trace a gradual increase in the number of specific cytoplasmic granules and an accompanying loss of affinity for basic stains. Also, as divisions occur, there are slight loss of size and increase of density of the nucleus.

3. The products of the last divisions of the myelocytes are the metamyelocytes. These cells develop without further division into polymorphonuclear leukocytes. Metamyelo-

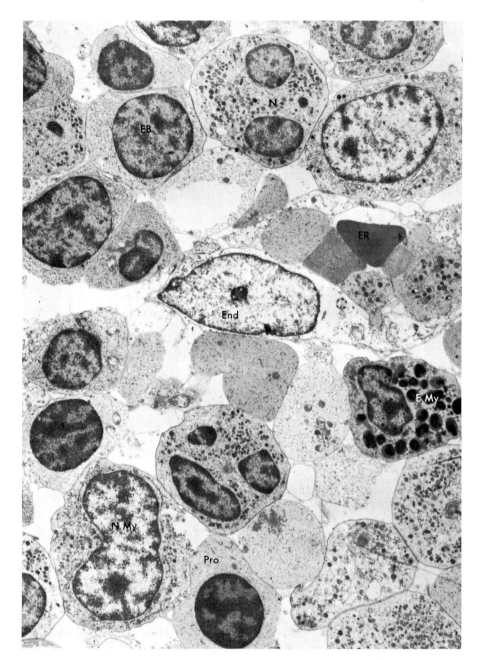

Fig. 6-8. Electron micrograph of bone marrow from cat. *EB,* Erythroblast; *EMy,* eosinophilic myelocyte; *End,* endothelial cell of capillary; *ER,* erythrocyte; *N,* neutrophil; *NMy,* neutrophilic myelocyte; *Pro,* proerythrocyte. (×5,500.)

cytes are, in fact, early stages of granulocytes that are not sufficiently mature to enter the circulation under normal conditions.

Juvenile leukocytes. In some pathological states, leukocytes enter the bloodstream before they are fully mature. During infections

and after tissue damage the total white blood cell count (leukocytosis) increases, and more cells with lobular nuclei appear in a blood smear. These immature cells are called band or stab cells because of their nuclear appearance, which resembles the forms normally seen in myelocytes and metamyelocytes. An increase in these forms in the blood is sometimes described as a *shift to the right* or a shift to younger forms.

Proerythroblasts, erythroblasts, normoblasts. As the primitive stem cell (CFU) divides, its daughters differentiate into erythrocytes. They decrease in size, lose their nuclei, and fill up their cytoplasm with hemoglobin. This process can be divided into three recognizable stages: the proerythroblast, the erythroblast, and the normoblast, although, as usual, such distinctions are rather arbitrary.

1. The proerythroblast is the earliest recognizable stage in the development of the red blood cell. It differs from the promyelocyte in the following ways. It is slightly smaller and has a more chromatic nucleus; hemoglobin is beginning to develop in its cyto-

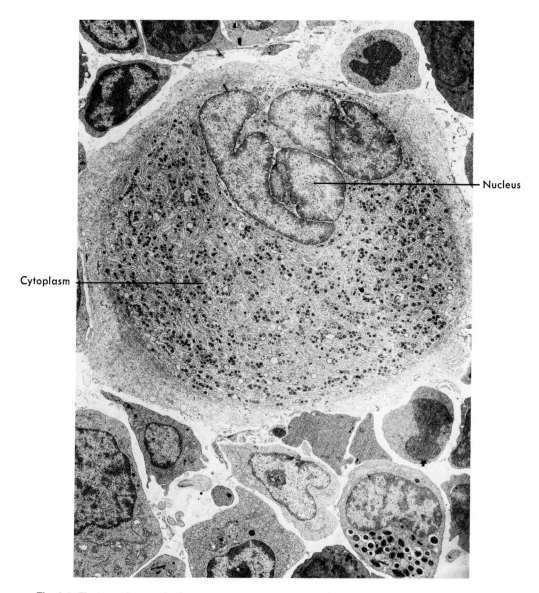

Nucleus

Cytoplasm

Fig. 6-9. Electron micrograph of a megakaryocyte from bone marrow of rat. Many of the granules are lysosomes. Also present is a light meshwork consisting of vesicles and tubules. (×4000.) (Courtesy Dr. H. Nakahara.)

plasm; at this stage the cytoplasm is basic, like that of the hematocytoblast and the promyelocyte, but the presence of hemoglobin gives it a slightly purplish or grayish tinge.

2. In the next stage, the erythroblast, a series of changes develops gradually as the cells divide. These changes are of two kinds: an increase in the amount of hemoglobin in the cytoplasm and a decrease in the size of the cell and its nucleus. The former change is expressed morphologically as a shift in color from the grayish blue of the proerythroblast toward the pink that is characteristic of the erythrocyte. When the pink color is fully developed, the cells are called normoblasts.

3. A normoblast is only slightly larger than an erythrocyte but differs from it in having a nucleus. Normoblasts undergo several divisions, during which their nuclei become progressively smaller and darker. Ultimately the nucleus of the normoblast is reduced to a compact, deeply staining mass, and, when this is extruded from its surface, the cell is a fully developed red blood corpuscle.

Giant cells or megakaryocytes. Megakaryocytes are the largest cells of bone marrow and the most readily recognized. They may measure more than 100 μm in diameter. They have a rather dense reddish cytoplasm and a polymorphic nucleus (Fig. 6-9). In size and color they resemble the osteoclasts, which will be found at the margin of the marrow. Osteoclasts, however, have many separate nuclei (polykaryocytes), whereas the parts of the nucleus of a giant cell are connected by strands of nuclear material. It is from the cytoplasm of the giant cell that the blood platelets are formed.

• • •

In addition to the cells just described, all types of blood corpuscles are to be found in bone marrow.

Development of blood cells in the embryo. Although the most important permanent source of blood cells is the red bone marrow, there are several other sites of blood formation that occur during embryonic development.

The first area in which this occurs is in the yolk sac of the embryo. Other sites of origin are the mesenchyme, thymus, liver, spleen, and lymph nodes.

Germinal centers of lymph nodes

Lymphoid tissue contains centers of lymphocyte production. For details, see Chapter 10.

7

Muscle

The cells of muscle are specialized for contractility; that is, they contain within themselves contractile proteins that can change in length, permitting the cells to shorten. The cells are often referred to as muscle *fibers,* to the lasting confusion of students who have just learned about the intercellular, noncontractile fibers of connective tissue that serve as binding and padding elements in the matrix.

Three types of muscle are usually distinguished: smooth muscle, skeletal muscle, and cardiac muscle.

Skeletal *(striated)* muscle is found in named muscle masses connected to the skeleton and is concerned with body movement.

Cardiac muscle (also striated) composes the contractile portion of the heart wall and is involved in the pumping of blood.

Smooth muscle is found as part of the walls of viscera, serving to alter the tone of the walls of hollow organs such as the stomach, bladder, and uterus and to effect the movement of materials through tubular organs (such as the gut, the urinary system, or the vascular bed). Small accumulations of smooth muscle cells also are found in the skin, where they are wrapped around hair follicles or surrounding ducts of exocrine glands. Isolated smooth muscle fibers can also be found in the tunica propria of the digestive tract.

All these muscle tissue types are composed of elongated cells with well-defined nuclei, a cytoplasm that stains red with eosin, and fibrils (myofibrils) in the cytoplasm. The myofibrils are made up of contractile proteins that run the length of the cell and are clearly visible at the light microscope level in skeletal and cardiac muscle but not in smooth muscle. The cell boundaries are distinct because of a coating of basement membrane–like material adhering to the plasma membrane *(sarcolemma).*

In examining the three basic muscle types, it is important to keep in mind certain fundamental differences among them. The muscle types differ in the mode of attachment of the individual cells to each other and in the connective tissue framework that provides support for the muscle mass and a sling to transmit the force of muscular contraction. They also differ in the nature of the surrounding connective tissue framework itself and in the extent and arrangement of the vascular bed, the lymphatic drainage, and the relationships between individual muscle cells and the nerve supply. Diversity will also be noted in the number and location of nuclei per cell, the visible details of the contractile apparatus (myofibrils), and the distinctness of the cell borders and the intercellular matrix at the light microscope level.

SKELETAL MUSCLE

Skeletal muscle cells (also called fibers) are cylindrical, prismatic-shaped cells that average 3 cm in length but vary from around 1 mm in the stapedius muscle to over 4 cm in long antigravity muscles such as the gluteus maximus. The fibers are grouped together into bundles called *fasciculi* that vary in size. They give a coarse grain to a cross section of a large muscle mass. The individual cells in a bundle attach to the investing connective tissue sheath but not to each other. They contract separately in response to their own individual motor nerve input. A single motor neuron contacts several muscle cells, the number varying with the muscle type from only a few in the delicately controlled eye muscles to several hundred in large, strong, mass-action muscles (gluteus maximus). The motor neuron and its associated muscle fibers are called a *motor unit.*

Within a muscle fascicle, some muscle fibers run from one end of the bundle to the other, some end within the bundle, and some start and finish within the bundle, never reaching the ends. The individual fibers connect to the delicate interior connective tissue meshwork of the bundle called the *endomysium.* Bundles are joined to each other by a coarser connective tissue sheath called the *perimysium,* and the whole mass is held together by an *epimysium.* All these connective tissue scaffolds are composed of a mixture of collagenous fibers, elastic fibers, and fibroblasts. In a muscle mass as a whole, the bundles may run parallel to each other from one tendon to the other, may attach at an angle to a centrally placed riblike shelf of connective tissue (pennate or featherlike arrangements), or may project out from a single central point as do the spokes of a wheel (the radial arrangement). The radial arrangement is the most powerful arrangement but has the least shortening distance, whereas the parallel arrangement is not powerful, but the distance over which the muscle can contract is considerable.

Muscle of exactly the same morphologic appearance as that of the skeletal muscle is found in various places where it is not attached to the bones. In such situations it has no surrounding connective tissue sheath but merges with the connective tissue about it. Such muscle is not truly skeletal, since it does not move parts of the skeleton. In the tongue, for instance, it is more accurately described by the name voluntary muscle. In other regions, muscle of this type is not, strictly speaking, either skeletal or voluntary. The wall of the esophagus contains, in its upper portion, striated muscle that is neither under the control of the voluntary centers of the nervous system nor attached to bone. It is morphologically indistinguishable from skeletal muscle, however, and is therefore called by the same name.

At the light microscope level single skeletal muscle fibers are multinucleate, containing many pale, elongate ovoid nuclei pushed against the sides of the cell. A cell may contain several hundred of these. The cell is encapsulated by a sarcolemma that is visible at the light microscope level because of its coating of amorphous ground substance. The cells are seen to be conspicuously striped (striated). In cross section the cytoplasm appears coarsely granular due to the many myofibrils contained within it (Fig. 7-1). These myofibrils constitute the contractile apparatus of the cell.

At relatively high magnification (high dry) some detail of the contractile apparatus can be seen, especially in the relaxed state. At this level it is possible to see alternate light and dark disks (Fig. 7-1). The dark disks are called anisotropic or A bands because they are darker stripes under polarized light; the light bands are called isotropic or I bands. In particularly good preparations each light band is seen to be crossed by a thin dark line called the Z band (from the German Zwischenschiebe or intermediate disk). The distance between two Z bands is called a sarcomere. At the light microscope level these bands look continuous across the cell, but in fact that appearance is due to the alignment of many individual columns of contractile protein within the cell, each column visible in cross section as a small dot in the cytoplasm (Fig. 7-1).

At the electron microscope level a muscle cell is dominated by the contractile apparatus and its investing membrane structures; the details of this arrangement will be described first. The function of a muscle cell involves changing its length. The functional unit of contraction is the *sarcomere*. When muscle

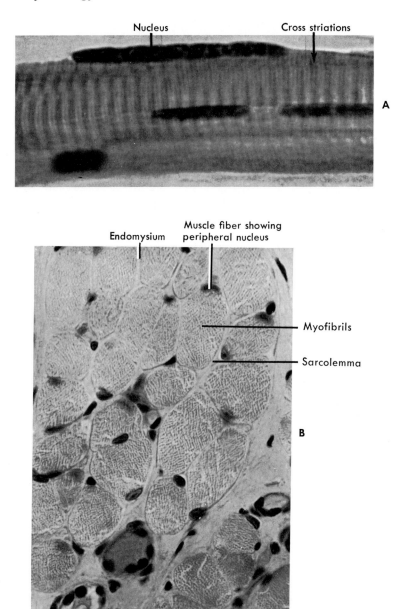

Nucleus   Cross striations

Endomysium   Muscle fiber showing peripheral nucleus

Myofibrils

Sarcolemma

Capillary   Perimysium

A

B

Fig. 7-1. Human striated muscle. **A,** Longitudinal section; **B,** transverse section. (**A,** ×2,000; **B,** ×640.)

fibers are treated with acid, the myofibrils fall apart at the Z lines. Local application of neural transmitters by means of a tiny glass capillary tube placed at the Z line results in a brief contraction of the region between two Z bands. Because of this, the distance between two Z bands has been called the structural and functional unit of the muscle contractile apparatus. On examination with the electron microscope, the myofibrils are seen to be made up of yet smaller linear structures, the *myofilaments,* clustered together in highly

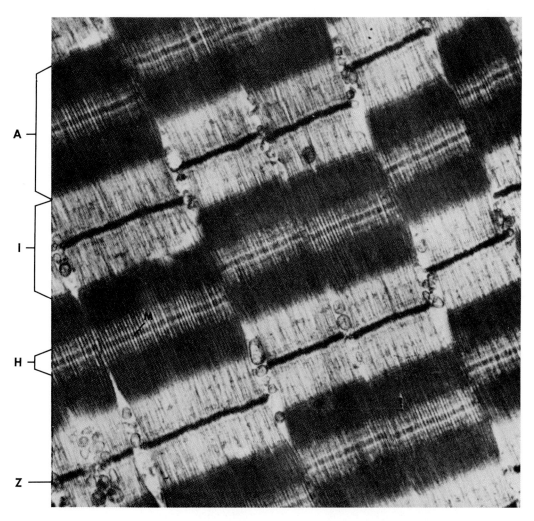

Fig. 7-2. Electron micrograph showing portion of several myofibrils of relaxed rabbit psoas muscle. Isotropic, *I,* bands are bisected by dark *Z* band. Anisotropic, *A,* bands are dark except for central light portion, the *H* band, which contains dark M band (unlabeled). (×25,000.) (Courtesy Dr. H. E. Huxley.)

organized arrays. There are two kinds of myofilaments (Figs. 7-3 and 7-4) that differ in their size and chemical composition. The *thick filaments* contain a protein called *myosin* and are approximately 10 nm in diameter and 1.5 μm long. They are the chief constituent of the A band. The *thin filaments* contain *actin* and two associated proteins called tropomyosin and troponin (Fig. 7-7), measure 5 nm in diameter, and extend about 1 μm in either direction from a Z line. They give rise to the I band of the light microscope level and extend to variable distances into

the A band. When a muscle contracts, the Z bands draw closer together, changing the banding pattern visible at the light microscope level. The explanation most widely accepted for muscle contraction is that the thin filaments "slide" into the thick filaments to shorten the sarcomere. The details of this process will be described later.

The sarcoplasm or cytoplasm fills the spaces between the myofibrils and is most abundant in the region of the nucleus. Located within the sarcoplasm are mitochondria, which are large, abundant, and most

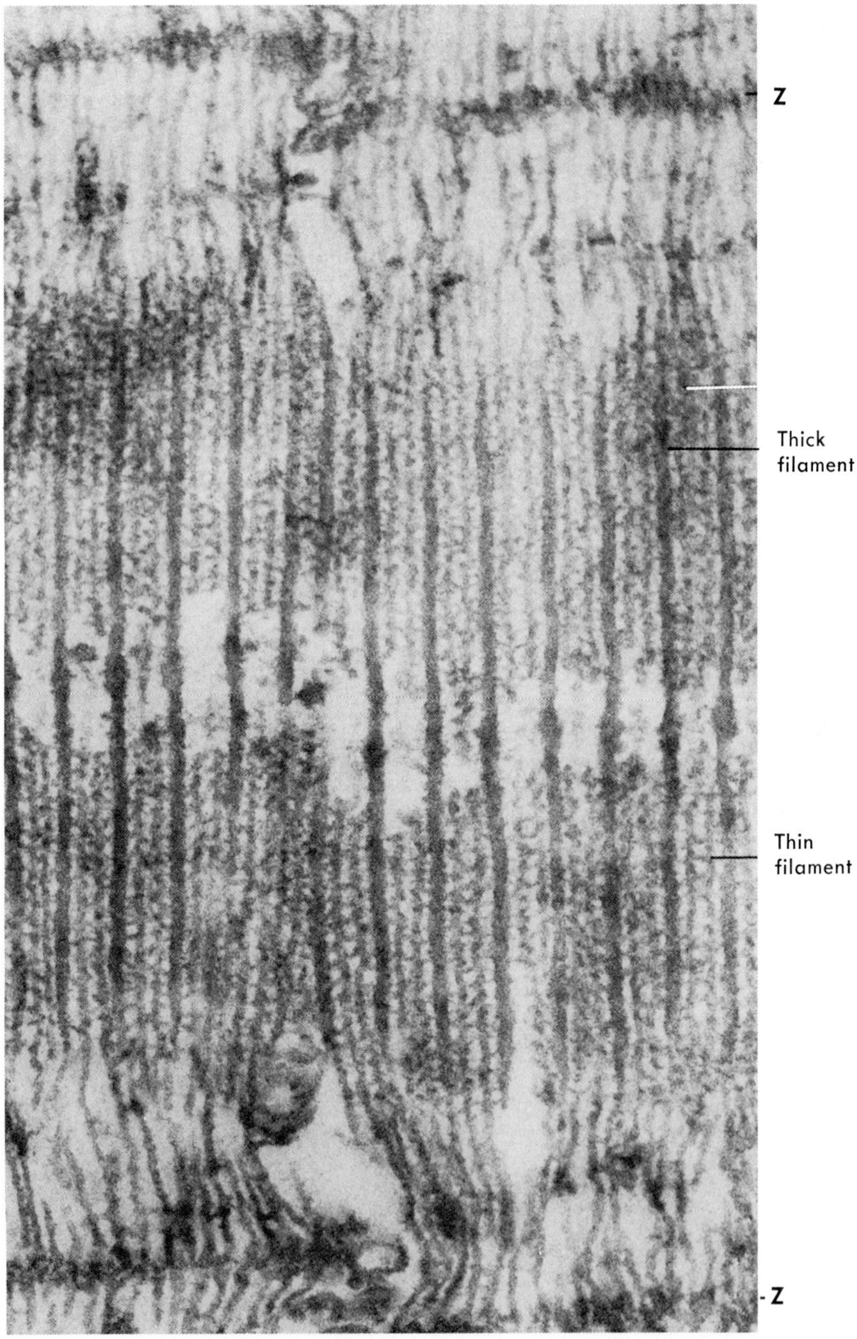

Fig. 7-3. Electron micrograph of longitudinal section of relaxed psoas muscle of a rabbit. Thick myosin filaments extend throughout length of A band; thin actin filaments are present in I band and extend into A band to H zone. This section shows that there are two thin filaments located between each thick filament. (×148,000.) (Courtesy Dr. H. E. Huxley.)

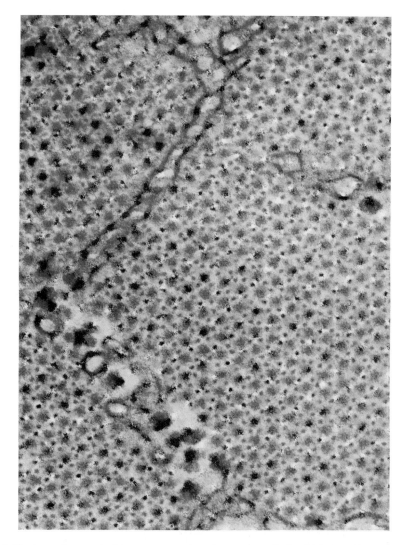

Fig. 7-4. Electron micrograph of transverse section of several myofibrils of A band of frog skeletal muscle. Thinner (actin) filaments have hexagonal pattern in reference to thicker (myosin) filaments. (×75,000.) (Courtesy Dr. H. E. Huxley.)

numerous at the poles of the nucleus. They also occur between the myofibrils, where they are usually arranged with their long axis parallel to the long axis of the myofibrils (Fig. 7-5). In addition, a small Golgi network is located at the pole of the nucleus, and lipid droplets and particles of glycogen occur between the myofibrils.

Sarcoplasmic reticulum

The sarcoplasmic reticulum, which corresponds to the endoplasmic reticulum of other cells, is visible only with the electron microscope. The membrane system is extremely intricate and is intimately associated with the initiation and cessation of muscle contraction. It is a continuous system of fine, membrane-bound, interconnecting cisternae forming a meshwork around each myofibril (Fig. 7-6).

The cisternae are arranged parallel to the long axis of the myofibrils and have frequent cross-connections. In the region of the A-I band junction the cisternae terminate in lat-

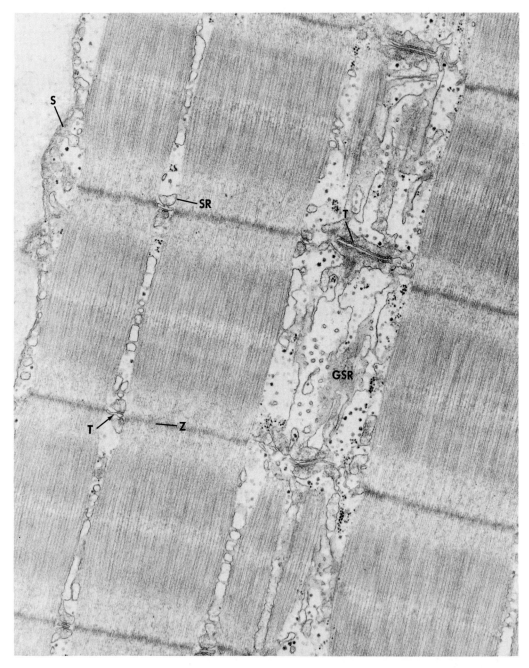

Fig. 7-5. Electron micrograph of longitudinal section of amphibian skeletal muscle showing sarcoplasmic reticulum and T system. *S,* sarcolemma; *SR,* sarcoplasmic reticulum in transverse section; *GSR,* grazing section through sarcoplasmic reticulum with terminal cisterns and adjacent T tubules; *T,* in transverse section; *Z,* Z band. (×32,000.) (Courtesy Drs. M. A. Cahill and D. E. Kelly.)

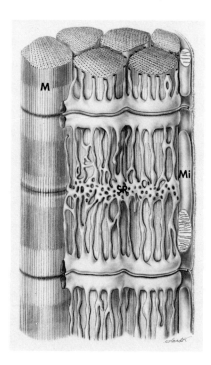

Fig. 7-6. Three-dimensional drawing of group of myofibrils, *M*, from skeletal muscle surrounded by a net sarcoplasmic reticulum, *SR. Mi,* Mitochondrion. Each myofibril is made up of many myofilaments. (From Bloom, W., and D. W. Fawcett. 1968. A textbook of histology. 9th ed. W. B. Saunders Co., Philadelphia.)

eral dilations that are separated from a similar dilated cisternae on the adjacent side of the A-I junction by a smaller transverse (T) tubule. This arrangement of the two cisternae and the centrally located T tubule is known as a *triad.* There are two triads in each sarcomere. The T tubules are not an integral part of the sarcoplastic reticulum but are invaginations of the sarcolemma. Their lumina open into the surrounding extracellular space (Fig. 7-5).

Contraction

When a muscle fiber contracts it becomes shorter and broader. This is also true for each sarcomere. The "sliding filament" explanation is now generally accepted as the mechanism that accounts for muscular contraction. Basically, this mechanism involves a change in the relative position of the actin and myosin filaments. During contraction the thin actin filaments that are attached to the Z line move into the A band. Although the filaments themselves do not alter in length, the sliding movements results in a change in appearance of the sarcomere, notably a partial or complete obliteration of the H band (Fig. 7-2). Furthermore, the myosin filaments come to lie in close proximity to the Z lines; the I bands and the sarcomeres decrease in width as this movement takes place. The contraction is dependent on interaction of actin and myosin to form an actomyosin complex.

The actin filaments are composed of two strands of fibrous actin that are coiled around each other to form a helix. Each of these strands is made up of globular subunits of G-actin (Fig. 7-7). Tropomyosin, troponin, and F-actin are recently described proteins associated with the actin filament. Troponin is a complex protein occurring at regular intervals along the helical chain of globular molecules and is attached to tropomyosin, a fibrous narrow molecule that winds around the two rows of G-actin as two continuous strands. Myosin filaments are composed of light and heavy meromyosin subunits. The light meromyosin units are arranged longitudinally and form the core of the myosin filaments. The heavy subunits consist of rods with globular heads that extend as cross-connections or bridges between the myosin and actin filaments. It has been suggested that cross-connections function as levers which attach to the actin filaments at specific activation sites normally shielded by troponin and tropomyosin except during contraction. Activation apparently induces the levers to exert a pull on the actin filament, causing it to undergo a sliding movement. When the contraction stimulus is discontinued, the lever falls back to its original position. Subsequent stimuli would result in a repetition of this process. Accordingly, the mechanism involves a pull on the actin filaments at successive sites by the cross-attachments originating in the thick myosin filament. This mechanism operates in a manner similar to that of a ratchet and wheel. The overall result of the actions referred to above consists in a successive sliding of the filaments and a shortening of the sarcomeres.

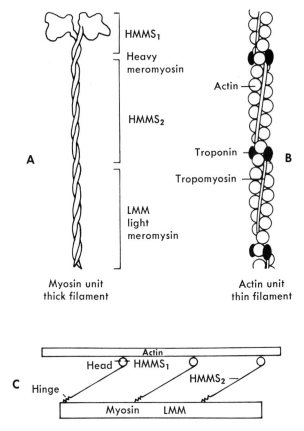

Fig. 7-7. Molecular structure of myofilaments. **A,** Thick filament; **B,** thin filament; **C,** association between thick (myosin) and thin (actin) filament. (Diagram prepared by Douglas Martin.)

Role of the T system

Stimulation of a muscle results in the contraction of all the myofibrils simultaneously to a maximum degree. This is known as the *all or none law*. The contraction occurs initially at the A-I junction, which it will be recalled is the location of the triads. It has been known for some time that muscular contraction is dependent (in part) on the presence of calcium ions in the sarcoplasm that surrounds the myofibrils. It was not until the discovery of the sarcoplasmic reticulum and the T system, however, that the role of calcium was elucidated. Stimulation of a muscle fiber results in the rapid depolarization of the surface, which then spreads to the interior of the fiber by way of the tubules of the T system; this in turn causes a rapid and copious release of calcium ions from the cisternal membranes

brought about by an increase in the permeability of the latter. The calcium ions thus released into the sarcoplasm bind to troponin, which shifts in position and opens active sites on the G-actin filaments, to which myosin then binds. Calcium is then returned to the sarcoplasmic reticulum, tropomyosin reblocks active sites on the G-actin, and the muscle relaxes. It is this sudden and copious release and subsequent binding of calcium ions to activation sites on the thin filaments that serves as a triggering effect to produce muscular contraction. The energy utilized in the contraction is derived from high-energy phosphates that eventually give rise to ATP; this is enzymatically split by ATPase in the H-m portion of myosin to yield energy utilized in activating the rachet mechanism, resulting in the sliding of filaments.

Blood and nerve supply

The muscle has an abundant supply of arteries that penetrate the epimysium and terminate as capillaries. Most of the capillaries are longitudinally arranged between the muscle fibers; however, many occur between the arteries, giving rise to plexuses. The veins usually follow the arteries and are characterized by the presence of valves. Lymph capillaries occur along with the blood vessels and in the connective tissue septa.

Each muscle has at least one nerve that pierces the epimysium in a region known as the *motor point*. The nerve consists of the following components: (1) motor fibers, (2) sensory branches to muscle spindles, (3) sensory fibers terminating in fascia, and (4) autonomic fibers that supply the blood vessels.

SMOOTH MUSCLE

Most smooth muscle is derived from mesenchyme, the cells of which are not originally different from those that give rise to the connective tissues. The muscle cells (myoblasts), however, soon assume elongate spindle shapes and elaborate a small amount of intercellular matrix, which gradually becomes obscured as the cells crowd together into sheets. Two muscle types are derived from ectoderm: the ciliary muscle of the eye and the modified contractile cells (myoepithelial cells) around certain glandular ducts.

Individual smooth muscle cells at the light microscope level appear as spindle-shaped cells in side view, with a single centrally located nucleus at the widest part of the cell. They vary in size from 20 μm or so in the muscle coat of blood vessels to 0.5 mm in the pregnant uterus. The nucleus is pale with granular chromatin and may appear folded or pleated if the cell was caught in contracture at the time of fixation (so-called *agonal contraction*). Several nucleoli are present. The cytoplasm is fairly homogeneous and eosinophilic and can be mistaken for collagen fibers by unsuspecting students. It may help to remember that smooth muscle is usually more bluish in appearance than collagen. Some cells in a mass appear darker than others, probably due to their state of contraction

when fixed. The contractile apparatus is not visible at the light microscope level in smooth muscle cells.

In transverse section the smooth muscle cells appear as disks of cytoplasm having various diameters. The largest of the disks are cut through the middle of the fibers and include the nucleus of the cell. The smaller sections pass through the ends of the fibers and therefore have no nuclei in them. The characteristics peculiar to smooth muscle in cross section are the small size and round shape of the individual fiber, the homogeneous appearance of the cytoplasm, and the fact that the nuclei are centrally located in the cells (Fig. 7-8).

The smooth muscle fiber is enveloped by a plasma membrane studded with vesicles believed to be concerned with pinocytotic activity. External to the membrane is a homogeneous coat or layer similar to the basal lamina commonly observed in epithelial cells. External to the basal lamina, scattered reticular fibers occur. In certain regions of the cell surface, specializations occur that suggest by their appearance and relation to adjacent cells that they may be specialized desmosomes.

The myofilaments are delicate structures usually oriented in the direction of the long axis of the cell. Mitochondria occur in the region of the nuclear poles, beneath the cell membrane, and also between the myofibrils. The endoplasmic reticulum and Golgi apparatus, located at the nuclear poles, are poorly developed and not closely related to the contractile apparatus spatially as are the intracellular membranes of striated muscle.

At the electron microscope level the cytoplasm is seen to contain fine filaments similar to the actin filaments of skeletal muscle (Fig. 7-9), varying in diameter from 2 to 8 nm. They are occasionally seen to originate in dark patches along the cell membrane and within the cytoplasm, which may be anchoring structures to transmit the force of their contraction into cell shortening. Thicker filaments resembling the myosin of skeletal muscle are also seen, but their orientation in relationship to the thin filaments has not

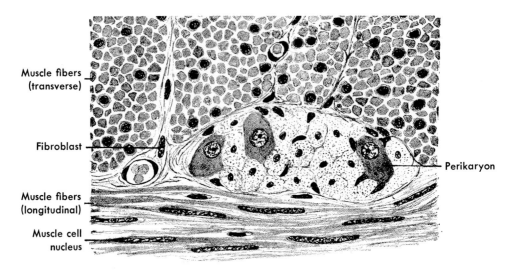

Muscle fibers
(transverse)

Fibroblast

Muscle fibers
(longitudinal)

Muscle cell
nucleus

Perikaryon

Fig. 7-8. Smooth muscle from wall of intestine of monkey showing longitudinal and transverse sections of fibers. Compare nuclei of muscle cells with those of fibroblasts of connective tissue among muscle fibers. Also illustrated are perikaryon, fibers, and supporting cells of Auerbach's nerve plexus.

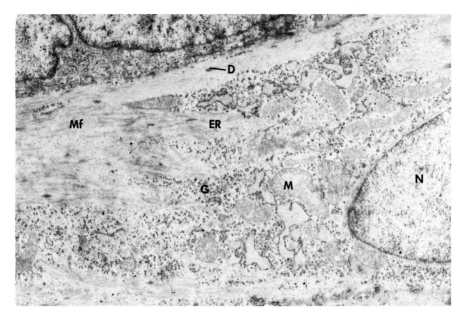

Fig. 7-9. Electron micrograph of portion of smooth muscle cells from small intestine of rat. *D,* Dense body; *ER,* cisternae of endoplasmic reticulum; *Mf,* myofilaments; *N,* nucleus; *M,* mitochondrion; *G,* glycogen. (×17,000.)

been worked out, and not all cells seem to have them, even when conditions are favorable for visualizing them (if the muscle is slightly stretched during fixation). This is in contrast to skeletal and cardiac muscle, which have well-organized arrays of thin and thick filaments. Since smooth muscle contains actin, myosin, troponin, and tropomyosin, it is assumed that its contraction is similar to that of skeletal muscle.

The intracellular membrane system (sarcoplasmic reticulum) is poorly developed in smooth muscle cells and is not associated with any organized contractile apparatus the way it is in skeletal and cardiac muscle. Clustered at the poles of the nucleus are patches of rough endoplasmic reticulum and Golgi apparatus, which become more prominent in hypertrophied muscle such as in the wall of the pregnant uterus. The cells contain mitochondria mostly at their ends. The mitochondria have a dense matrix and fewer cristae than do most cell types. Running near the cell surface is a thin layer of endoplasmic reticulum that is often associated with small vesicles. The latter resemble pinocytotic vesicles (called caveolae) that seem to open onto the cell surface. This membrane system and its associated vesicles may play a role in contraction by coupling electrical stimulation of the cell surface with the release of calcium and the initiation of muscular contraction (see description in the discussion on skeletal muscle).

Smooth muscle cells group together in a variety of ways. Sometimes they are found singly or in small groups in a spiral wrapping around blood vessel walls or as strands associated with hair follicles in the skin. More commonly they form sheets of cells all roughly parallel and woven into bundles, often braided together in sacklike organs (the uterus, bladder, or stomach), wrapped as distinct layers (in the gut), or in a spiral fashion (in the bronchial tree). The individual cells in a sheet are arranged parallel to each other in slightly staggered fashion and are held together by fine reticular fibers and collagen. Compared to other muscle types, the connective tissue is sparse.

Smooth muscle cells are held together by gap junctions and by an outer coating of glycoprotein similar to that of a basement membrane. A gap junction (*nexus*) is similar to an occludens type of cell connection except that a narrow space of about 2 nm remains between the apposed cell membranes. Crossing the gap are structures, visible after freeze fracture, that may permit passage of information (ions and small molecules) between the cells. This arrangement may explain why groups of smooth muscle tend to contract together in orderly waves.

Most smooth muscle is not under voluntary control, although recent experiments indicate that this can be accomplished by learning procedures if an adequate signal is given to the subject about the state of contraction of the muscle to be controlled. The cells are innervated by the autonomic nervous system. There are two basic neural arrangements—the multiunit type and the visceral type.

1. In the multiunit type of arrangement each muscle cell receives a direct innervation and has an organized neuromuscular contact (motor endplate) on its surface. This arrangement is rare but can be seen in the ductus deferens (where rapid, coordinated contraction of the tubular wall is required for rapid expulsion of sperm during ejaculation) and in the ciliary body of the eye (where rapid adjustments are needed for accomodation of lens shape for near vision).

2. The more common neuromuscular arrangement is the visceral type in which nerve fibers run along sheets of muscle cells, making organized contacts with only a few of the individual cells. Stimulation at one point along the muscle sweeps along the muscle sheet, passing from cell to cell perhaps across gap junctions, and induces a wavelike undulation through the smooth muscle mass. This can be seen sometimes as *contraction bands* after fixation where regions of dark and light staining can be seen running across a muscle sheet.

When a nerve fiber does contact a smooth muscle cell in such a sheet, it does not form an organized neuromuscular junction of the type seen in skeletal muscle (Chapter 8). Instead, the nerve fiber expands into a varicosity that rests on the cell surface, with a gap of 10 to 20 nm or more between the nerve and the muscle. When the nerve is stimulated, it releases packets of transmitters into this cleft, which then diffuse across to stimulate the muscle cell.

CARDIAC MUSCLE

Cardiac muscle is found only in the walls of the heart and in the major veins as they enter the heart. The functional peculiarity of cardiac muscle is its ability to contract rhythmically and continuously as a result of the inherent activity of heart muscle cells. Mor-

phologically cardiac muscle can be readily distinguished from smooth and skeletal muscle, although it shares some of the characteristics of each.

A slice through the muscular wall of the heart reveals the cells arranged as branching networks with some connective tissue around them containing a capillary bed and a lymphatic drainage system more prominent than those in other muscle types (Fig. 7-10). The nuclei are centrally located, usually one per cell. The striations caused by the contractile apparatus are less distinct than in skeletal muscle. The cell boundaries are also less noticeable than in skeletal muscle except at certain points where prominent transverse

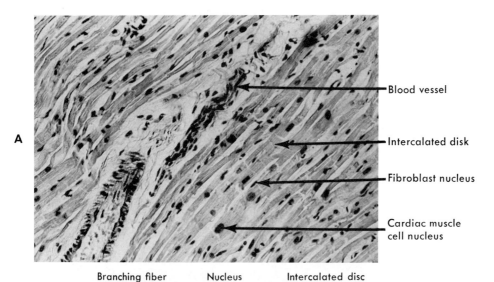

A

- Blood vessel
- Intercalated disk
- Fibroblast nucleus
- Cardiac muscle cell nucleus

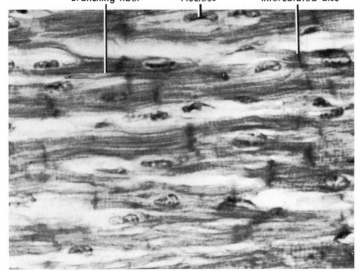

Branching fiber   Nucleus   Intercalated disc

B

Fig. 7-10. Longitudinal sections of cardiac muscle. **A,** Human. **B,** Dog. (**A,** ×250; **B,** ×400.)

markings can be seen that are different from the striations of the main part of the cell bodies. These are the *intercalated disks*. They are peculiar to cardiac muscle and often appear as steplike formations in the fiber network. They show up better in tissue treated with silver stains. They are found at the position of the Z band of skeletal muscle, and they form a specialized intercellular junction. The individual fibers of the muscle sheet appear continuous (like a syncytium) and are often irregular in shape rather than smoothly spindle-shaped, as in skeletal or smooth muscle.

The presence of transverse intercalated disks, single centrally located nuclei in weakly striated cells, and branching fibers is diagnostic of cardiac muscle.

In both transverse and longitudinal section the position of the nuclei differentiates skeletal muscle from cardiac muscle (Fig. 7-10). In distinguishing cardiac muscle from smooth muscle, one must observe the extent and character of the cytoplasm. The fibers of cardiac muscle are thicker than those of smooth muscle, having diameters of from 9 to 20 μm. It is possible to see in cross sections the cut ends of the myofibrils; these give the cytoplasm a granular appearance except in the region close to the nucleus, which is occupied by membranes and lipid.

The contractile apparatus is similar to that of skeletal muscle, although the number of myofibrils per cell varies from one region of the heart to another (Fig. 7-11). The transverse T system of ventricular muscle is bet-

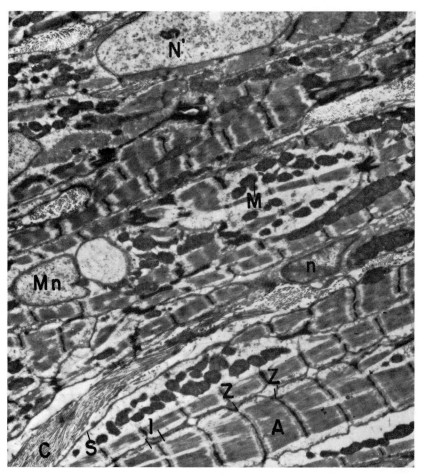

Fig. 7-11. Electron photomicrograph of cardiac muscle of snake. *A,* A disk; *C,* collagen fibrillae; *I,* I disk; *M,* mitochondrion; *Mn,* muscle cell nucleus; *N′,* nucleolus; *n,* nucleus of fibroblast; *S,* sarcolemma; *Z,* Z disk. (×6,000.) (Courtesy Dr. F. Gonzales.)

Table 2. Most important diagnostic features of muscles

Type	Nucleus	Myofibrils	Sarcolemma and external coating	Shape and size
Smooth				
Longitudinal section	Central	Faint; no striation	Very thin	Spindle
Cross section	Central	Invisible	Very thin	Circular, 7 μm
Skeletal				
Longitudinal section	Peripheral	Well-marked striations	Definite sheath	Uniform thickness
Cross section	Peripheral	Visible as dots in groups	Definite sheath	Rounded polygons, 17 to 87 μm
Cardiac				
Longitudinal section	Central	Lightly striated	Thin sheath	Branching
Cross section	Central	Visible as dots	Thin sheath	Round, 9 to 20 μm

ter developed than in skeletal muscle but is absent in the impulse-conducting system of the heart (see discussion on Purkinje system in Chapter 9) and in the atrial muscle. The sarcoplasmic reticulum is less well-developed than in skeletal muscle and is more irregularly arranged. It extends down the entire myofibril column rather than being interrupted at the sarcomere boundary, as in skeletal muscle. This can permit greater spread of a stimulus along the contractile columns than in skeletal muscle. The sarcoplasmic reticulum forms junctions along the T system near the Z lines of the sarcomeres. Although the T tubules are wider than in skeletal muscle, the cisternae are not expanded. Presumably all these specializations involve the unusual functional properties of cardiac muscle, which is a continuously active muscle mass, undergoing contractions at the rate of about 70/min for a lifetime; skeletal muscle is usually active only intermittently.

Appropriate to the high energy requirements of cardiac muscle cells, they are packed with numerous mitochondria near the nucleus, just under the sarcolemma and in rows between the myofibrils. They have many closely packed cristae and are often associated with lipid droplets, one energy source for muscular contraction. The cells also contain a large amount of glycogen arranged not in aggregates as in other tissues, but as individual accumulations, especially near the nucleus and the sarcolemma.

The site of contact between the ends of adjacent cardiac muscle cells is highly specialized and forms an intercalated disk. The cells in adjoining columns are not usually aligned together but are out of register, forming a steplike appearance. Along the disk zone the apposing membranes are thrown into folds that interlock and are reinforced by occludens junctions, desmosomal junctions, and nexus junctions. In addition to the disks, the cells are connected laterally by tight junctions and desmosomes. The unusual reinforcement at the ends of the cells forming the disks may serve to keep the sheet from breaking apart during the wringing action of the heart wall in its pumping cycle. It also serves as the site of attachment of the contractile apparatus of the cell, since myofilaments are seen to insert into the dark fibrillar material bordering the disks.

COMPARISON OF MUSCLE TYPES

The differences described between types of muscle are summarized in Table 2.

8

Nervous tissue

The most complex tissue in the body is nervous tissue. This great complexity has evolved from the ability of nerve cells (neurons) to communicate with each other and with other cell types (muscle cells, gland cells). All cells that form functional communities are in communication with each other by way of electrical signals and chemical messages that assist in maintaining the integrity of the cell community as a whole. These signals control growth, repair, and the relative positions of cells. Nervous tissue, however, has as its *major function* the elaboration of chemical messages (neural transmitters and hormones) and the development of channels of communication for the coordination of body functions. All tissues reflect their history by revealing a varying capacity for adaptation to new conditions throughout life. Nervous tissue has specialized in this adaptability as well, leading to the poorly understood functions of learning and memory. Although many features of neural organization are genetically programmed, the fine details of cellular contacts and the formation of functional circuits or cell populations appear to be influenced by the conditions prevailing when the cells acquire their first contacts. Nerve cells have lost the ability to move and to reproduce and usually have only limited powers to repair damage. Description of the cells that form nervous tissue can only attempt to point out some of the common features and try to give some idea of the incredible variety of cell sizes, shapes, and microstructure.

The nervous system can be divided into a peripheral nervous system and a central nervous system (CNS). The peripheral nervous system gathers information from the body surface, from special sense organs, and from the viscera and transmits signals to the central nervous system. It also contains output channels that convey a stream of signals to effector organs in the body (muscle and glands, the motor system), which react to changes in the internal and external environment. Between the incoming signals and the outgoing commands there is a mass of nervous tissue involved in comparing inputs, in processing, and in decision-making. This mass of tissue is called the central nervous system and is located for the most part within the spinal cord, brain stem, and cerebral cortex (Fig. 8-2).

To begin, the organization of a portion of the spinal cord will be examined inasmuch as many of the features of neural organization are illustrated in a relatively simple manner in this structure. The spinal cord on cross section appears as an oval profile with a central, gray H-shaped pattern of nerve cells and their processes (the *neuropil*) and a surrounding ring of white matter; in the latter the main conducting pathways linking different parts of the spinal cord with each other and with higher centers of the central nervous system are located (Fig. 8-3). Penetrating the dorsal surface of the cord on either side is a bundle of nerve fibers called the *dorsal root*. Most of the fibers passing into the cord through the dorsal root carry sensory in-

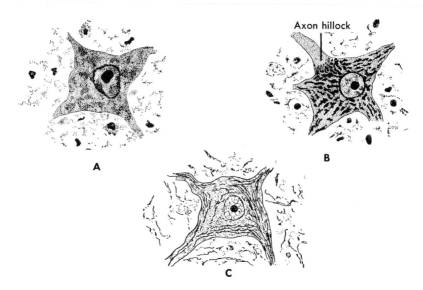

Fig. 8-1. Perikarya of motor neurons in spinal cord stained in three different ways. **A,** Hematoxylin and eosin; **B,** toluidine blue, to show Nissl substance; **C,** silver nitrate, to show neurofibrils.

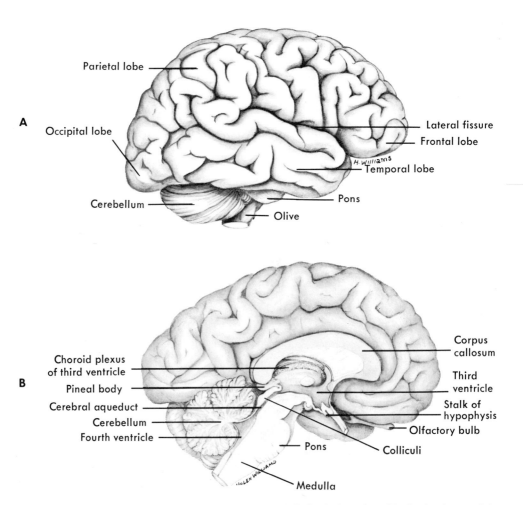

Fig. 8-2. A, Lateral view of brain (male, 45 years of age). **B,** Sagittal section of brain showing medial aspect of left half. (From Francis, C. C, and A. H. Martin. 1975. Introduction to human anatomy. 7th ed. The C. V. Mosby Co., St. Louis.)

Fig. 8-3. Spinal cord of cat. (Low magnification.)

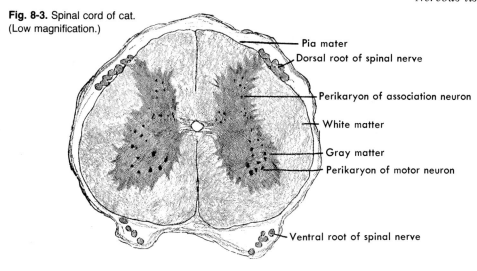

Pia mater
Dorsal root of spinal nerve
Perikaryon of association neuron
White matter
Gray matter
Perikaryon of motor neuron
Ventral root of spinal nerve

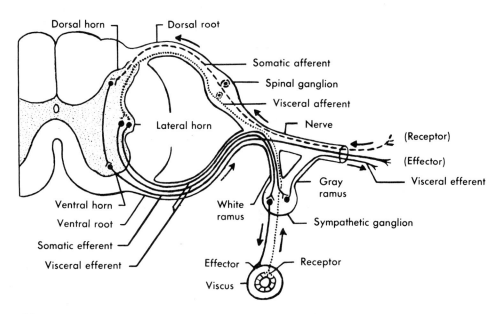

Dorsal horn
Dorsal root
Somatic afferent
Spinal ganglion
Visceral afferent
Nerve
(Receptor)
(Effector)
Lateral horn
Visceral efferent
Gray ramus
Ventral horn
White ramus
Sympathetic ganglion
Ventral root
Somatic efferent
Visceral efferent
Effector
Receptor
Viscus

Fig. 8-4. Diagram showing relationship of somatic and visceral neurons to spinal cord, sympathetic ganglia, and viscera. (From Bevelander, G. 1971. Outline of histology. 7th ed. The C. V. Mosby Co., St. Louis.)

formation from the body surface, muscles, and joints and the viscera. The dorsal root is thus a sensory channel. The nerve cells in this root are specialized conducting cells. Their information-receiving ends (*dendrites*) are located in the periphery whereas their cell bodies (*somata or perikarya*) are located in clusters outside the spinal cord in structures called *ganglia* (Fig. 8-4). Leading from the cell bodies, long conducting processes called *axons* arise that convey information

into the spinal cord along the dorsal root. Some of these processes travel through the gray matter and end directly on motor neurons. The points of contact between the incoming sensory fibers and the motor neurons are called *synapses*, and individual motor neurons may be covered with thousands of these. Most incoming sensory fibers do not reach motor neurons directly. Instead, they branch into a pool of interconnecting neurons called *interneurons* that perform many integrative functions. Built into the circuitry of the spinal cord are a number of stereotypic responses called *reflexes*. The most familiar reflex is the monosynaptic stretch reflex or *knee jerk reflex* that can be elicited when a tendon is tapped, causing a sudden stretch of a muscle. The result is a reflex contraction of the muscle to restore its length to normal. The linkage of neurons required for this reflex consists of an incoming group of sensory neurons conveying the information that the muscle has been stretched and a pool of motor neurons that control the contraction of the muscle cells. No interneurons are required, and the reflex is referred to as monosynaptic. For other reflexes, varying numbers of interneurons are needed to channel the incoming information to related motor neurons in order to achieve coordinated muscle responses.

The local reflex circuits of the spinal cord, such as the monosynaptic knee jerk reflex and similar reflex circuits in the brain stem that are associated with eye muscles, facial muscles, and so forth are coordinated and modified by impulses reaching the motor cells from higher centers in the brain stem and cortex. To achieve this kind of whole body integration, the nervous system utilizes many long, communicating pathways called *fiber tracts* in which the nerve fibers transmit impulses of a similar nature. Fig. 8-5 shows examples of several such tracts in the spinal cord. The corticospinal pathways conduct impulses from the cerebral cortex. Perhaps 10%

of the nerve fibers in these tracts end directly on motor neurons; the remainder, on interneurons that link the motor neurons together in local circuits. The result provides a mechanism by means of which the higher centers control motor function. Similarly, the vestibulospinals and reticulospinals are pathways linking other motor-coordinating centers in the brain stem to the motor neurons. In addition to these descending tracts, there are ascending tracts that carry information to higher centers for processing. For example, in the dorsal columns (fasciculus gracilis, cuneatus) (Fig. 8-5) there are accumulations of axons that carry information from the body surface. It is not necessary in this context to describe all the interconnections between the local reflex circuits of the spinal cord or brain stem and other parts of the central nervous system, but it should be obvious that many different kinds of neurons are necessary to accomplish the various tasks involved in collecting, routing, processing, and utilizing information.

At its most primitive level, the central nervous system may be divided into (1) a spinal cord that coordinates body responses below the level of the neck and (2) a hindbrain, midbrain, and forebrain that serve functions of the head and neck area. The hindbrain is associated with the ears, the midbrain with the eyes, and the forebrain with the sense of smell (olfaction); each area has accumulated a mass of gray matter (interneuronal circuits, cortex) to process special sensory informa-

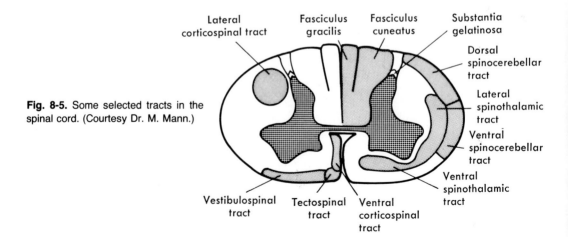

Fig. 8-5. Some selected tracts in the spinal cord. (Courtesy Dr. M. Mann.)

Lateral corticospinal tract

Fasciculus gracilis

Fasciculus cuneatus

Substantia gelatinosa

Dorsal spinocerebellar tract

Lateral spinothalamic tract

Ventral spinocerebellar tract

Ventral spinothalamic tract

Vestibulospinal tract

Tectospinal tract

Ventral corticospinal tract

tion. The information from the ear (hearing and equilibrium) funnels into cell clusters called *nuclei* in the medulla and pons (Fig. 8-2) and into the cerebellum. Information from the retina reaches nuclei in the midbrain and is relayed through the roof structure of the midbrain called the inferior colliculi (Fig. 8-2). The forebrain has acquired the most remarkable increase in associative tissue, resulting in the expansive cerebral hemispheres of man. All of these areas (cerebellum, colliculi, cerebral hemispheres) contain orderly arrangements of many layers of different cell types. We will consider the anatomy of these areas later (Chapter 21).

In summary, neurons can be divided into three basic groups on the basis of structure and function:

1. *Sensory (first order or afferent)* neurons, which are so situated and constructed as to respond to stimuli arising from within or outside the organism and to send impulses to the central nervous system

2. *Association (second order, intercalated, or internuncial)* neurons *(interneurons)* which serve as links between sensory neurons and neurons of the third group

3. *Motor (efferent or third order)* neurons, which convey impulses to muscles or glands, stimulating them to activity

The sensory and motor neurons have long axons and are referred to as Golgi type I neurons; the association neurons have elaborately branched dendrites and short axons and are called Golgi type II neurons. Examples of some of these cells are shown in Fig. 8-6.

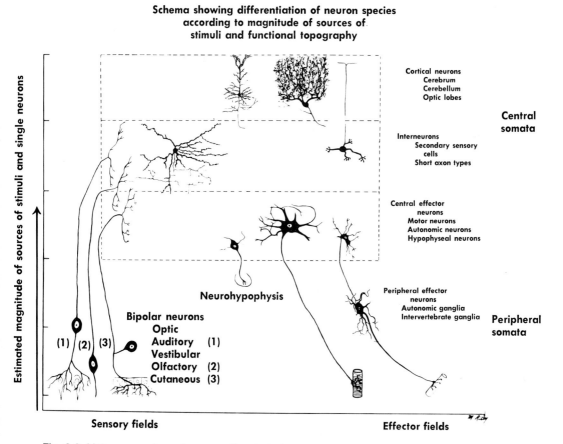

Schema showing differentiation of neuron species according to magnitude of sources of stimuli and functional topography

Estimated magnitude of sources of stimuli and single neurons

Cortical neurons
Cerebrum
Cerebellum
Optic lobes

Central somata

Interneurons
Secondary sensory cells
Short axon types

Central effector neurons
Motor neurons
Autonomic neurons
Hypophyseal neurons

Neurohypophysis

Bipolar neurons
Optic
(1) (2) (3) Auditory (1)
Vestibular
Olfactory (2)
Cutaneous (3)

Peripheral effector neurons
Autonomic ganglia
Intervertebrate ganglia

Peripheral somata

Sensory fields

Effector fields

Fig. 8-6. Major neuron types in mammalian central nervous system, arranged according to general role, hierarchical level, and probable magnitude and diversity of sources of synaptic connections. (From Bodian, D.: Cold Spring Harbor Symp. Quant. Biol. **17:**1, 1952.)

BASIC UNIT OF COMMUNICATION— THE NEURON

Two basic classes of cells are found in nervous tissues. These cells are *neurons* and *glia*. Neurons are the basic units of communication and are extremely variable in size and shape. Glia appear to be the structural elements that hold neuronal tissue together, influence information transfer, and the like (see later). The extensions of these cells in space are extremely important in determining how the communities of cells in the nervous system communicate with each other. The nucleus of a neuron is contained within the cell body or *perikaryon* (Fig. 8-1). Extending from the perikaryon are a variable number of cell processes, usually branched. Most neurons are highly elongated and polarized so that one set of cellular processes, the *dendrites*, receive information and another set of processes, the *telodendria*, transmit this information to the next cell in the chain. Dendrites are often complexly branched and form a treelike arbor (the *dendritic tree*). Much of the diversity of form found in neurons is due to the variation in

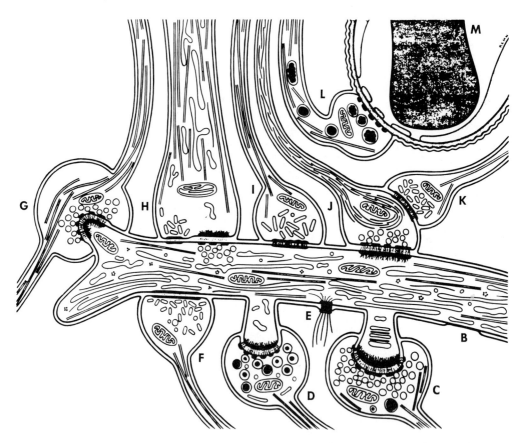

Fig. 8-7. Scheme of the ultrastructural morphology of synapses, showing various junctional structures, grouped around a dendrite, *A*. The tight junction, *B*, and the desmosome, *E*, are without synaptic significance. Excitatory synaptic boutons are shown, *C* and *G*, containing small spherical translucent vesicles. *D*, A bouton with dense-cored, catecholamine-containing vesicles; *F*, an inhibitory synapse containing small flattened vesicles; *H*, a reciprocal synaptic structure between two dendritic profiles, inhibitory toward dendrite *A* and excitatory in the opposite direction; *I*, an inhibitory synapse containing large flattened vesicles. *J* and *K*, Two serial synapses; *J* is excitatory to the dendrite; *K* is inhibitory to *J*. *L*, A neurosecretory ending adjacent to a vascular channel, *M*, surrounded by a fenestrated endothelium. All the boutons in this diagram are of the terminal type except *G*, which is a *bouton de passage* (From Warwick, R., and P. L. Williams [eds.] 1973. Gray's anatomy, 35th [British] ed. W. B. Saunders Co., Philadelphia; Longman's Group, Ltd., Harlow, England.)

dendritic branching. The terminal branches of the neuron form either an array of terminal expansions (synaptic bulbs or boutons, Fig. 8-7) or a single, unbranched process. The site of contact between one nerve cell and another is called a *synapse*. The dendritic tree and perikaryon of a nerve cell may be covered with thousands of these synapses. If the information transmitted across a synapse is sufficient to activate the cell, a propagated nerve impulse is generated at a point on the cell surface called the *axon hillock*, and from there a wave of electrical activity is conveyed along the *axon* (Fig. 8-1) to the terminal boutons. The axon, which can vary in length from micrometers to meters, is capable of conducting a nerve impulse at a speed approaching 100 M/sec in some large axons. The conducting axons surrounded by their sheaths are called *nerve fibers*.

As a result of recent studies of neuron fine structure and electrical activity, there has been a revolution in our concepts concerned with information processing and transfer between nerve cells. The classic neuron is visualized as a conducting channel, a one-way, information-transmitting, cellular system specialized to convey information over considerable distances. Many neurons do fit this concept, but it is becoming clear that there is another class of neurons with extensive dendritic trees in which incredibly complex information processing can occur that does not lead to long distance communication. Neurons of this other class form local circuits. Especially good examples of these latter circuits occur in the retina and in the olfactory bulb (Chapter 21). These neurons develop rather late in embryonic life and may provide a pool of cells that are modifiable and may be involved in the translation of experience into new circuits and capacities in the brain, thus providing the basic substrate for learning and memory. The interwoven processes of these cells are called *neuropil*. The neuropil is considered to be much more than a passive information-receiving region. In fact, the dendrites in local circuits are probably engaged in information processing that involves small, nonpropagated electrical activity and exchanges of chemical messages between the cell processes. Information entering such a network will be greatly modified before it leaves the local circuit.

The nervous system as a whole is integrated (1) by combining polarized conducting neurons and many local circuits that process information in a variety of ways and (2) combining information from many sources to form images of the condition of the body, its position in space, and a repertoire of responses designed to maintain the body in an optimal condition.

PERIKARYON

During development, embryonic nerve cells are elongated spindle-shaped rather unremarkable cells. The first major changes occur as threadlike extensions from the nucleated cytoplasmic mass (perikaryon) develop.

1. The cell ceases to divide.

2. The organelles associated with protein synthesis (ribosomes and endoplasmic reticulum) increase as the cell processes grow but remain for the most part within the perikaryon. The cell body thus becomes the metabolic center of the nerve cell.

3. The cell is faced with the problem of transporting proteins made in the perikaryon through the long cell processes, especially the axon, to the terminals. The most distant region of the cell process may be several meters from the perikaryon. There appears to be an elaborate process of axoplasmic transport of materials along the axons. If the axon is severed from the perikaryon, the protein-synthesizing machinery (referred to as *Nissl substance* in neurons) regresses temporarily (a process called *retrograde chromatolysis*) and then begins to reorganize. Protein synthesis again occurs, and a new axonal process sprouts from the amputated stump of the axon. The severed portion of axon that has lost contact with the cell body degenerates *(Wallerian degeneration)* and fragments; this process extends to the terminal endings as well. The process of degeneration can be traced with special staining meth-

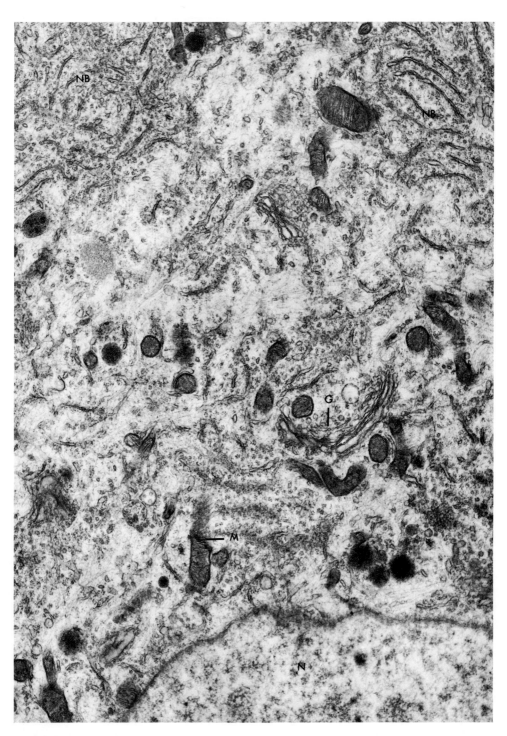

Fig. 8-8. Electron micrograph showing part of motor neuron of spinal cord of rat. In addition to characteristic organelles in this cell, such as nucleus, *N;* Golgi apparatus, *G;* and mitochondrion, *M,* several Nissl bodies, *NB,* are also shown. These last structures are composed of parallel cisternae of endoplasmic reticulum and numerous ribonucleoprotein particles, some in contact with membranes of the reticulum, others dispersed in cytoplasmic matrix. (×17,300.) (Courtesy Dr. R. Yates.)

ods *(Marchi and Nauta methods)* and the tracing of anatomical pathways by following the severed axons has been the source of much of our information concerning the manner in which the cells of the nervous system are linked together.

In light microscope preparations stained with basic dyes such as toluidine blue or cresyl violet, the cytoplasm of neurons displays an intensely basophilic component, the Nissl substance (Fig. 8-1, *B*). This material is most striking in the large motor neurons of the spinal cord and brain stem where the Nissl substance appears as large rhomboid blocks of material. In the cell bodies of sensory neurons of the dorsal root (sensory) ganglia, the Nissl substance looks like fine dust particles scattered through the cytoplasm. Different cell types have such predictable Nissl patterns that at one time the shape and distribution of the Nissl material was the basis for an elaborate classification system for neuron types. Nissl substance occurs in dendrites as well as cell bodies but not in axons. In large cells the region of the axon hillock is pale, giving a visual clue to the site of origin of the axon. At the electron microscope level (Fig. 8-8) Nissl substance corresponds to the rough endoplasmic reticulum pervading the entire cytoplasm of the perikaryon and the major dendrites. In motor neurons the rough endoplasmic reticulum is arranged in orderly stacks of nearly parallel broad cisternae that are studded with ribosomes. Ribosomes also lie free in the cytoplasmic matrix between the cisternae where they often are arranged in small clusters or rosettes. The protein-synthetic machinery of nerve cells differs in this regard from other protein-secreting cells such as those in the exocrine pancreas. It may be that the difference in architecture of the neurons is correlated with the size and complexity of the molecules made by neurons.

The Golgi apparatus of neurons at light microscope levels appears as a tangled webbing of interlocking strands and small vacuoles surrounding the nucleus in a halo. At the electron microscope level (Fig. 8-8) this structure consists of a complex of broad, flat cisternae associated with several small vesicles. The large cisternae usually occur in closely packed stacks of 5 to 7 plates without ribosomes of either the attached or free variety. Associated with the Golgi apparatus region is an assortment of dense inclusions of various shapes and sizes, which are probably lysosomes. In many epithelial cells the Golgi apparatus is confined to a single region, usually near the apical pole of the nucleus, but in nerve cells the Golgi apparatus extends throughout the cytoplasm into the dendrites, but not the axons.

Nerve cells also contain structures called multivesicular bodies, spherical profiles surrounded by a unit membrane. They occur throughout the cell body, dendrites, and axons, but are especially prominent near the Golgi apparatus. They may represent packaging for cellular debris that will then be degraded by the lysosomal enzymes. Nerve cells also tend to accumulate *lipofuscin*, a pigmented material considered to be a by-product of the wear and tear of aging, as it tends to accumulate in nerve cells as they age.

The mitochondria of nerve cells are similar to those in other vertebrate cells (Fig. 8-8) and may vary in size and shape from plump, sausage-shaped organelles 0.5 μm or more in width to long narrow organelles less than 0.1 μm wide and several micrometers long. The mitochondria are apparently in constant motion, changing size, shape, and cell position rapidly. They tend to migrate from the perikaryon into a cell process and then return. The mitochondria appear to follow within tracks associated with long parallel microtubules and neurofilaments that may function as conveyor belts to which cellular organelles or particulate matter can bind and be transported for varying distances. These transport channels can move materials rapidly and may be more prominent in nerve cells because of the need for communication between the cell body and its long processes. Microtubules appear in electron microscope preparations as long tubular elements 20 to 26 nm in diameter. In cross section each tubule exhibits a dense wall about 6 nm thick surrounding a lighter core and a dense center. Neurofilaments are thinner, averaging 10 nm in diameter and in cross

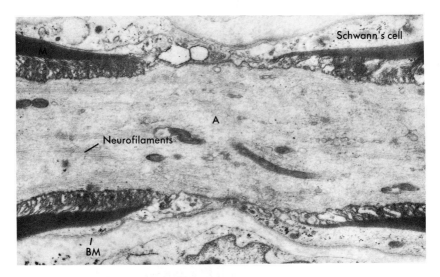

Fig. 8-9. Electron micrograph of longitudinal section of human myelinated nerve fiber in region of node of Ranvier. *A,* Axis cylinder; *BM,* basement membrane of Schwann cell; *M,* myelin. Note that myelin is lacking in region of node. (×17,000.)

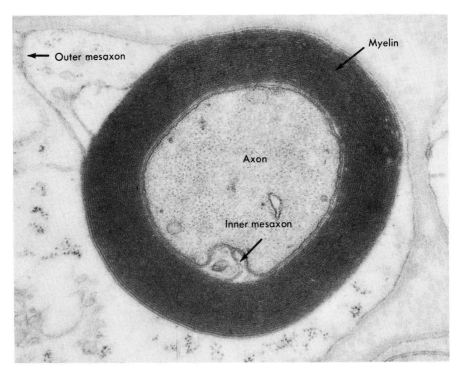

Fig. 8-10. Electron micrograph of transverse section of myelinated nerve from gingiva of monkey. (×38,000.)

section also show a tubular appearance with a dense outer layer and a lighter inner core.

The perikaryon contains a dense network of neurofilaments and microtubules that appear as fairly orderly parallel areas in loose bundles which surround other organelles (Nissl bodies and mitochondria). In the cell processes (both dendrites and axons) the microtubules and neurofilaments clearly form parallel, prominent arrays (Figs. 8-9 and 8-10). It is probable that the *neurofibrils* (Fig. 8-1, *C*) of light microscopy are clumped microtubules and neurofilaments.

Neurons usually have a large, round, centrally located nucleus. In small neurons only a thin film of cytoplasm coats the nucleus, but in larger neurons it is surrounded by a thicker margin of cytoplasm. The interior of the nucleus lacks chromatin particles and is typically vesicular.

Most neurons have a conspicuous, large, spherical nucleolus that may occupy as much as one third of the nuclear volume. There is usually only one nucleolus, which may contain clear round vacuoles in an otherwise intensely staining matrix. Nerve cells do not divide once they reach maturity; accordingly, the neuron population is stable. Many neurons have twice the usual complement of DNA, that is, they are tetraploid. This may provide an adaptation to compensate for the failure of neurons to divide.

DENDRITES

Dendrites are extensions of the perikaryon of a neuron and contain inclusions similar to those occurring in the perikaryon. Dendrites, however, lack a myelin sheath. At the light microscope level they can be distinguished from axons that do not contain Nissl substance and may or may not have a visible myelin sheath. Dendrites usually have irregular contours consisting of projecting spines or thorns, whereas axons are smooth. Most neurons have many dendrites and are referred to as multipolar. Some neurons have two processes projecting from the cell body; these cells are called bipolar (Fig. 8-6). An example of the latter is the bipolar cell in the retina. Sensory ganglia are populated by cells in which the bases of the two cell processes have fused to form one process that subsequently branches into two. These neurons are called unipolar. The two processes—one carrying impulses toward the cell body—are indistinguishable, since they have the structural features of axons. Unipolar cells therefore do not have processes resembling the dendrites of multipolar neurons.

The most striking features of dendrites are neurotubules that appear to be arranged in orderly patterns which are occasionally interrupted by other cellular organelles (neurofilaments, endoplasmic reticulum, mitochondria, Golgi apparatus, vesicles, and multivesicular bodies).

Most of the synaptic connections between cells occur on the dendrites either on the main trunk of the process or on projecting spines. Spines become more prominent distal to the main stem of the dendrite as it emerges from the perikaryon.

AXON

In multipolar neurons the axon originates from a cone-shaped elevation called the *axon hillock*. This region is often pale in stained preparations due to a lack of Nissl substance (Fig. 8-1). This staining difference, however, is barely noticeable in small neurons. At the base of the hillock the microtubules change orientation and funnel into the axon. Another feature of the axon hillock is the presence of a dense material coating the plasma membrane in the vicinity of the hillock. A similar undercoating lies beneath the plasma membrane at the nodes of Ranvier in myelinated axons (Figs. 8-9 and 8-11). Neither of these features occurs in sensory ganglion cells where the cell process leaves the perikaryon. This may be due to the fact that this initial segment is not the site of initiation of an action potential, whereas at other initial segments (first part of an axon as it emerges from the axon hillock before it is coated with myelin) and at the nodes of Ranvier, action potentials are generated.

Beyond its site of origin in the axon hillock, the axon contains mitochondria, neurofilaments, microtubules, smooth endoplasmic reticulum, vesicles, and multivescular bodies, but no granular endoplasmic reticulum

Node of Ranvier

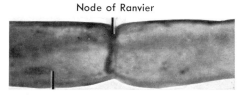

Nerve fiber

Fig. 8-11. Nerve fiber, teased preparation. (Silver stain; ×160.)

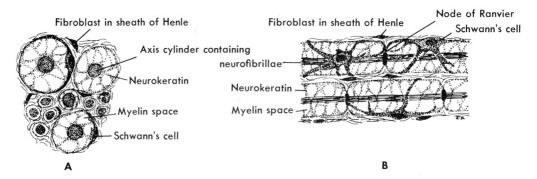

Fibroblast in sheath of Henle

Axis cylinder containing
neurofibrillae

Neurokeratin

Myelin space

Schwann's cell

A

Fibroblast in sheath of Henle

Node of Ranvier

Schwann's cell

Neurokeratin

Myelin space

B

Fig. 8-12. Nerve fiber. **A,** Transverse section; **B,** longitudinal section.

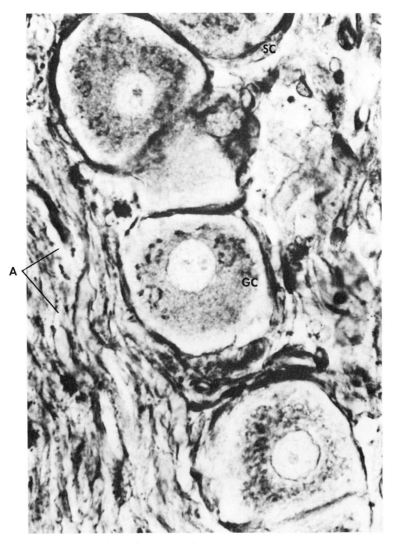

Fig. 8-13. Portion of sensory ganglion showing several neurons and nerve fibers. Golgi method. *A,* Axons; *GC,* ganglion cell; *SC,* satellite cell. (Approx. ×640.) (From collection of Dr. T. Thorsan.)

or free ribosomes. Fewer tubules and filaments are present in axons than in dendrites. It is believed that the parallel arrangement of microtubules and neurofilaments may play a role in axoplasmic flow. At the light microscope level the axon cytoplasm itself is called the *axis cylinder*; it appears to be filled with *neurofibrils* embedded within an *axoplasm* (Fig. 8-12). Neurofibrils probably consist of clumped neurofilaments and microtubules. The axoplasm shrinks considerably in routine preparations so that it frequently appears as a thin acidophilic core in hematoxylin and eosin preparations.

Many axons have branching collaterals, some of which may make contact with the perikaryon from which it originates.

CELLULAR SHEATHS OF NEURONS

The axons and cell bodies of neurons in the peripheral nervous system are surrounded by sheaths formed by cells derived from the neural crest. The cells enveloping the cell body are called *satellite cells* (Fig. 8-13), and those surrounding the axons are called *Schwann cells* (Figs. 8-12 and 8-14), but they are essentially the same in structure and function.

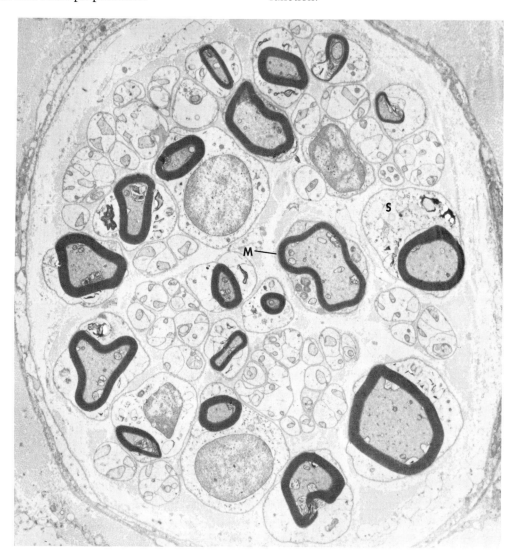

Fig. 8-14. Electron micrograph of transverse section of small nerve trunk. *M*, Myelin sheath; *S*, Schwann cell. (×2,500.)

Sometimes the sheath formed by these cells is a simple wrapping of cell cytoplasm that envelopes the cell body and axon in an indentation of a Schwann cell or satellite cell. The axon, because of its length, is covered with a row of similar cells, each segment of the axon lying in an invagination of the ensheathing cell (Fig. 8-15). Nerve cell bodies and axons with such thin film of cytoplasm are called *nonmyelinated* because the sheath is barely visible at the light microscope level. In special preparations it can be observed and is then referred to as the *neurilemma.* More complex laminated wrappings can also be formed around axons. This *myelin sheath* is visible at the light microscope level because it takes up osmic acid, and such axons

are called *myelinated.* A myelinated nerve fiber is enclosed along its length by a series of Schwann cells, each of which envelops its length of axon in a spirally arranged sheet of plasma membrane (Fig. 8-10). The region where two Schwann cells abut is called a *node of Ranvier* (Figs. 8-9 and 8-11), and the distance covered by a single Schwann cell is known as an *internode.*

The internodal distance ranges from approximately 300 μm in the smallest fibers to 1,500 μm in the largest. The internodal region is arranged in a series of concentric subcellular compartments that separate the axoplasm from the connective tissue that sheaths the nerve in the periphery. First, there is the Schwann cell membrane, next a thin film of Schwann cell cytoplasm, then several layers of Schwann cell sheaths, an outer thicker layer of cytoplasm and finally the Schwann cell membrane and its basal lamina. At a node, myelin is lacking, and at the light microscope level the site appears as an interruption in the sheath (Figs. 8-9 and 8-11). It is at this site that action potentials are generated. The elongated nuclei of the Schwann cells are located approximately halfway between each node and appear to lie in indentations of the myelin.

In fixed preparations of peripheral nerves the myelin of each internode may unravel slightly, producing oblique incisions called the *Schmidt-Lanterman clefts.* These clefts were once thought to be artifacts but are now recognized as inclusions of Schwann cell cytoplasm within the myelin. Their significance is unknown.

The perikarya of most neurons in the peripheral nervous system are covered by a complete coating of satellite cell cytoplasm. The nuclei of these satellite cells appear bean or crescent shaped and rest on flattened portions of the neuronal surface (Fig. 8-13).

The sheath of satellite cells extends along the axon as it leaves the perikaryon (Fig. 8-13). The relationship between the perikaryon and its satellite cells varies in different neuron populations. In autonomic ganglia the satellite cell sheath is incomplete, and the ganglion may be exposed for

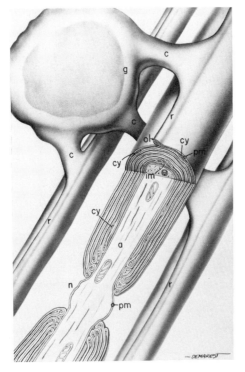

Fig. 8-15. Diagram of myelinated axons, showing how processes, *c,* of a neuroglia cell, *g,* enwrap axons, *a,* by means of a spiral membranous fold, which ultimately becomes packed at intervals of 13 to 18 nm. *cy,* "Trapped" cytoplasm of glial cell; *im,* inner mesaxon and inner loop of plasma membrane; *n,* bare portion of axon or node of Ranvier; *ol,* outer loop of plasma membrane; *pm,* plasma membrane; *r,* external ridge of myelin sheath. (From Bunge, M. B., R. P., Bunge, and H. Ris. 1961. J. Biophys. Biochem. Cytol. **10:**67-94.)

variable distances, whereas in dorsal root ganglia the cells are entirely covered with a protective sheath.

FINE STRUCTURE OF THE MYELIN SHEATH

Unmyelinated axons may have a variety of relationships with reference to Schwann cells. Individual axons of less than 1 μm in diameter indent the surface of the Schwann cell and lie in a separate trough or groove in the Schwann cell cytoplasm. As many as five to twenty axons may be ensheathed by one Schwann cell, but each axon is covered by a chain of such cells running along its length. In the autonomic nervous system several axons may be in a single groove within a Schwann cell.

In myelinated axons the axis cylinder is surrounded by a phospholipid-containing component that appears black when treated with osmic acid (osmophilia). When the myelin is removed by fat solvents, certain stains indicate that myelin is penetrated by a protein framework called *neurokeratin* (Fig. 8-12). In light microscope sections stained for either fat or neurokeratin, myelin sheaths appear as tubes surrounding a shrunken axis cylinder. Axons measuring more than 1 μm in diameter have myelin sheaths. Electron microscopy has shown that the myelin sheath consists of a system of concentric lamellar membranes approximately 3 nm thick, varying in number from a few to fifty or more (Fig. 8-10). The membrane is derived from the Schwann cell membrane, which wraps around the nerve fiber in concentric layers. White or myelinated fibers conduct impulses at a more rapid rate than do gray or unmyelinated fibers. This explains why somatic reflexes (involving myelinated fibers and skeletal muscle) are more rapid than visceral reflexes (involving slightly myelinated fibers and smooth muscle fibers).

In the central nervous system the oligodendrocytes form myelin by wrapping their plasma membranes around the nerve fiber in a manner similar to that described for the peripheral nervous system (Fig. 8-15).

SYNAPSE

The term synapse means "to fasten together," and refers to a site where processes of neurons come into functional contact with each other or with muscle or gland cells. At the light microscope level, synapses can be visualized by the use of silver stains, which outline the profile of the expanded terminal boutons that form the *presynaptic element*. The area of specialized cell surface contacted by the terminal bouton is referred to as the *postsynaptic membrane*, and the space between these two elements is the *synaptic cleft* (Fig. 8-16). Information can traverse the cleft either in the form of chemicals released from the presynaptic terminal (chemical synapses) or as an electrical signal (electrical synapse). Of the two types, chemical synapses have been more extensively studied. All chemical synapses in the central nervous system contain three elements: a presynaptic element, a postsynaptic element, and a synaptic cleft 20 to 40 nm wide. Presynaptic elements exhibit an accumulation of synaptic vesicles that contain neural transmitters. The presynaptic element is usually an axonal terminal; however, contacts between dendrites (*dendrodendritic synapses*) as well as those between cell bodies (*somatosomatic*) and between axons (*axoaxonic*) have been demonstrated. Beneath the presynaptic ending one may observe the postsynaptic membrane, with dark filamentous or granular material condensing in the adjacent cytoplasm. This dense material may underlie the entire zone of contact or be limited to small areas.

Various attempts have been made to classify different synaptic types on the basis of structure. However, no scheme has proved entirely satisfactory. Cell contacts may be made on dendrites, cell bodies, or axons.

PERIPHERAL NERVES

Nerves or nerve trunks are groups or bundles of fibers (axons, dendrites, and their collaterals) bound together by connective tissues and invested with blood capillaries. Nerves per se do not include perikarya. A

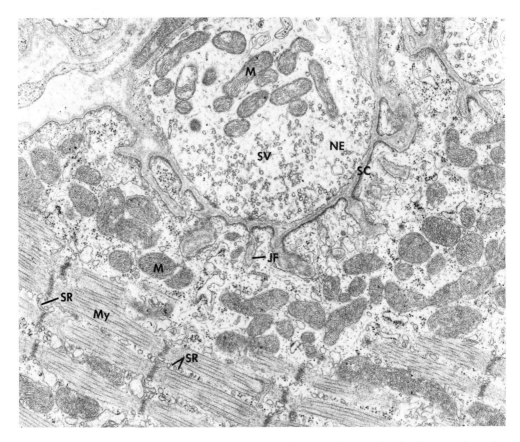

Fig. 8-16. Electron micrograph of myoneural junction of extraocular muscle showing axonal termination. Underlying muscle is "fast" or "twitch" type. Sarcolemma is thrown into junctional folds, *JF*. *M,* Mitochondria; *My,* myofibrils; *NE,* nerve ending; *SC,* synaptic cleft; *SR,* sarcoplastic reticulum; *SV,* synaptic vesicles. (×35,000; reduced ⅓.) (Courtesy Drs. M. A. Cahill and D. E. Kelly.)

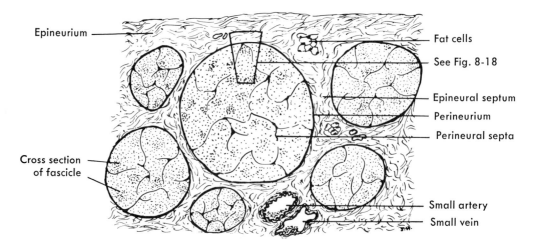

Fig. 8-17. Portion of transverse section of nerve trunk.

single discrete bundle of nerve fibers and connective tissue is called a fascicle (Figs. 8-17 to 8-19). Some of the larger nerve trunks are composed of numerous fascicles, with an attendant increase in the amount of connective tissue and capillaries. The terminology used to designate the topography of the connective tissue associated with the nervous system is similar to that established for connective tissues found in skeletal muscles.

In nerve trunks comprised of several fascicles, the entire structure is enclosed by a loosely arranged covering of collagenous and elastic fibers known as the epineurium (Figs. 8-17 and 8-18). In the large nerve trunks the epineurium is frequently prominent and contains many blood vessels. It also may give rise to extensions, known as epineural septa, occupying spaces between adjacent groups of fascicles. As the nerve trunk divides, the epineurium is reduced until it can no longer be distinguished from fine areolar tissue (Figs. 8-17 and 8-18).

A single fascicle is held together by a concentrically arranged layer of dense collagenous fibers called the perineurium. The perineurium varies from a thick prominent structure in large nerves to a very thin one in

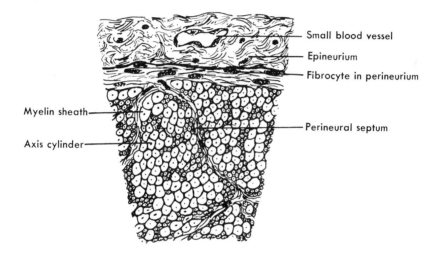

Myelin sheath

Axis cylinder

Small blood vessel

Epineurium

Fibrocyte in perineurium

Perineural septum

Fig. 8-18. Medium-power view of nerve fibers and surrounding connective tissue.

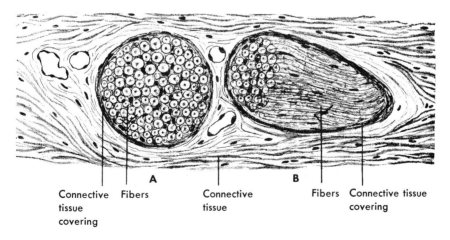

Connective tissue covering

Fibers

A

Connective tissue

B

Fibers

Connective tissue covering

Fig. 8-19. Myelinated nerve fibers forming small trunks in areolar tissue. **A,** Cut transversely; **B,** cut tangentially.

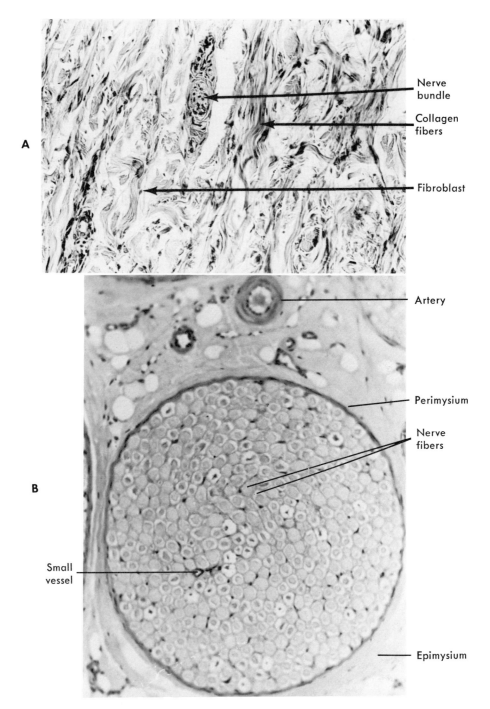

A

Nerve
bundle

Collagen
fibers

Fibroblast

Artery

Perimysium

Nerve
fibers

B

Small
vessel

Epimysium

Fig. 8-20. A, Dense fibrous tissue, irregularly arranged, from dermal layer of skin. Note nerve bundle.
B, Transverse section of nerve showing fibers and surrounding connective tissue. (×240.)

small nerves. Branches or trabeculae of the perineurium (perineural septa of some authors) penetrate the fascicle and give rise to the endoneurium, which in turn separates the individual nerve fibers. The endoneurium is composed of fine connective tissue sheaths that completely enclose and are intimately associated with the neurilemma of individual fibers. These sheaths are known as the sheaths of Henle or endoneural sheaths (Fig. 8-18).

Small nerve trunks occurring in connective tissue are distinguishable from the fibers of connective tissue by the following features (Fig. 8-20). In longitudinal section, nerves appear as groups of fine fibers arranged regularly and parallel. The myelin sheaths may be completely dissolved; if this is true, each axis cylinder is then separated from its neighbor by a space bounded by the neurilemma sheath. The axis cylinder and neurokeratin are less eosinophilic (or more basophilic) than the surrounding connective tissue fibers. Sections through nerves containing a majority of nonmyelinated fibers are somewhat more difficult to distinguish and may even be confused with smooth muscle fibers. In nonmyelinated fibers the neurilemma sheaths are irregular and nearly in contact with the somewhat basophilic axis cylinders.

PERIPHERAL GANGLIA

The cranial and spinal ganglia (Figs. 8-21 and 8-22) are aggregations of afferent neurons situated on the sensory roots of their respective nerves. Each ganglion is enclosed by a connective tissue capsule that is continuous with the epineurium and perineurium of the peripheral nerve, which divides into trabeculae to provide a framework for the cell bodies. The neuron perikarya of the ganglion are found in clusters separated by small amounts of connective tissue and bundles of

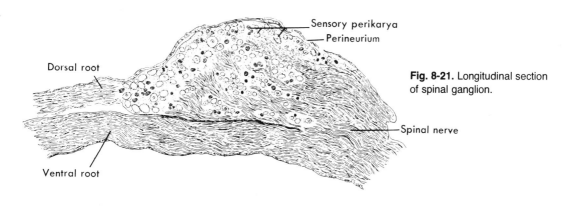

Fig. 8-21. Longitudinal section of spinal ganglion.

Dorsal root — Sensory perikarya — Perineurium — Spinal nerve — Ventral root

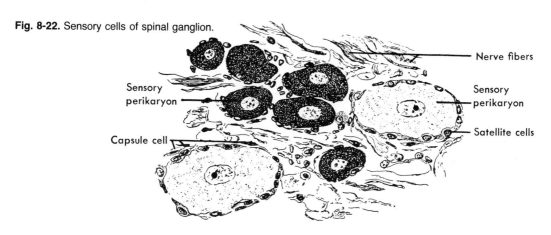

Fig. 8-22. Sensory cells of spinal ganglion.

Sensory perikaryon — Capsule cell — Nerve fibers — Sensory perikaryon — Satellite cells nerve fibers. Each cell is covered with two sheaths. The outer one, being collagenous, is laid down by fibroblasts. The inner sheath consists of a film of satellite cell cytoplasm. Satellite cells are derived from the same neural ectoderm as are the sensory neurons. The satellite cell sheath is complete, and the nuclei of the cells appear tightly attached to the neuron perikarya (Fig. 8-23). Most of the ganglion cells are unipolar, and in the case of the larger ganglion cells, the process is coiled and looped over the cell body to form a tangled configuration that is called a *glomerulus*. The smaller, darker-staining ganglion cells usually do not have this coiled structure.

The autonomic ganglia (Fig. 8-24) form

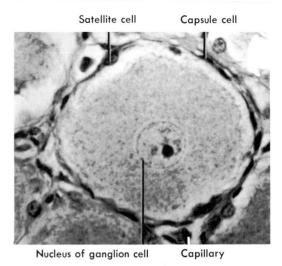

Satellite cell   Capsule cell

Nucleus of ganglion cell   Capillary

Fig. 8-23. Sensory neuron from spinal ganglion of monkey. (×640.)

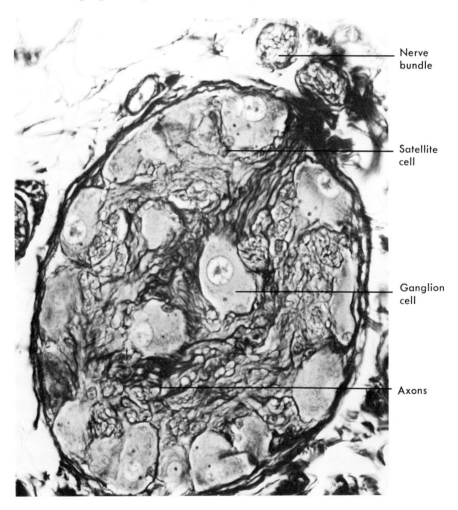

Nerve bundle

Satellite cell

Ganglion cell

Axons

Fig. 8-24. Section through autonomic ganglion (celiac plexus). (Golgi method.) (From collection of Dr. T. Thorsan.)

chains along the spinal cord or clusters of cells associated with the cranial nerves. The basic structure of an autonomic ganglion is similar to that of a sensory ganglion, but the cells are multipolar and are less variable in size (25 to 45 μm) than are those of spinal ganglia. Many of the cells have eccentrically placed nuclei and often more than one nucleolus. Binucleate cells are not uncommon. In contrast, the cells of spinal ganglia (Fig. 8-23) range from 15 to 100 μm in size and contain centrally placed nuclei with a prominent nucleolus. The satellite cells of autonomic ganglia do not completely invest the perikarya and may appear drawn away from the cell surface.

NERVE FIBER ENDINGS
Motor endings

The motor endings are the terminal parts of the efferent neurons, which are in contact with either muscles or glands. Striated muscles may exhibit two types of motor endings.

1. The motor end plate, shown in Fig. 8-25, consists of a terminal ramification of a naked fiber that ends on a mass of granular modified sarcoplasm. These structures appear in whole mounts as elevated areas,

which measure from 40 to 60 μm in diameter. In the region of the end plate the fiber terminates in several bulbous expansions, and the region between the nerve and the muscle fiber is devoid of the Schwann cell covering. Where the nerve fiber terminates, it indents the muscle fiber and forms a synaptic gutter. The nerve terminal contains numerous vesicles and mitochondria (Figs. 8-16 and 8-26).

2. In some cases the motor terminations consist of a simpler bulblike arrangement of small loops that end on the surface of the sarcolemma.

The efferent fibers that supply cardiac muscle, smooth muscle, and glands are part of the autonomic nervous system. These fibers are usually nonmyelinated and often terminate in nodular thickenings. In muscle these terminations end near the nucleus of the muscle fiber; in glands the fibers reach to the base or sides of the gland cell where they end freely in an expanded terminal loop.

Receptors

Receptors can be classified according to the type of energy they normally respond to (the so-called *adequate stimulus*). The usual classes of receptors are mechanoreceptors,

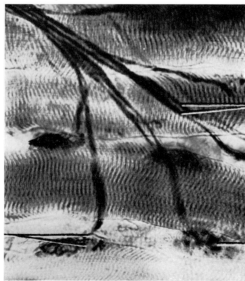

Myelinated fibers

Naked fibers

End plate

Fig. 8-25. Motor end plate. (Whole mount silver preparation.)

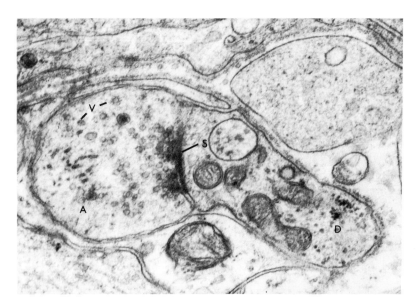

Fig. 8-26. Electron micrograph of axon-dendritic synapse of sympathetic ganglion of guinea pig. *A,* Axon showing presynaptic vesicles, *V; D,* dendrite; *S,* synaptic cleft. (×32,000.) (Courtesy Mrs. N. Sulkin.)

thermoreceptors, chemoreceptors, and photoreceptors which respond to stretch or pressure, temperature, chemicals, and light, respectively. These classes can also be defined in terms of their body position as exteroceptors, enteroceptors and proprioceptors that respond to external stimuli, visceral and vascular stimuli, and changes in the locomotor system (that is, muscle, tendons, and joints), respectively. There is a final group of receptors called *nociceptors* that respond to noxious and potentially damaging stimuli.

Many receptor cells are unremarkable in appearance except that they may have specialized organelle populations or distributions related to their specialized sensory functions. Mitochondria tend to be abundant, and the cytoplasm may have numerous small, dense, core granules, presumably containing neurotransmitters. There may also be an abundant Golgi apparatus and vesicular population designed to enhance the renewal and repair of the receptor surface. In many receptor endings, particularly in mechanoreceptors sensitive to stretch or pressure, cell resilience may be enhanced by a large accumulation of fine microfilaments within the matrix of the cytoplasm.

Many receptors are surrounded by or embedded in specialized nonsensory cells that assist in trapping or focusing the stimulus energy.

Aside from those located in specialized organs, such as the eye and ear, the sensory endings, terminations of afferent fibers, consist of the following types: free endings, encapsulated endings, and muscle spindles.

Free endings. Free endings are the simplest type from the structural standpoint. They consist of terminal branches of delicate fibers that often show slight enlargements. These endings have been observed in stratified epithelia, tendon, and other connective tissue.

Encapsulated endings. Encapsulated endings are characterized by the presence of a central naked fiber or several branches embedded in tissue fluid, which is enclosed within a connective tissue capsule. From their structure and location, one may infer that these might function as pressure receptors. There are several varieties of encapsulated endings: (1) the tactile corpuscles of Meissner, (2) the genital corpuscles, (3) the bulbous and cylindrical corpuscles of Krause, and (4) the lamellar corpuscles of Pacini (Fig.

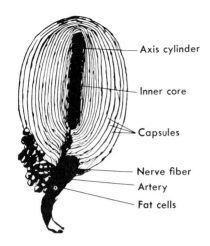

— Axis cylinder

— Inner core

— Capsules

— Nerve fiber
— Artery
— Fat cells

Fig. 8-27. Small lamellar corpuscle from mesentery of cat. Nuclei of capsule cells appear as thickenings. Myelin of nerve fiber may be traced to the inner core. (×50.) (From Bremer, F., and H. Weatherford. 1948. A textbook of histology. The Blakiston Co., New York.)

8-27). The last named are so large as to be visible with the unaided eye.

Muscle spindles. Most muscles have sensory fibers that terminate about slender bundles of muscle fibers, which are poorly developed. The terminal parts of the nerve fibers are arranged spirally around these muscle cells. This complex of nerve and muscle is enclosed within a dense connective tissue sheath and is known as a muscle spindle. Structures analogous to muscle spindles also occur in tendons.

NEUROGLIA (GLIA)

The other cell type in neural tissue is the glial cell. The nervous system is composed almost entirely of cells—neurons and neuroglia—with a thin film of extracellular fluid but lacks a connective tissue framework. The nuclei of glia cells are prominently stained by basic dyes, but the details of their shapes and locations can only be seen with metallic impregnation techniques (Fig. 8-28).

At the light microscope level there appear to be two categories of glial cells—the *macroglia* and the *microglia*. The macroglia are the astrocytes and the oligodendrocytes. These cells originate from neuroectoderm, but they have only one type of cell process.

They do not from synapses, and they remain able to divide throughout life, especially when the nervous system is damaged. After injury, they may participate in repair. The microglia are assumed to be derived from mesoderm.

The connective tissue framework of nerve trunks has previously been described, but the central nervous system does not have such an internal support. On the other hand, the meninges and an abundant arterial system (the latter containing relatively large amounts of elastic fibers and some collagenous fibers) form a tough external support for the central nervous system. Internally the support supplied by the presence of blood vessels is slight, and a type of interstitial cell known as an astroglial cell forms a pericapillary barrier that prevents the encroachment of blood vessel connective tissue on nerve cells. The astroglia (collectively referred to as neuroglia) form a part of the so-called internal support of the central nervous system. The microglia, another class of glial cells, are believed by some authors to belong to the reticuloendothelial system and consist of inactive macrophages that do not aid in tissue support. Many investigators are of the opinion that the main internal support of the central nervous system is provided by the hydrostatic pressure of tissue fluid. Although glia may serve as mechanical support, they may also influence neuronal transmission and neural metabolism.

Astroglia

The most common type of neuroglia cell is the astroglia. These are branching cells, some of which (*fibrous*) (Fig. 8-28, *A*) have long, slender processes. Other astroglia cells (*protoplasmic*) (Fig. 8-28, *B*) are similar to the fibrous ones except that the processes are considerably thicker and perhaps more branched. Although different features have been described for the two types, the chief morphologic difference between them appears to be whether the processes are thick or thin, since they both contain neuroglia fibers within the processes. In either kind of astroglia the cells have specialized processes

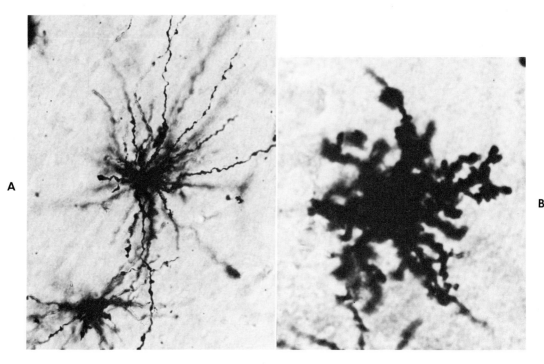

Fig. 8-28. A, Fibrous astrocyte. **B,** Protoplasmic astrocyte. (Golgi method; ×500.) (From collection of Dr. T. Thorsan.)

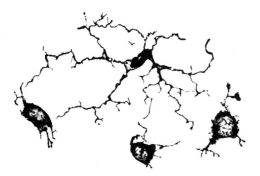

Fig. 8-29. Neuroglia cells from brain of rabbit. Microglia (above) and oligodendroglia. (Stained by Penfield's method.) (From Bremer, F., and H. Weatherford. 1948. A text-book of histology. The Blakiston Co., New York.)

that are in close contact with the walls of the blood vessels of the nervous system. These *sucker feet* have been thought to enable the cell to derive nourishment from the blood; it is also stated, however, that their function is to provide a special limiting membrane around the vessels (Fig. 8-28).

Oligodendria

A second type of neuroglia cell is the oligodendria (or oligodendroglia). These cells have short beaded processes but no neuroglia fibrils. Their nuclei are smaller and darker than those of the astroglia cells. They are grouped around nerve cells and are aligned in rows along the fiber tracts in the brain and spinal cord where they function to produce myelin sheaths.

Microglia

A third type is the microglia, the smallest of the neuroglia cells. They have deeply staining nuclei, are irregular in shape, and have no fibrils or sucker feet. They are said to be phagocytic. Oligodendria and microglia are illustrated in Fig. 8-29.

Other types

The ependyma or layer that lines the central canal of the nervous system forms the fourth group of neuroglia cells. These are elongated cells that are arranged in a layer-like columnar epithelium. They contain fibrils and are sometimes ciliated.

It is of interest to note that these supporting cells, although similar in appearance and function to the simpler mesenchymal derivatives such as reticular tissue, are for the most part ectodermal in origin. This is certainly true of the ependyma and of the astroglia, which form the greater part of the tissue. The microglia are probably mesodermal in origin; the oligodendria are said to be ectodermal.

9

Circulatory system

The circulatory system is made up of the blood vascular system and the lymph vascular system. The *blood vascular system* consists of (1) the heart, a muscular organ that pumps the blood; (2) arteries that convey the blood to the organs and tissues; (3) the *capillaries*, small channels that anastomose, divide, and provide for interchange of various substances between blood and tissue fluid; and (4) veins that return blood to the heart.

BLOOD VASCULAR SYSTEM

The several components of the blood vascular system all have a similar and continuous lining that consists of a single layer of endothelial cells. In capillaries the endothelial layer forms the chief structural component of the wall. In the heart, arteries, and veins additional coats of muscle and connective tissue are added to the lining. The discussion will begin with the capillaries and then describe the structural elements that are gradually added to the basic endothelial cell wall of the capillaries as the vessels enlarge to form the major components of the arterial and venous system.

Capillaries

Capillaries are delicate endothelial tubes having a diameter of 7 to 9 μm. They form networks whose distribution is correlated with the metabolic activity of the tissue or organ in which they occur. Kidney, liver and lungs—organs having a high metabolic activity—exhibit a pattern in which capillaries are numerous and closely aligned. In regions such as the serous membranes (Fig. 9-1), capillaries are more sparsely distributed.

The capillary wall consists of a single layer of flat endothelial cells separated from a thin layer of connective tissue by a basement membrane. The cells are arranged so that their long axis is parallel with the long axis of the capillary (Fig. 9-2). In surface view they appear to be arranged in a mosaic with serrated edges. The cytoplasm is clear or finely granular. The nucleus is somewhat elongated and centrally located. The cells are thicker in the region of the nucleus, and in fixed preparations the nucleus appears to bulge into the lumen. The capillary wall usually consists of from one to three cells. Large capillaries have three to five cells. Capillaries are invested by a thin sheath of collagen or reticular fibers and a discontinuous layer of pericapillary cells. The basement membrane visible with the light microscope consists of a *basal lamina* of amorphous material and fine reticular fibers. Pericapillary cells include *fibroblasts, histiocytes,* and *pericytes.* Pericytes are irregular branching cells resembling fibroblasts. Pericytes are invested by a basal lamina and are distributed at intervals along the capillary walls. It was formerly believed that pericytes were contractile; recent studies have shown that this is not true.

The electron microscope has revealed structural details of the capillary wall that have led to the separation of capillaries into two groups: *continuous* and *fenestrated.* The *continuous* type of capillaries occur in several sites such as lung, muscle, and skin. The cy-

Capillary

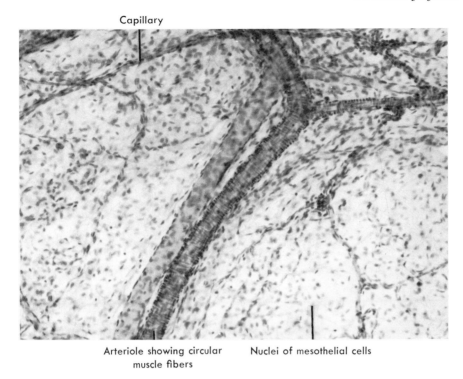

Arteriole showing circular   Nuclei of mesothelial cells
muscle fibers

Fig. 9-1. Stretch preparation of mesentery, surface view showing arrangement of vascular elements. (×40.)

Nucleus of endothelial cell of capillary

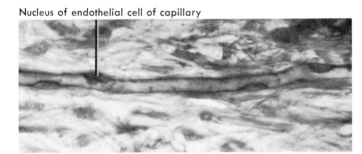

Fig. 9-2. Longitudinal section of capillary. (×640.)

toplasm of the endothelial cells is thick in the region of the nucleus, but attenuated in other regions. It contains organelles common to most other cells as well as numerous *pinocytotic vesicles* or *caveoli*. The vesicles arise by invagination of the cell membrane during the process of cell drinking known as pinocytosis. The vesicles thus formed are bound by a unit membrane and measure 60 to 70 nm in diameter. They migrate to the opposite side of the cell wall and discharge their contents into the surrounding space, thus providing an avenue for the transport of macromolecules across the endothelium.

The cells making up the endothelial sleeve are fitted together in an irregular, patchwork fashion. The edges of adjoining cells overlap or interdigitate and are separated by spaces around 200 Å (20 nm) wide, filled with an amorphous material of low-electron density. At intervals, the cell membranes close into macula occludens junctions, which are discontinuous fusions of the contiguous membranes that leave a 20 nm channel for the passage of fluids between the capillary lumen and the tissue spaces.

In a few regions of the body, the wall of the capillary becomes a barrier to restrict the passage of large molecules into the tissue fluid from the capillary. An example of this arrangement is found in the brain, where most brain tissue (with the exception of regions such as the median eminence of the hypothalamus) resides behind a *blood-brain barrier*. Such regions can be defined easily because they are not stained by a supravital dye such as trypan blue injected into the vascular bed.

The basis for the blood-brain barrier and other similar barriers (blood–cerebrospinal fluid, blood-testis) lies in the specialized structure of the capillary bed. The endothelial cells are joined by ribbonlike zonula occludens instead of by the seamlike intermittent maculae occludens, and the endothelial tube is completely encased in a substantial basement membrane.

The *fenestrated* type of capillaries occur in regions such as the intestinal villi, kidney glomeruli, and endocrine glands, organs where exchanges between the blood and extracellular fluid are extensive (Fig. 9-3). The thin regions of the cell are perforated by numerous pores that have a diameter of 30

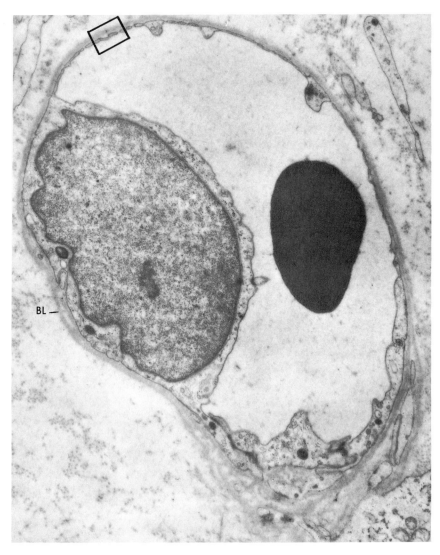

Fig. 9-3. Electron micrograph of a fenestrated capillary cut transversely. Wall of capillary consists of attenuated endothelial cell whose nucleus projects into lumen. Cytoplasm of endothelial cell contains many pinocytotic vesicles and is invested by delicate basement membrane (lamina), *BL*. (×11,000.)

to 80 nm. The pores are closed by a thin diaphragm and the basal lamina of the endothelial cell (Fig. 9-4).

Some of the endothelial cells are held together in a relatively simple end-to-end arrangement; others overlap to form oblique or S-shaped junctions. In most junctions there is an appreciable gap occupied by electron-dense material.

Sinusoidal capillaries are larger in diameter than ordinary capillaries and occur in endocrine glands such as the thyroid, anterior pituitary, and adrenal cortex. The endothelial cells are reduced in size, have pores, and are invested by an attenuated adventitia. *Sinusoids* occur in organs such as the liver, spleen, and blood-forming organs. They have a diameter larger than those of the sinusoidal capillaries. The lining cells are phagocytic and belong to the reticuloendothelial system. An example of this kind of lining cell occurs in the liver and is known as the von Kupffer cell. The lining cells of the sinusoids, in contrast with those of the sinuses, have wide intercellular spaces and lack a continuous basal lamina.

Capillaries and small venules account for most of the exchange that takes place between blood and surrounding tissues. Several factors are involved in exchange and they vary in different locations and in diverse physiological conditions. Transfer of substances from capillaries to tissues is influenced by blood pressure. The osmotic pressure of the blood facilitates reabsorption. Exchange across the vascular wall is also car-

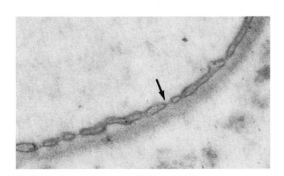

Fig. 9-4. Electron micrograph of part of endothelial cell of capillary shown in area represented by box in Fig. 9-3. Arrow indicates pore. (×27,000.)

ried on by pinocytotic vesicles through pores in the cell wall and in the region of cell junctions.

The venules appear to be particularly sensitive to agents such as bradykinin that increase the passage of macromolecules from the capillary bed into tissue fluid, and leakiness at this site in the bed seems to contribute substantially to the fluid buildup (edema) caused by these agents.

Arteries

Arteries are composed of three coats or tunics:

1. The inner coat or *intima* consists of an inner endothelial lining, an intermediate layer of connective tissue, and an external band of elastic tissue.

2. A middle coat or *media* consists chiefly of circularly arranged smooth muscle cells interspersed with varying amounts of connective tissue.

3. An external coat or *adventitia* is composed almost exclusively of collagenous and elastic connective tissue.

Arteries are usually classified as large, medium, and small, depending on the amount and arrangement of the several component tissues in the different tunics. In this system of vessels there is a gradual change of structure as the caliber increases. These changes however, are not abrupt and cannot be accurately correlated with the size of the vessels.

Arterioles and small arteries. Vessels having a diameter of 20 to 100 μm are usually included in this group. The intima consists of an endothelial lining and an attenuated internal elastic membrane. The media is made up of one to five layers of smooth muscle cells with a few scattered elastic fibers. The adventitia is thinner than the media and consists of loosely arranged collagen and elastic fibers that blend with surrounding connective tissue. The arterioles exhibit, though in attenuated form, the three coats typical of arteries (Figs. 9-5 and 9-6).

As blood flows through the arterioles toward a capillary bed, it enters a series of smaller channels called the metarterioles and finally, in some tissues such as skeletal mus-

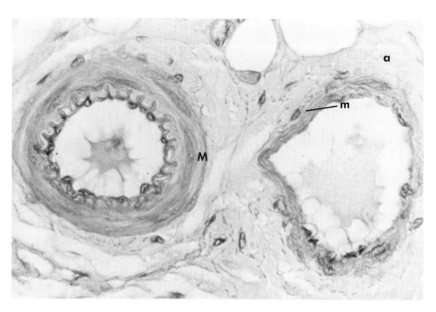

Fig. 9-5. Vascular elements. Left, small artery showing prominent internal elastic membrane and muscular media, *M;* right, small vein with relatively thin media, *m,* and extensive adventitia, *a.* Upper portion, several small vessels. (×640.)

cle, flows past a *precapillary sphincter* into the capillary bed. The arterioles have a strong, muscular coat whose state of contraction (and hence diameter) is controlled by a dense innervation from the sympathetic division of the autonomic nervous system. The metarterioles are wrapped by a few highly active smooth muscle fibers. The precapillary sphincter is a region where a single muscle cell winds around the capillary wall. Both the metarterioles and precapillary sphincters have only sparse innervation, but the contractility of the muscle spiraling around the vessel walls is extremely sensitive to local conditions in the tissue, such as the levels of oxygen, carbon dioxide, hydrogen ions, or electrolytes whose concentrations vary with the metabolic status of the tissue. These local factors are major controllers of blood flow through individual capillary beds, adjusting the degree of flow to the local metabolic demands of the tissue. Central control and the routing of blood into or past larger vascular beds in tissues and organs is exercised through the dense mat of innervation of the arterioles and venules, which regulates the pressure head across the capillary bed

and the channel size available for the passage of blood (lumen diameter). Arterioles can be thought of as "stopcocks" to control the amount of blood perfusing a particular capillary bed. The entire channel from the 100 μm vessels down to where the muscle wrapping disappears at the entry to the capillary bed is sensitive to circulating humoral agents such as the catecholamines (epinephrine and norepinephrine), bradykinin, and angiotensin. The regulation of blood flow thus involves a constantly shifting balance of neural control, local regulation by metabolic conditions, and circulating humoral agents.

Small arteries are usually considered to be those that connect arterioles with medium-sized arteries. As these vessels increase in caliber, there is usually a corresponding increase in the thickness of the various coats (Figs. 9-5 and 9-6). This is especially true in the case of the media, which in vessels 150 μm in diameter may contain three or four layers of muscle cells and a few scattered elastic fibers. The adventitia contains elastic fibers adjacent to the external surface of the media. As these vessels increase in diameter, they show all the structural features present

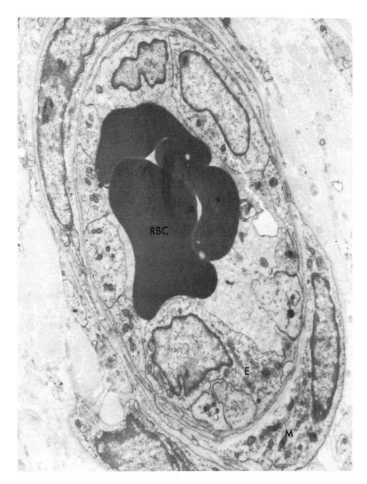

Fig. 9-6. Electron micrograph of transverse section of arteriole. Vessel wall is made up of several endothelial cells, *E,* surrounded by single layer of smooth muscle cells, *M,* and lumen contains red blood cells, *RBC.* (×4,500.)

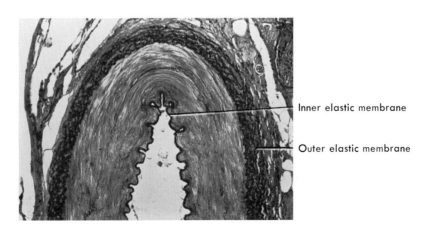

Inner elastic membrane

Outer elastic membrane

Fig. 9-7. Medium-sized artery showing distribution of elastic tissue. (Verhoeff's method; ×125.)

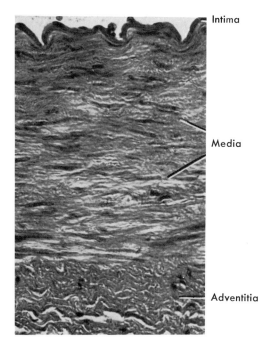

Intima

Media

Adventitia

Fig. 9-8. Medium-sized artery. (Hematoxylin and eosin stain; ×240.)

in medium-sized arteries: an intima with an inner elastic membrane, a muscular media interspersed with elastic fibers, and a connective tissue adventitia exhibiting an internal and external elastic membrane.

Medium-sized arteries. Most of the named arteries such as the axillary, mesenteric, splenic, and radial are included in this group. These arteries have relatively thick walls due to the large amount of muscle present in the media (Figs. 9-7 to 9-9). They are known as muscular or distributing arteries in contrast with the so-called elastic arteries (large arteries) such as the aorta, which are adapted for large-volume flow.

The arterial blood vessel wall is made up of three definite layers.

1. The innermost layer or *intima* consists of endothelial cells that rest on an intermediate layer made up of delicate elastic and collagen fibers and scattered fibroblasts and an internal elastic membrane that consists of a thick fenestrated band which in some vessels

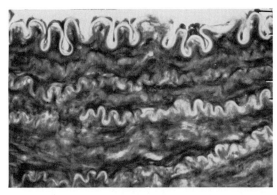

Endothelial nucleus

Inner elastic membrane

Fine collagenous fibers

Elastic fiber in media

Fig. 9-9. Medium-sized artery showing intima and media. (×400.)

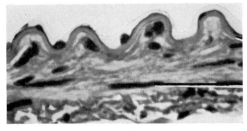

Inner elastic membrane

Smooth muscle cell nucleus

Fig. 9-10. Longitudinal section of luminal portion of small artery. (Hematoxylin and eosin stain; ×640.)

is split and appears double (Figs. 9-10 and 9-11). This membrane is in intimate contact with the inner boundary of the media.

2. The *media*, the thickest layer, consists of from twenty to forty layers of circularly disposed muscle fibers. Between the muscle fibers there are small and varying amounts of collagen, reticular and elastic fibers, and fibroblasts. In vessels of large caliber there is a network of elastic fibers, the external elastic membrane located at the junction of the media and the adventitia (Fig. 9-7).

3. The *adventitia* is made up of a thick coat of connective tissue consisting of collagenous and elastic fibers arranged for the most part in a longitudinal direction. The elastic fibers are located adjacent to the media, whereas the outer part of the adventitia blends with the surrounding connective tissue.

Aorta (elastic-type arteries). The intima of the aorta is lined with short polygonal endothelial cells. Below this lining is a layer con-

taining fine collagenous and elastic fibers and also a few scattered fibroblasts. The deeper portion of the intima also contains collagenous as well as longitudinally oriented muscle and elastic fibers. The internal elastic membrane consists of two or more lamellae that blend with similar membranes of the interna and media; hence it is difficult to identify.

The second coat or media is by far the thickest layer, forming approximately four fifths of the thickness of the wall (Fig. 9-12). It consists of a mixture of circularly arranged smooth muscle and elastic fibers. The latter predominate and mingle, on the one hand, with the elastic fibers of the intima and, on the other, with those of the outermost layer or adventitia. The smooth muscle fibers unite to form branching bands and, like the elastic fibers, appear spirally arranged. The muscle fibers are enclosed or surrounded by delicate reticular fibers.

The adventitia is a comparatively thin coat

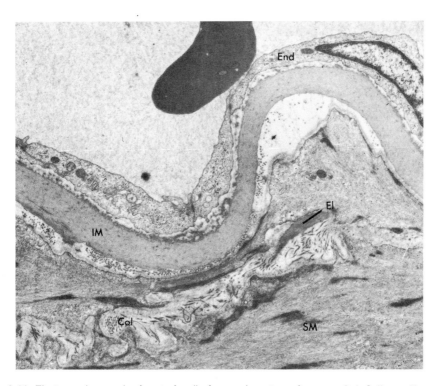

Fig. 9-11. Electron micrograph of part of wall of muscular artery of mouse. *Col,* Collagen fibers; *El,* elastic fiber; *End,* endothelium bordering lumen; *IM,* inner elastic membrane; *SM,* smooth muscle. (×10,000.)

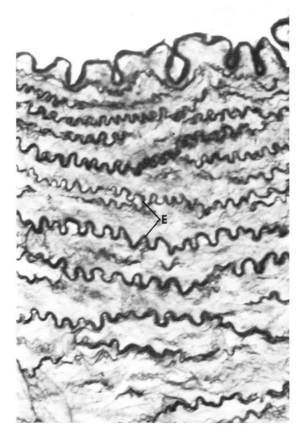

Fig. 9-12. Section of part of wall of aorta showing relative amount and distribution of elastic fibers, *E,* in this vessel. (Voerhoeff's method; ×500.)

of connective tissue. Elastic fibers are concentrated at the outer border of the media, forming the external elastic membrane. Collagenous fibers merge with those of the connective tissue surrounding the vessel and are arranged in longitudinal spirals. In the adventitia and the outer portion of the media are small nutrient vessels (vasa vasorum) and nerves (nervi vasorum).

The aorta and a few other similar vessels are sometimes called arteries of the elastic type. The common iliacs, carotids, and pulmonaries belong in this group.

The composition of the walls of the arteries influences pulse pressure in the vascular bed. In old age the arterial walls lose much of their elastic and muscular tissues, which are replaced by relatively unyielding fibrous tissue and calcified plaques. As a result, the blood pressure changes induced during contraction of the heart are not damped and the arterial pressure can rise very high during systole (contraction of the heart) and fall very low during diastole (filling of the heart). These pressure extremes are prevented in a highly elastic, compliant vascular bed, and blood flow is steadier.

Veins

The veins, by which blood returns from the capillaries to the heart, have walls that are composed largely of collagenous connective tissue, with muscle and elastic fibers much less prominent than they are in the arterial wall. Because of the reduced amount of elastic tissue, veins do not retain their shape after death and appear in sections as irregularly rounded structures. In general,

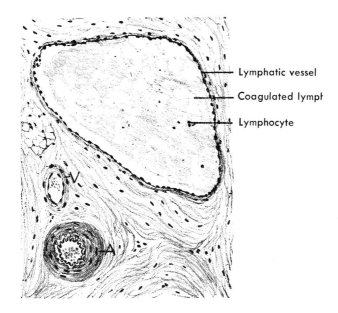

Fig. 9-13. Lymphatic artery and vein from hilum of lymph node. *V*, Vein; *A*, artery.

the wall of a vein is not so thick as that of the accompanying artery, but its lumen is larger.

The organization of the wall into three coats is frequently indistinct. Tracing the system back from the capillaries toward the heart, one may observe small veins and venules, medium caliber veins, and large veins.

Small veins and venules. Small veins and venules occur in the connective tissue of organs (Fig. 9-13). The first addition to the endothelium that changes the vessel from a capillary to a venule is not muscle but collagenous fibers. These and the accompanying fibroblasts are oriented longitudinally with respect to the vessel. As the caliber of the venule increases, its wall includes first muscle and then, in still larger vessels, scattered elastic fibers. The elements are arranged as in arteries but in different proportions. The larger vessels of this group have three coats: the intima consists of endothelium, subendothelial collagenous fibers, and scattered elastic fibers. The latter do not form a complete membrane and are not present in sufficient number to cause the scalloping of the border of the lumen, which is characteristic of arteries. The media is a thin coat of muscle interspersed with collagenous fibers. The adventitia, which consists of collagenous tissue, is the thickest of the three coats.

Medium-sized veins. Veins of medium caliber exhibit many of the characteristics just described (Fig. 9-14). The adventitia of collagenous fibers is the thickest of the coats. The muscle of the media and the elastic tissue of the intima increase somewhat in amount, but there is no inner elastic membrane (Figs. 9-14 and 9-15). In some veins of this group longitudinal muscle fibers occur in the intima and in the adventitia. In the latter coat, there may be a complete layer of longitudinal muscle fibers placed next to the circular muscle fibers of the media. This is not, however, a common occurrence.

Large veins. Large veins show an increase in the amount of longitudinal muscle in the adventitia and a slight increase in the amount of elastic tissue in the intima. The elastic tissue, however, is not as prominent, even in the largest veins, as it is in small arteries. The circular muscle of the media is reduced in veins of this group and is lacking entirely in a few of them.

Some veins, particularly those of the extremities, also contain valves. They consist of a thin connective tissue membrane. The surfaces of the valves are covered by endothelium, which is reflected from the internal surface of the intima.

Medium-sized artery

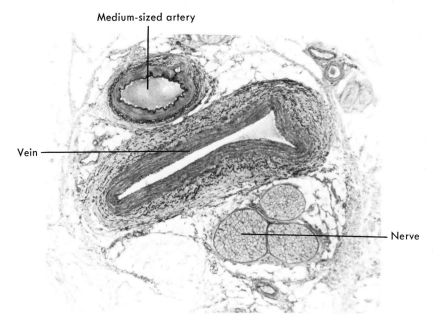

Vein

Nerve

Fig. 9-14. Section showing typical arrangement of a medium-sized artery, vein, and nerve. (Hematoxylin and eosin.)

Comparison of veins and arteries

The difference between the smaller arterial and the venous vessels lies in the amount of muscle and connective tissue present in each. Muscle is the predominant tissue in arterioles; in the venules there is little muscle and the walls consist mainly of endothelium and connective tissue. The larger vessels of the two groups may be distinguished by the following: intima, media, adventitia, and size and shape of vessels.

Intima. In arteries the presence of a complete inner elastic membrane is a distinguishing feature. This membrane contracts after death, throwing the intima into small folds and allowing the endothelial nuclei to project into the lumen of the vessel. In the veins the endothelium remains smooth. The entire intima of some veins extends into the lumen at intervals in large folds or reduplications, which serve as valves to prevent the backflow of the blood.

Media. The media is the thickest coat of any artery and consists of muscle interspersed with elastic tissue. In veins the media is a thin coat of muscle; it usually con-

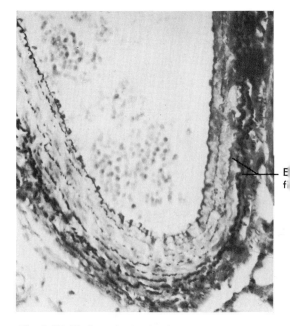

E
f

Fig. 9-15. Medium-sized vein showing distribution of elastic tissue.

tains all circular fibers, but occasionally has longitudinal fibers. It has more collagenous white fibers than does the media of an artery and includes elastic tissue only in the largest vessels in the system.

Adventitia. In arteries the adventitia is less important than the media. It contains the outer elastic membrane, and there are seldom any muscle fibers in it. The adventitia of the vein is its thickest coat and often contains several longitudinal muscle fibers.

Size and shape of vessels. The lumen of the vein is larger than that of the accompanying artery, but its wall is thinner. Because of the relatively large amount of elastic tissue, arteries retain their round shape in sections more often than do the veins. The latter are likely to be collapsed in section.

Vascular and nerve supply of blood vessels

Many arteries and veins have a blood and lymph supply. Small nutrient vessels, the *vasa vasorum*, enter the adventitia and reach the deep layers of the media in a capillary network. Networks of lymphatics occur in the adventitia of large arteries and veins. Unmyelinated axons (vasomotor) derived from sympathetic ganglia penetrate the wall of the vessels and terminate in the muscle cells of the media. Myelinated fibers that terminate in the vessel walls are sensory in function.

HEART

The heart is a specialized portion of the vascular system and develops from an enlargement of two veins in the embryo. It has three coats—endocardium, myocardium, and epicardium.

Endocardium

The endocardium, which corresponds to the intima of the vessels, includes an endothelial lining and a relatively thick subendothelial layer, which is made up of connective tissue, smooth muscle, and elastic fibers. The valves of the heart are folds of the endocardium in which the fibroelastic elements are prominent. The annuli fibrosi are rings of dense connective tissue that surround the openings from one chamber to another. A *subendocardial layer* of loose connective tissue binds the endocardium to the underlying myocardium. This layer contains numerous blood vessels, nerves, and branches of the conduction system of the heart.

Myocardium

The myocardium or muscular coat corresponds to the media of the vessels. It is made up of interlacing bundles of muscle. The tissue, however, is not like that of the media of the vessels. It is muscle of specialized type, cardiac, found nowhere else in the body. In the atria the muscle fibers are arranged in bundles that form a latticelike structure. In the ventricle some of the muscle fibers on the internal surface appear as isolated bundles. They are known as the trabeculae carnae. Connective tissue occupies the spaces between the muscle. Cardiac muscle is arranged in sheets that enclose the ventricles and atria in a spiral fashion. Most of these fibers are attached to the *cardiac skeleton,* a central supporting structure of the heart. The nature of this muscle has been discussed in Chapter 7.

Epicardium

The epicardium is the visceral portion of the pericardial sac enclosing the heart. Its covering consists of a single layer of flattened mesothelial cells. Subjacent to the mesothelial cells is a fibrous layer containing scattered elastic fibers. The epicardium is attached to the myocardium by a layer of vascularized areolar connective tissue, the subepicardial layer.

Valves of the heart

The atrioventricular valves, the *tricuspid* and *mitral,* consist of reduplications of endocardium and a plate of connective tissue beginning at the collar of tough fibrous tissue surrounding the roots of the major vessels *(the annulus fibrosa)* and reinforced by strands of dense ligamentous tissue. The core of the valve consists mostly of dense cartilage-like (chondroid) tissue containing small spindle-shaped or rounded cells. Outside the core is a covering layer of endocardium that is thickened on the atrial side of each valve flap to resist the mechanical pressures that occur when the valves close. The connective tissue core is penetrated by the fibrous chordae tendineae that hold the valve flaps to the papillary muscles of the ventricles. Small slips of muscle penetrate into the bases of the valves. Normal valves do not contain capillary beds.

The semilunar valves are similar in structure except that they are thinner, have no chordae tendinae, and have a thicker chondral plate to provide more reinforcement in the absence of the chordae. Varying amounts of elastin are found, depending on the need for resilience in the valves.

Cardiac skeleton

The cardiac skeleton consists of dense connective tissue and serves as the site of attachment for the valves. There are three components: the *annuli fibrosi*, the *trigona fibrosa*, and the *septum membranaceum*. The annuli fibrosa enclose the origins of the aorta,

pulmonary artery, and the atrioventricular canals. The trigona fibrosa consists of fibrous tissue located between the arterial foramina and the atrioventricular canals. The membraneous septum is the membraneous part of the interventricular septum and serves as an attachment for some cardiac muscle fibers.

Impulse-conducting system

The heart contains modified cardiac fibers whose function is to coordinate the heartbeat by regulating the time of contraction of the atria and ventricles. The impulse that coordinates contraction normally begins at the *sinoatrial (SA) node*, which is located in the right atrium at the point of entry of the superior vena cava. From the sinoatrial node, the impulse spreads over the atrial muscle to the atrioventricular node, located in the posterior portion of the interventricular septum. From this point a bundle of modified cardiac muscle cells (the Purkinje fibers) bifurcates and a separate branch passes down through the subendocardial tissue of the right and left ventricles. The cells within the

Purkinje fibers

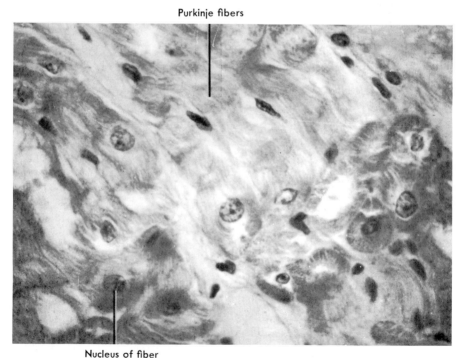

Nucleus of fiber

Fig. 9-16. Purkinje fibers of heart. (×640.)

two nodal regions are spindle-shaped, highly branching cells separated from each other by bits of connective tissue. The bundles of Purkinje fibers *(bundles of His)* in the ventricular walls are indistinct in the human heart but can be distinguished from ordinary cardiac muscle by their foamy-appearing cytoplasm, reduced number of myofibrils, and increased cellular diameter. Comparison of cardiac muscle in Fig. 7-6 with that shown in Fig. 9-16 illustrates the marked reduction in the number of myofibrils occurring in the Purkinje fibers.

Vascular and nerve supply of the heart

Two coronary arteries supply the blood to the heart. These vessels penetrate the myocardium where they break up into capillary plexuses. The blood is returned by way of cardiac veins that empty into the right atrium by way of the coronary sinus. Lymph vessels are abundant in the myocardium. They are also present in the subendocardial and subepicardial regions. The nerve supply is derived from the vagus and the sympathetic division of the autonomic system. These two systems are antagonistic. The vagus fibers decrease the rhythm of the SA nodes and slow transmission of cardiac impulses into the ventricles. The sympathetic fibers increase heart action by accelerating the discharge of the SA node and increasing the excitability of heart muscle and the force of the contraction of both the atria and the ventricles.

LYMPHATIC SYSTEM

The lymphatic system consists of lymph capillaries and vessels but is unlike the blood vascular system in that it does not form a complete circuit through which the fluid leaves and returns to a central propelling organ. Lymph capillaries begin blindly in the connective tissues from which they collect tissue fluid. The latter passes as lymph from the capillaries to larger vessels, which join together, forming ultimately the thoracic duct and the right lymphatic duct. The thoracic duct is the larger of the two, since it alone receives lymph drainage from the abdomen. It empties its contents into the bloodstream at the junction of the left internal jugular and left subclavian veins. In some cases there is a right lymphatic duct opening into the corresponding veins on the right side of the body, but the single duct on this side is often replaced by several smaller lymphatics.

Lymphatic vessels are thin walled and less conspicuous than the blood vessels (Fig. 9-13). The structure of the larger lymphatics most nearly resembles that of the veins, but, rather than containing blood, they are filled with a granular coagulum containing a few lymphocytes. The large lymphatics are composed of three coats: (1) an intima of endothelium and subendothelial tissue, (2) a media of circular muscle with little elastic tissue, and (3) an adventitia of loose connective tissue with scattered bundles of longitudinal muscle. They have numerous valves and are distinguishable from veins chiefly through the absence of blood in them.

10

Lymphoid system

The lymphoid system is made up of a collection of distinct organs (thymus, spleen, lymph nodes, tonsils) and a more diffusely arranged meshwork of lymphocytes (diffuse lymphoid tissue) widely distributed beneath the moist epithelial membranes of the digestive and respiratory tracts. Wherever it is found, lymphoid tissue consists of reticular cells and fibers that provide a framework for the support of an accumulation of lymphocytes and macrophages. In certain regions, lymphocytes tend to cluster together in concentrations called *nodules*. These nodules can be found in lymph nodes, the tonsils, and the spleen and are also widely distributed along the digestive tract where they are referred to as *Peyer's patches.*

CELLS OF THE IMMUNE SYSTEM

Mammals have a highly developed immune defense system involving circulating antibodies *(humoral immunity)* and direct cellular responses *(cell-mediated immunity).* These integrated chemical and cellular responses provide the basis for the ability of mammals to defend themselves against a wide range of antigens (foreign proteins). The development of cell-mediated immunity depends on the activity of the thymus, where a class of lymphocytes called T cells are produced. A second class of lymphocytes called B cells are required for humoral immunity. In birds an organ called the bursa of Fabricius is required for the development of B cells, but the site of B cell maturation in mammals has yet to be identified. Since the

discovery of these two classes of lymphocytes, it has been necessary to reinterpret many immune responses in terms of interactions between B and T cells. In this chapter the structure of lymphoid tissue and the lines of defense against disease will be considered. We will first consider what cell types are found in lymphoid tissue, then try to give some idea of how they may interact in a typical immune reaction, and finally describe the organization of lymphoid tissue.

Lymphocytes

One of the main morphological features of lymphocytes is that they are round cells with a high nucleus-to-cytoplasm ratio. At the light microscope level the nucleus frequently appears to be round, but under higher magnification it is seen to be indented. The cytoplasm has a few mitochondria, a small Golgi apparatus region, and a few lysosomes. In a living preparation, lymphocytes are motile and tend to stretch into a "hand mirror" shape. When classified on the basis of size, lymphocytes are a heterogeneous population, which for convenience is divided into small, medium, and large, although size ranges overlap considerably. They are widely distributed throughout the body; they form a large proportion of the white blood cells of the blood and peritoneal fluid and the great majority of cells in lymph and in the lymphoid organs.

Another way of classifying lymphocytes is on the basis of their primary site of origin. T cells are formed in the thymus. B cells may

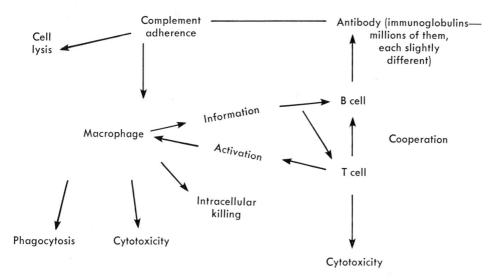

Diagram 1. Cellular interactions involved in the immune response. Illustrated here are the ways that cellular and humoral immune defenses interact to destroy bacteria. The cells involved are lymphocytes (B and T cells) and macrophages. T cells can activate macrophages, which in turn can process foreign proteins, which will induce B cells to manufacture antibodies that participate in cell breakdown *(lysis)*.

be derived from bone marrow in mammals, although conclusive evidence for this is lacking. The cells that give rise to T cells are called T immunoblasts and can be distinguished from B cell precursors by their rich polyribosome content. B immunoblasts have abundant endoplasmic reticulum. The two populations can also be distinguished on the basis of their surface chemistry, the antigenic determinants coating the cell surface. The B cell line gives rise to *plasma cells*, which contain abundant endoplasmic reticulum and secrete antibodies.

Macrophages

Macrophages are usually large cells with a simple round eccentrically placed nucleus and a bulky cytoplasm filled with vacuoles. Generally, these cells are actively phagocytic, and at the electron microscope level their cytoplasm can be seen to contain lysosomes, phagosomes, and bits of partly digested material. There has been some controversy about the origin of these cells, but the most widely supported view is that tissue macrophages are derived from circulating macrophages, which in turn originate in bone marrow.

The reticular cells of lymphoid tissues appear to be specialized macrophages adapted for long-term retention of antigen on their surface. It seems clear that in addition to their general scavenger function, macrophages help process foreign proteins (antigens), and they may also take part in the immune reaction at the tissue level by a series of interactions with B and T cells (Diagram 1).

Polymorphonuclear cells

A general description of these cells was given in Chapter 6. The immune functions of these cells are poorly understood. Many contain proteolytic enzymes and can engulf (phagocytize) bacteria. They tend to accumulate at sites of tissue injury and may be concerned with removing cellular and tissue debris. In allergic reactions they may increase tissue damage by releasing agents that disrupt the local blood flow (vasoactive amines) and by releasing chemicals that attract more polymorphs to the site.

CELL INTERACTIONS

The main features of a typical immune reaction are shown in Diagram 1. Note especially the cooperation between T and B cells and the communication between both types of lymphocytes and the tissue macrophages. The upper part of the diagram shows the humoral component of the immune response: the surfaces of foreign materials are coated with antibodies and other proteins called complement to aid in immune recognition and disposal by macrophages and to induce breakdown of cells when the invading element is cellular. The lower part of the diagram illustrates the cell-mediated aspects of the immune response.

CLASSIFICATION OF LYMPHOID TISSUES

It is useful to divide the various accumulations of lymphoid tissue into primary or central organs, where lymphocytes are produced and where they undergo development (the thymus and mammalian equivalent of the bursa of Fabricius in birds), and secondary or peripheral organs, where foreign materials are extracted from body fluids and immune responses are initiated (lymph nodes, spleen, Peyer's patches, tonsils). The tissues of the secondary lymphoid system, although anatomically discrete, are strategically placed accumulations of lymphocytes along the most likely channels of invasion of the body. There is a constant traffic pattern of lymphocytes leaving the primary organs to seed the secondary organs and then leaving the secondary organs to circulate in blood and lymph.

PRIMARY LYMPHOID ORGANS

Primary lymphoid organs are concerned for the most part with the production of B and T cells (populations of lymphocytes) in an environment protected from antigens, and are dependent on a steady flow of stem cells (lymphocyte precursors) to provide a stock for continuous production. A tentative scheme for the sources of these stem cells is shown in Diagram 2. In the embryo the yolk sac is the first site of hemopoietic stem cell production. The site of blood cell formation then shifts to the fetal liver and spleen and finally to bone marrow, where it persists in adult life. The main primary lymphoid organ in mammals is the thymus; a

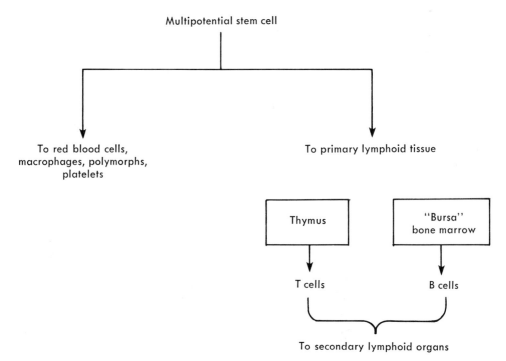

Diagram 2

steady stream of stem cells flows into the thymus throughout embryonic and adult life to provide replacements for lymphocytes lost by cell death or emigration from the thymus. Within the thymus the stem cells differentiate into T cells, but further functional changes, including changes in surface antigens, will occur after the cells leave the thymus and seed the secondary lymphoid organs.

Mammalian lymphocytes that arise independently of the thymus are called B cells on the basis of their similarity to cells that arise from the bursa of Fabricius in birds, a lymphoid organ associated with the gut. The mammalian B cell may be produced in the liver and spleen in embryos and in the bone marrow in adults.

Thymus

The thymus develops as an outgrowth from the pharyngeal wall of the embryo and has a framework of epithelial (endodermal) rather than connective tissue (mesenchymal) origin. Later in development the groundwork becomes infiltrated with lymphocyte stem cells from the various blood cell–producing sites of the embryo. In the adult the thymus lies in the thorax just below the sternum. Its size varies greatly with age. It is largest in relationship to total body weight at birth, and although it continues to enlarge until puberty, it does so at a slower rate than does the body as a whole so that its relative weight declines. At puberty the thymus begins to involute, and it is gradually infiltrated with fat cells.

The thymus usually consists of two lobes joined together by connective tissue. The lobes are surrounded by a connective tissue capsule that gives off several septa which partially divide each lobe into lobules (Fig. 10-1). Each lobe consists of a cortex and a medulla. Often a lobule is so cut that its connection with the medullary region of the central core is not apparent and it looks as though a mass of the lighter medullary tissue were completely surrounded by cortex. If the lobule is small, it has an appearance similar to that of a germinal center (see lymph nodes for definition of this structure). There are however no germinal centers in the thymus, an organ that is not directly involved in antigenic recognition. The peripheral part of each lobule appears denser and stains more intensely than the medulla due to local accumulations of small lymphocytes (Fig. 10-2, A). This region is known as the cortex. The abundance of the lymphocytes in this region tends to obscure the presence of the reticular cells. The deepest part of the cortex contains a different lymphocyte population and is called the *paracortical zone.*

The capsule of the thymus may contain blood vessels, but lymphatics are lacking. No afferent lymph vessels enter the thymus, and

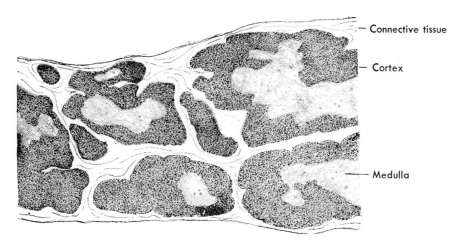

— Connective tissue

— Cortex

— Medulla

Fig. 10-1. Thymus of monkey. (Hematoxylin and eosin stain.)

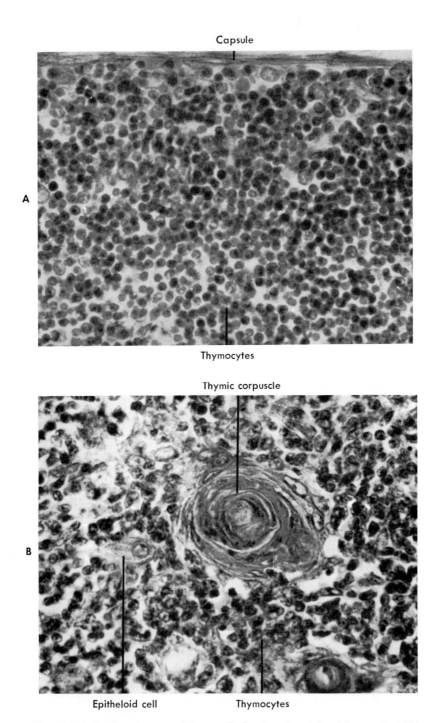

Capsule

A

Thymocytes

Thymic corpuscle

B

Epitheloid cell   Thymocytes

Fig. 10-2. A, Section of cortex of thymus. **B,** Section of medulla of thymus. (×640.)

accordingly, there is no mechanism for filtering lymph. The reticular connective tissue of the thymus differs from that found in other lymphatic organs. The reticular fibers are less numerous and occur chiefly around blood vessels to form the blood thymus barrier. The reticular cells are large and irregularly shaped and have pale-staining nuclei (Fig. 10-3).

The cells that give rise to lymphocytes, that is, lymphoblasts *(immunoblasts)* in the cortex, are larger and stain less intensely than the small lymphocytes in the medulla. The developing T stem cells in the cortex are protected from circulating antigens in the bloodstream by the thymic capillary bed, which is sheathed by a continuous epithelium that provides channels through which the capillaries run. To reach a T stem cell, an antigen would have to pass through a capillary wall and its basement membrane coating. It would then have to pass through

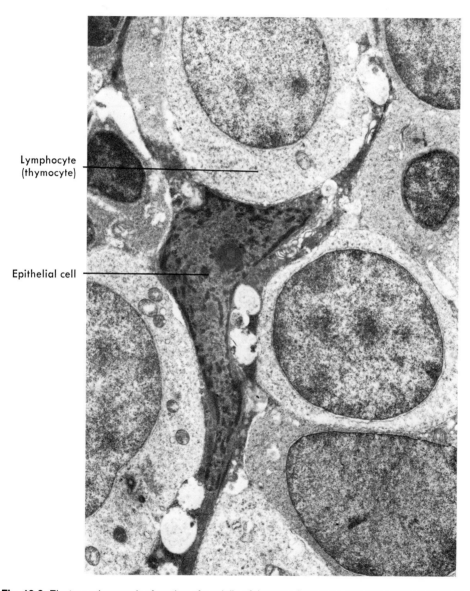

Lymphocyte (thymocyte)

Epithelial cell

Fig. 10-3. Electron micrograph of portion of medulla of thymus of monkey. (×7,000.) (Courtesy Dr. H. Nakahara.)

a perivascular space containing macrophages and then through the epithelial cell layer that sheaths the blood vessel wall. This barrier is fully formed in the adult thymus but is incomplete in the embryo, which generally is not exposed to foreign proteins. In contrast, secondary lymphoid tissue (lymph nodes and spleen, for example) is so constructed that it provides the greatest possible exposure of lymphocytes to circulating antigens. Due to its lack of lymphatic drainage and its elaborate barrier system, the thymus is organized to screen out antigen and to provide a sterile environment for the differentiation of T cells. This barrier system does not extend into the medulla, which is specialized to provide a channel for the entry of differentiated T cells into the bloodstream for circulation to secondary lymphoid tissues.

Lymphocytes leave the thymus by migrating into the medulla where the capillary bed is no longer sheathed by epithelial cells, and there the lymphocytes enter the blood by migrating through the walls of postcapillary venules.

Another component of the medulla is the *thymic* or *Hassall's corpuscle* (Fig. 10-2, *B*). This structure consists of a group of cells ranging from 12 to 180 μm in diameter. These structures contain a hyaline center stained red with eosin, which seems to be derived from degenerating cells, since it may contain several pyknotic nuclei. Around this center are compressed cells concentrically arranged in a type of whorl. Except for the hyaline center with its degenerating nuclei, the corpuscle somewhat resembles the small arteries that ramify through the thymic

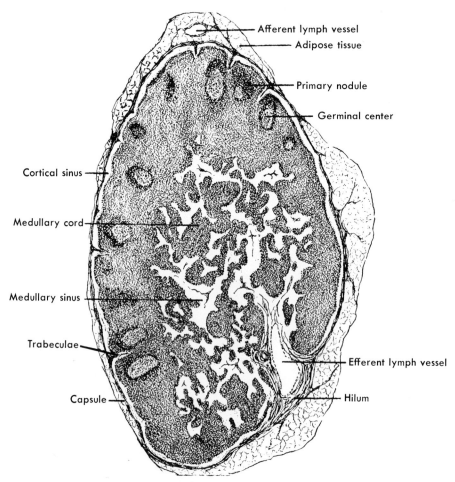

Fig. 10-4. Lymph node of cat. (Hematoxylin and eosin stain.)

medulla. Morphologically, Hassall's corpuscles seem to be undergoing the same changes that occur in keratinized epithelium elsewhere in the body. Because the lymphocytes are less concentrated, the underlying reticular framework of epithelial cells is more visible in the medulla. In the cortex the thymocytes (lymphocytes) can obscure the details of the framework of the organ (Fig. 10-2, *A*). In addition to the lymphocytes and reticular cells, the thymus also has free macrophages, mast cells, and plasma cells in the connective tissue capsule and septa.

SECONDARY LYMPHOID ORGANS
Lymph nodes

A lymph node (lymph gland) is a mass of lymphatic tissue enclosed in a capsule of connective tissue. Many such nodes are scattered along the course of the lymph vessels of the body, the most conspicuous groups lying in the cervical region, the axilla, and the groin. Each node is a small bean-shaped organ (from 1 to 25 mm in diameter) having an indented hilum (Fig. 10-4). The nodes are whitish in color in a fresh specimen. When stained with hematoxylin and eosin, a section of a node appears as a mass of purple tissue enclosed in a capsule that sends trabeculae toward the center of the node from its convex surface. The framework of the node consists of a meshwork of reticular cells held together by desmosomes and arranged on a lattice of reticular fibers. These fibers are connected to the capsule and its trabeculae. The node is placed in the channel of an afferent lymph vessel (Fig. 10-5), which breaks up into a number of branches that empty into a sinus lying beneath the capsule (the subcapsular sinus) (Fig. 10-7). This sinus drains directly into the efferent lymph vessels, which leave the node to provide an overflow mechanism,

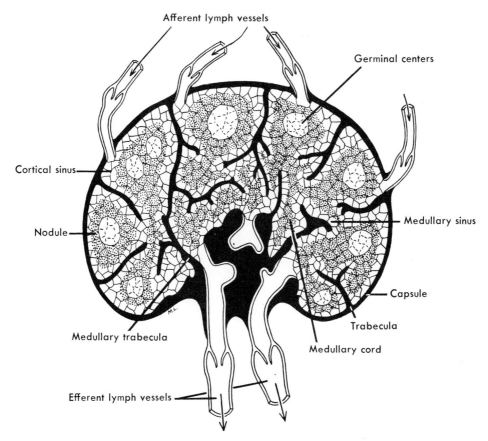

Fig. 10-5. Diagram showing relation of lymph node to lymphatic vessels. This diagram does not indicate arterial and venous supply of lymph node. (Redrawn from Maximow and Bloom.)

and into sinuses that penetrate the substance of the node. These intermediary sinuses drain into the deeper part of the node, the medulla. Valves in these vessels prevent lymph from reversing direction.

A lymph node, like the thymus, has a cortex and medulla. In the lymph node these zones are a specialization: the cortical zone allows for lymphocyte entry and production and antigenic stimulation; the medulla, for lymphocyte reentry into the lymph stream. Unlike the cortex of the thymus, the outer zone of a lymph node is made up of loosely packed areas of lymphocytes (diffuse cortex) and a denser aggregation (lymphoid follicles or nodules). (Fig. 10-6). The diffuse cortex contains a capillary bed supplied by arteries that penetrate the node along the trabeculae (Fig. 10-7). In this capillary bed are postcapillary venules lined with high cuboidal epithelium, which play a role in the recirculation of lymphocytes. These specialized capillaries are the port of entry for circulating differentiated lymphocytes to seed the lymph node. After passage through the node, the lymphocytes pass into the efferent lymphatics and eventually return to the blood by way of the thoracic duct, a total transit time of about 14 hours. Similar recirculations occur in other secondary lymphatic tissues, the estimated times varying with the tissues. A given lymphocyte may reenter the spleen on the average of four or five times a day.

The lymph node has a dual function. It is the site for the production and accumulation of lymphocytes, and it is also a biological filter where macrophages remove particulate matter from the entering lymph. The *cortical region* contains nodules that consist of a germinal center containing a population of large,

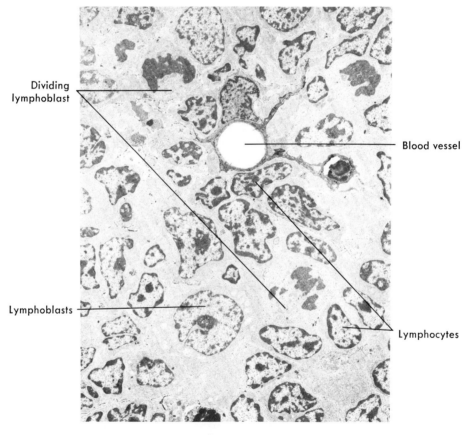

Fig. 10-6. Section of part of germinal center of lymph node of mouse showing several lymphocytes, lymphoblasts (some are dividing), and blood vessel. (×3,000.) (Courtesy Dr. H. Nakahara.)

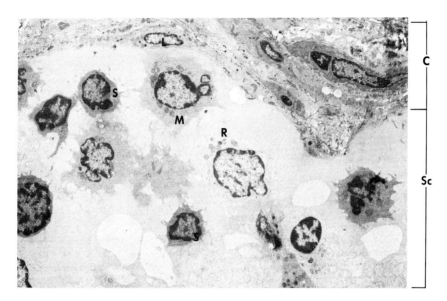

Fig. 10-7. Electron micrograph showing periphery of lymph node of rat. *C,* Capsule; *Sc,* subcapsular sinus; *L (white),* lining (littoral) cell; *M* and *S,* medium and small lymphocyte, respectively; *R,* reticulo-cyte. (×2,500.) (Courtesy Dr. H. Nakahara.)

Capsule

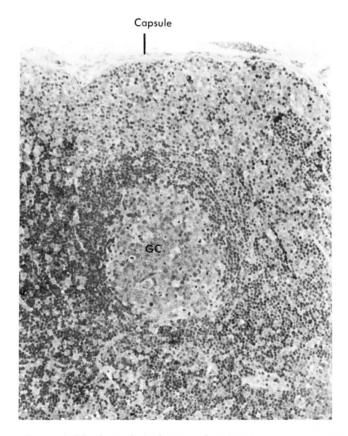

Fig. 10-8. Photomicrograph (plastic section) of cortex of cat lymph node showing germinal center, *GC.* (×160.)

pale-staining lymphoblasts, reticular cells, and macrophages surrounded by a rim of B lymphocytes (Figs. 10-8 and 10-9). The whole structure is referred to as a secondary follicle or nodule. The small lymphocytes are the most numerous cell types in follicles. In lymphatic tissue they have a somewhat different appearance than they do in blood smears or in ordinary connective tissue. In lymphatic tissue the nucleus of small lymphocytes contains clumps of chromatin that produce a mottled nuclear staining. In blood and connective tissue the nucleus appears more uniformly staining. The medium-sized lymphocytes are less numerous than the small variety and may be observed among clusters of small lymphocytes. The nuclei of medium-sized lymphocytes contain small particles of chromatin. They exhibit a small amount of basophilic cytoplasm and typically one or two nucleoli. Occasionally these cells may be observed in mitosis. Large lymphocytes are the least numerous and are widely scattered in lymph nodes, including the medullary cords. They are spherical, measure up to 15 to 20 μm in diameter, and

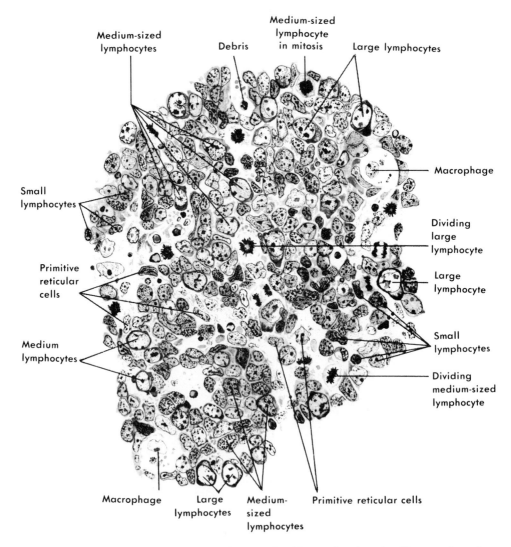

Fig. 10-9. Portion of actively lymphocytopoietic nodule of human lymph node. (Hematoxylin-eosin-azure II; ×750.) (From Bloom G., and D. W. Fawcett. 1968. A textbook of histology, 9th ed. W. B. Saunders Co., Philadelphia.)

have a clear pale nucleus with distinct nucleoli. The cytoplasm of these cells is more abundant than that in other lymphocytes and is basophilic. Their numbers vary with the functional state of the node, and they may be absent altogether.

The basic framework of lymphatic tissue consists of reticular cells and fibers. The cells are of two types: (1) primitive reticular cells and (2) phagocytic fixed macrophages. The primitive reticular cells are members of the reticuloendothelial system. They have large, vesicular irregularly shaped nuclei and cytoplasm with numerous cellular extensions. They may on occasion become free macrophages. The reticulum also contains undifferentiated cells that may give rise to phagocytic cells or lymphocytes. Other cells occasionally seen in lymph nodes are plasma cells and blood cells.

The *medulla* of lymph nodes is composed of sinuses and cords. The medullary cords (Figs. 10-10 and 10-11) originate in the diffuse cortex and penetrate into the medulla, where they interdigitate between the sinuses. They contain blood vessels, macrophages, and a variable number of lymphoblasts and plasma cells, depending on how much stimulation the node has received. Cells can move freely into the medullary sinuses, which are lymph-filled spaces lined by macrophages. Medullary sinuses are like peripheral sinuses in structure and lie between the medullary cords and the strands of trabeculae (Fig. 10-10). The medullary trabeculae are composed chiefly of dense collagenous fibrous tissue that radiates from the hilum. The trabeculae contain blood vessels. In the tissue of the hilum, efferent lymph vessels are prominent.

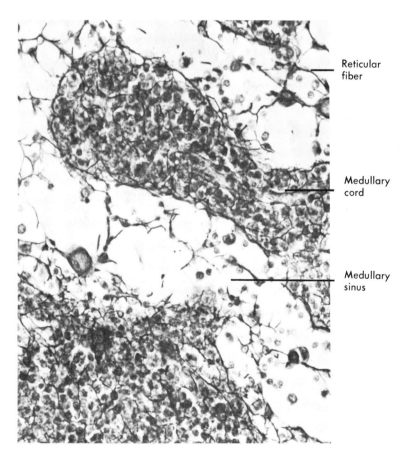

Reticular fiber

Medullary cord

Medullary sinus

Fig. 10-10. Photomicrograph of part of medulla of lymph node of dog stained to show reticular fibers. (×400.)

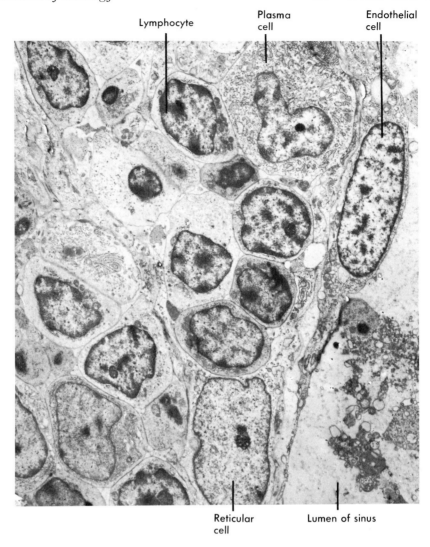

Fig. 10-11. Electron micrograph of part of medullary cord of lymph node of cat in region of medullary sinus. (×4,800.)

Peyer's patches and gut associated lymphoid tissue

Peyer's patches can be viewed as modified lymph nodes beneath the intestinal epithelium (Fig. 14-25). They contain the main features of a lymph node, including a diffuse cortex, lymphoid follicles with germinal centers, and a capillary bed with specialized postcapillary venules to permit entry of lymphocytes into the lymphatic tissue. As in lymph nodes, there is a separation of T cells and B cells.

In addition to Peyer's patches there are many lymphocytes scattered within the lamina propria of the small intestinal villi and beneath the epithelial cells of the intestinal mucosal surface. As a population, these diffuse accumulations, along with the more organized nodules found in the gut wall, are referred to as gut-associated lymphoid tissue (GALT) and are concerned with defending the body against foreign materials that penetrate the body across moist epithelial membranes. The lymph nodes inserted in the lymphatic drainage from the various viscera (and from the surface of the body) serve as a

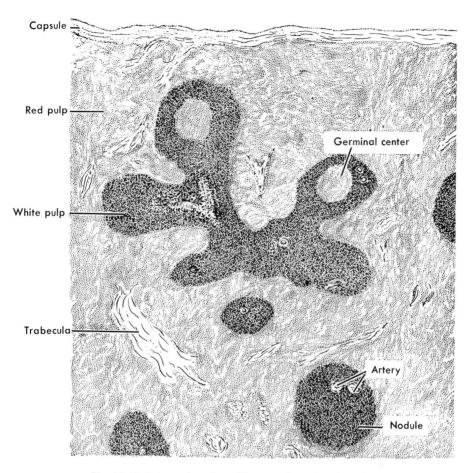

Capsule

Red pulp

Germinal center

White pulp

Trabecula

Artery

Nodule

Fig. 10-12. Spleen of monkey. (Hematoxylin and eosin stain.)

second line of defense against foreign materials.

Spleen

The spleen is the largest of the lymphoid organs. It is a mass of lymphatic tissue measuring 5 to 6 inches in length and 4 inches in width in man. The spleen differs from lymph nodes in that it is inserted as a filter in the blood vascular system rather than in the pathway of a lymphatic drainage. In addition to its role in immunity, it is concerned with storage and removal of worn-out erythrocytes and recycling of the iron contained in the hemoglobin of erythrocytes. In the fetus the spleen is also a blood-forming organ. Its role in immunity is to screen foreign material in the circulating bloodstream. Since the spleen is a biological fil-

ter, it is not surprising that there are a number of structural similarities between it and the organization of a lymph node. The major difference, as already noted, is that the spleen filters blood whereas the lymph node filters lymph.

Under low magnification the greater part of a section of the spleen appears reddish in color when stained with hematoxylin and eosin. This area is the red pulp. Scattered through this reddish mass are small patches that appear white in the living state but stain purple with hematoxylin and eosin (Fig. 10-12). These patches are called white pulp, the lymphatic tissue of the spleen. The white pulp follows and surrounds the blood vessel supply, and a section through a portion of white pulp contains a central arteriole. Unlike the arrangement in lymph nodes, there is no cortical or medullary area of the white pulp. Within the white pulp are zones of diffuse lymphoid tissue and germinal centers (follicles). Structures comparable to the medullary sinuses of lymph nodes do not exist in the spleen but cord-like elements in the red pulp are present; they contain lymphoblasts and plasma cells, which resemble the cell populations of the medullary cords of lymph nodes. This arrangement is sometimes referred to as *Billroth* or *pulp cords.* Although the pulp appears like ropelike cords of tissue in section, it should be remembered that the reticular meshwork is, in fact, a continuous sheet of spongy tissue and that the sinusoids tunnel through this spongy tissue. The white pulp is separated from red pulp by marginal zones (Fig. 10-17).

The general arrangement of capsule and trabeculae of the spleen is similar to that of a lymph node; that is, a series of trabeculae run in from the surrounding capsule on the convex surface and strands of connective tissue radiate inward from the hilum. Since sections of the spleen are usually prepared from small pieces of the organ, this arrangement may not be readily observed.

Blood enters the spleen at the hilum, and the arteries continue in the trabeculae for some distance. They enter the pulp while they still have the coats common to small arteries: intima, media, and adventitia. In the pulp the vessels ramify, and it is usually at the point of branching that the nodules are found. After passing through the nodules, the arteries enter the red pulp as the penicilli, in which three parts may be distinguished. The first part (arteriole of the pulp) is of fine caliber and the longest division of the penicillus. This divides into a number of vessels called the sheathed arteries, and these, in turn, divide into two or three

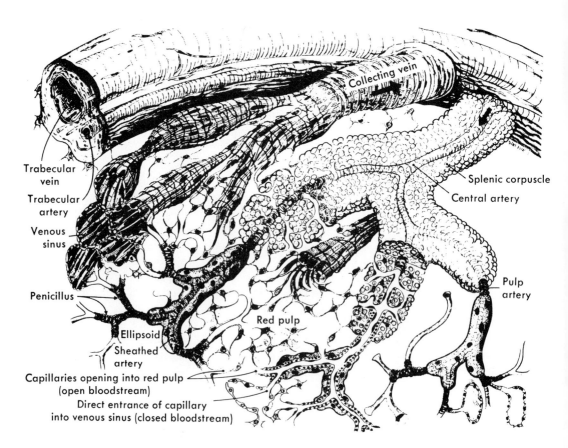

Fig. 10-13. Stereogram of spleen, illustrating concepts of open and closed circulation. (From Elias, H., and J. E. Pauly. 1966. Human microanatomy, 3d ed. F. A. Davis Co., Philadelphia.)

branches exhibiting the structure of capillaries, which may connect with the venous sinuses of the red pulp (Fig. 10-13).

Several theories exist concerning the course of the blood after it passes through the arterial capillaries. According to one view, it goes directly into the reticular meshwork of the red pulp, rather than passing by way of a continuous endothelial tubule to the venules. This is the *open circulation theory.* Other workers believe that no such "dumping" of corpuscles into the reticulum occurs and that the arterial capillaries lead to capillaries, which, in turn, connect with the venules. This is the *closed circulation theory.* The *mixed circulation theory* suggests that some arterioles open directly into the pulp whereas others connect with venules through capillaries.

The venous circulation begins with the splenic sinus, which is composed of an openwork endothelium through which corpuscles may pass readily. From the splenic sinuses, venules lead away and join each other, running back to the trabeculae. Blood leaves at the hilum. The circulation of the blood in the spleen is diagrammed in Fig. 10-13. Under the high power of the microscope the details of structure that may be seen are the capsule and trabeculae, red pulp, and white pulp.

Capsule and trabeculae. The capsule and trabeculae consist of dense, white connective tissue with a few scattered elastic fibers and smooth muscle, which is similar to the corresponding structure in the lymph node. The capsule of the spleen, however, since the organ borders on the body cavity, is covered by mesothelium, which appears as a layer of

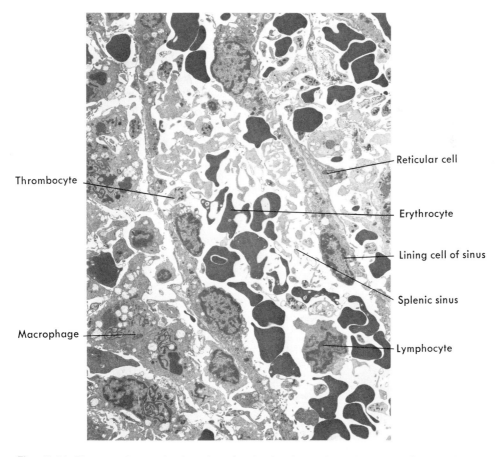

Fig. 10-14. Electron micrograph of portion of red pulp of rat spleen. (×2,000.) (Courtesy Dr. H. Nakahara.)

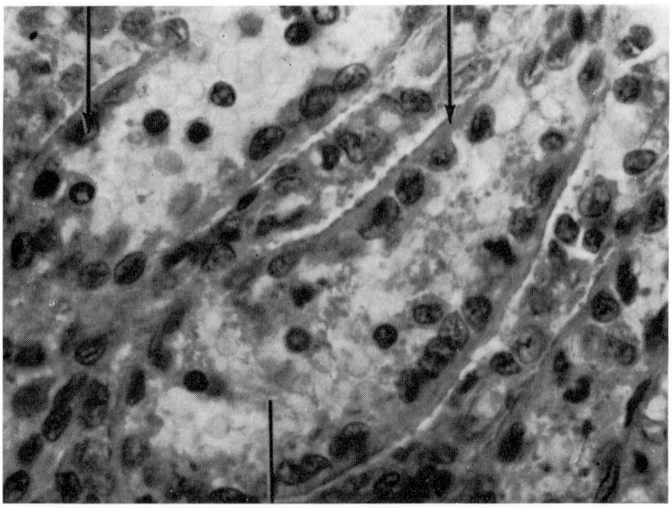

Reticuloendothelial cells   Basement membrane

Lumen of sinus containing cells undergoing phagocytosis

Fig. 10-15. Section of spleen showing splenic sinuses. (×640.)

squamous epithelium. This is often destroyed in preparing the specimen.

Red pulp. The framework of the red pulp is reticular tissue. It contains all types of blood cells, which have passed into it either from the open ends of the arterioles or through the walls of the sinuses (Fig. 10-14). The numerous erythrocytes that are present give this part of the organ its red color in both fresh and stained specimens (Fig. 10-12).

Among the reticular cells and corpuscles will be found free macrophages. These cells have vesicular nuclei and stain readily with eosin. They ingest fragments of worn-out erythrocytes, which may be seen in their cytoplasm. The macrophages are distributed throughout the red pulp.

Two kinds of blood vessels in the red pulp are of unusual structure. The more prominent of these are the splenic sinuses (Fig. 10-15). These vessels are the beginning of the venous system. They may be recognized as small spaces in the pulp, surrounded by a ring of endothelial-like cells whose nuclei project into the lumina of the vessels. Ordinarily, endothelial cells are closely joined, and their nuclei are flattened so as to project only slightly into the lumen of the vessels that they surround. In the splenic sinus these

cells, known as reticular cells, are loosely grouped, and the lack of tension of the cytoplasm permits the nuclei to extend into the vessel. These cells are surrounded by a loose arrangement of reticular tissue, forming a latticework through which the corpuscles may pass (Fig. 10-16). The inner (luminal) surface of the sinus is occupied by scattered lining cells that have a prominent nucleus. They are phagocytic and belong to the reticuloendothelial system.

The other type of blood vessel peculiar to the red pulp is the sheathed artery (second portion of the pencillus). Sheathed arteries are of capillary diameter and consist of endothelium plus a thin covering of concentrically placed cells, which are probably reticular. The vessels are inconspicuous elements of the red pulp in human beings and require special stains for adequate demonstration.

White pulp. The white pulp, like the red, has a groundwork of reticular tissue but differs from it in containing large numbers of lymphocytes, as well as monocytes and plasma cells. It thus resembles the medullary cords of a lymph node. It surrounds the arteries from the point where they leave the trabeculae to their division into penicilli, actually invading and replacing the adventitial

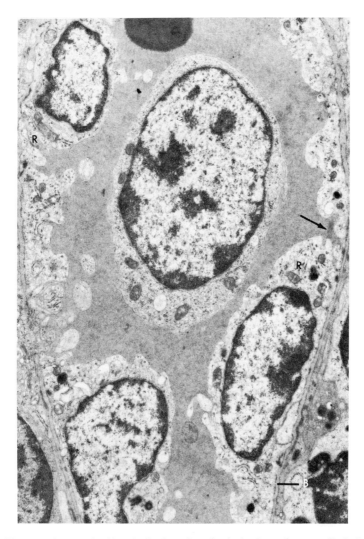

Fig. 10-16. Electron micrograph of longitudinal section of splenic sinus of mouse. Reticular (endothelial) cells, *R,* that line the sinus are elongated and are loosely applied one to the other. They rest on a basement membrane, *B,* which is interrupted at intervals (arrow). (×10,000.)

connective tissue of the vessels (Figs. 10-12 and 10-17). Elastic fibers belonging to the walls of the arteries are scattered through the white pulp. At various points, particularly where the vessels branch, the white pulp contains nodules that form extensions of its substance, asymmetrically placed with respect to the artery. In fetal life and childhood the nodules contain germinal centers; these persist into adult life in some animals, but not in man.

It will be remembered that all kinds of red and white blood cells are formed in the spleen during embryonic life. One would therefore find in embryonic spleens the precursors of the corpuscles, including giant cells. These, like the germinal centers of the nodules, may persist into adult life in some forms.

Tonsils
Palatine tonsil

The tonsils are masses of lymphoid tissue embedded in the lining of the throat between the arches of the palate. Three groups—the pharyngeal, palatine, and lingual tonsils—form a ring of tissue surrounding the pharynx. Their arrangement is best under-

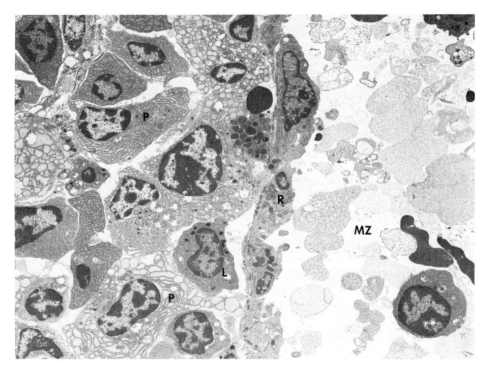

Fig. 10-17. Electron micrograph of portion of white pulp from rat spleen. Plasma cells, *P,* are very abundant. *L,* lymphocyte; *MZ,* marginal zone; *R,* reticular cell. (×3,000.) (Courtesy Dr. H. Nakahara.)

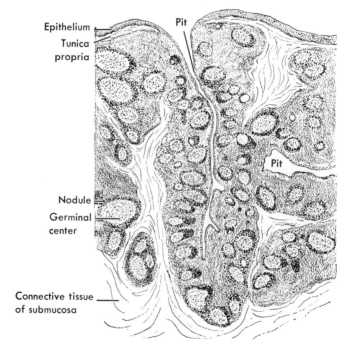

Fig. 10-18. Human palatine tonsil. (Hematoxylin and eosin stain.)

stood by reference to the structure of the wall of the pharynx. This consists of a layer of stratified squamous epithelium resting on a tunica propria of reticular or fine areolar tissue (Fig. 10-18). Beneath the tunica propria lies the submucosa of coarser areolar tissue, which contains scattered mucous glands. The tonsil develops between the tunica propria and the submucosa. As it enlarges it elevates the former and depresses the latter. The epithelium of the mucosa does not go smoothly over the surface of the tonsil but dips down in numerous deep pits or fossae. Under the low power of the microscope the tonsil appears as a mass of lymphoid tissue, bordered on one side by stratified squamous epithelium and surrounded on the other sides by areolar tissue, which forms a tough capsule immediately around it. The mucous glands sometimes found in the areolar tissue outside the capsule are not part of the tonsil, but belong to the pharyngeal wall. Noticeable features of the organ are its deep pits lined with stratified squamous epithelium and the presence of numerous germinal centers. The latter are usually grouped around the pits, but there is no division into cortex and medulla.

The pits (crypts) surrounded by lymphatic tissue are partially separated from each other by connective tissue derived from the capsule. Lymphocytes, mast cells, and plasma cells occur in this connective tissue; heterophilic leukocytes may also be present, which indicates a mild inflammatory condition. In the deeper regions of the crypts an infiltration of lymphocytes displaces the epithelium of the crypts to a considerable degree. Some of these cells pass through the epithelium and are eventually found in the saliva as the salivary corpuscles.

The lumina of the crypts often contain accumulations of living and degenerating lymphocytes, desquamated epithelial cells, detritus, and microorganisms.

Pharyngeal tonsil

The pharyngeal tonsil is a median aggregation of lymphoid tissue that lies in the wall of the nasopharynx. In this region the epithelium, as is characteristic of the nasopharynx, is chiefly of the pseudostratified, ciliated, columnar variety. Patches of stratified squamous epithelium also occur and become more numerous in the adult. The lymphoid tissue is similar to that of the palatine tonsil. The capsule of this organ is thin and contains many fine elastic fibers, which radiate into the core of the folds.

Lingual tonsil

The lingual tonsil is located in the root of the tongue. The surface epithelium is of the stratified squamous variety and forms the covering of the numerous crypts that occur in this tonsil. The lymphoid tissue is similar to that found in the other tonsils except that the lymph nodules may contain germinal centers.

The tonsils generally reach their highest state of development in childhood and then usually undergo involution. Unlike the lymph nodes, the tonsils do not possess lymphatic sinuses, and hence lymph is not filtered through them. They do, however, possess lymph capillaries, which end blindly about the outer surface of the tonsil; the only established function of the tonsils is the formation of lymphocytes.

SUMMARY AND COMPARISON OF THE LYMPHOID ORGANS

Thymus. The thymus is divided into cortex and medulla and is composed chiefly of epithelial cells and thymocytes, which resemble lymphocytes. The medulla contains thymic corpuscles, a diagnostic feature that distinguished the thymus from other lymphatic tissue. The cortex is a dense mass of thymocytes and epithelial tissue.

The thymus produces a humoral agent (hormone) that is effective in stimulating the production of lymphocytes in lymphoid organs. It is also responsible for establishing and regulating immunological reactions.

Lymph node. The lymph node consists of a cortex and a medulla. The cortex contains nodules that may have germinal centers, a peripheral sinus, and sinuses surrounding the trabeculae. The medulla is composed of cords, sinuses, and trabeculae. The capsule and trabeculae are of dense connective tissue, with scattered fibers of smooth muscle in the former. The lymph node filters lymph, produces new lymphocytes, has the phagocytic action of removing impurities from the lymph, and is also involved in immunological reactions.

Spleen. The spleen is composed of red and white pulp but not a cortex and medulla. The red pulp contains all types of blood cells and venous sinuses. The white pulp surrounds arteries and includes nodules that have no germinal centers in adult man. The spleen—a filter of blood—is phagocytic, forms new lymphocytes, and influences the metabolism and distribution of the erythrocytes.

Tonsil. The tonsils are masses of lymphoid tissue embedded in the wall of the pharynx. They are covered by stratified squamous epithelium, which dips into the substance of the organ, forming the pits. Lymph nodules with germinal centers are grouped around the pits. There are no sinuses.

11

Glands

In the following chapters, glands will be a prominent feature of each of the several organs to be considered. Accordingly, a general survey of typical characteristics of glands will be given at this juncture.

Glands are composed of epithelial cells, which perform the highly specialized function of producing *secretions*. These cells remove raw materials from tissue fluid or lymph and from them synthesize substances that ordinarily are not utilized by the gland cell itself to any great degree. The secretory products are released on free surfaces or into the blood-lymphatic complex of vessels for distribution to sites where the secretion products are utilized. Some glandular secretions are stored until the demands of the organism require the substance involved. In others, the secretions are elaborated and released either continually or intermittently.

Excretion, sometimes used interchangeably with secretion, is a process by which the end products of carbohydrate, fat, protein, and mineral metabolism are removed from the internal medium of the organism. Thus liver cells can remove decomposition products of hemoglobin from the blood and convert them into bile salts and bile pigments, which are then passed into the bile system and eventually into the small intestine. Bile salts utilized in lipid absorption and digestion are resorbed and reutilized several times. Bile salts may accordingly be considered to be secretion products. By contrast, the bile pigments not utilized in the body are eliminated with the fecal mass. These pigments may be considered to be excretions produced by a secretory mechanism. Certain cells in kidney tubules are capable of adding substances to urine by secretory processes. The sweat glands secrete a modified tissue fluid that serves several functions, at least one of them being excretory in function. Even the salivary glands are partially excretory by virtue of their ability to remove salts, thiocyanate ion, and urea from the body fluid. *Elimination* is the process by which excretions, secretions, and undigested food residue are expelled by the organism.

ENDOCRINE GLANDS

The endocrine glands, or glands of internal secretion, may have ducts in the embryonic state, but in the adult ducts are absent and the glands are accordingly classed as ductless glands. The secretions of endocrine glands may be stored or carried directly into blood capillaries, and it is by means of the latter that they are transported throughout the body to so-called target organs. The secretions of endocrine cells are called *hormones*, and in concert with the nervous system they regulate and coordinate the activities of all the cells in the body. Some hormones stimulate or suppress the activities of one or more specific glands or organs. Others, such as thyroxin, regulate the activities of most cells of the body.

Hormones have a varied chemical composition. Some are proteins (insulin), some modified amino acids (thyroxin), and others are modified sterols (adrenal steroids, estrogens, androgens). Some endocrine glands have a dual function. The pancreas, for example, elaborates the hormones insulin and glucagon as well as pancreatic juice, which contains a mixture of enzymes and sodium bicarbonate, and is accordingly classed as one of the *mixed glands* (that is, both endocrine and exocrine in function).

In glands with known endocrine function there are three major cell arrangements: clumps, follicles, and cords. All these cell associations are specialized to bring secretory cells as close to the blood supply as possible, since blood is the delivery channel for hormones.

Clumps. In the clump type of arrangement, secretion and utilization are of approximately the same magnitude. The secretion is stored within the epithelioid cells themselves and is released on demand into the abundant capillary network that permeates the clump. Examples of this type are the islands of Langerhans in the pancreas and the so-called interstitial cells in the testes. Clumps may be composed of small or large groups of irregularly shaped cells, but they do not form hollow spheres or tubes.

Follicles. A follicle consists of a cylinder or sphere of cells enclosing a cavity containing the stored secretion product. In the thyroid (for example, see Fig. 20-2), which consists of many follicles, the cells are usually cuboidal and exhibit a deeply staining secretion in the lumen called the colloid substance. Increased demand for the secretion results in a transfer of a hormone from the lumen to the abundant capillary network surrounding each follicle. Depletion of the colloid reserves results in collapse of the follicle, followed by a crowding of the cells, which appear columnar in transverse section. (See Fig. 20-2.) Since a depleted reserve initiates active secretory activity by the cells, the columnar form is associated with the active or secretory phase of these glands. In the embryo the follicles originate as clumps of epithelioid cells. These cells produce se-

cretions that are stored in cavities formed between the cells, which give rise to the space known as the "lumen" of the follicle. The thyroid is unique in its ability to store a large supply of hormone extracellularly.

Cords. In the cord the epithelioid cells are arranged in rows. The liver cords consist of two rows of cells closely aligned, whereas the adrenal cortex exhibits many subparallel rows of cells. Secretions are stored within the cells and transferred to the abundant capillary network as required. This arrangement ensures that no cell is very far from a capillary into which it can deliver its secretions.

Epithelioid cells. By definition, epithelia line cavities. With the exception of the follicular arrangement, endocrine gland cells do not line cavities. Prominent cuboidal or polygonal cells may occur in small or large irregular masses or in cords but invariably lack a cavity. (See Figs. 19-6, 20-8, and 20-14.) For this special situation the term *epithelioid* (epithelium-like) was introduced. When epithelioid cells occur, one is led to suspect an endocrine function; however, physiologic demonstration of endocrine activity is necessary before an endocrine role can be definitely ascribed to these cells.

EXOCRINE GLANDS

Exocrine glands, or glands of external secretion, retain connections with surfaces. Unicellular glands, for example, mucous cells, discharge their secretions directly on a free surface. Multicellular glands, for example, the salivary glands, discharge by way of a system of simple or branching ducts.

Ducts

There are several types of ducts: secretory, excretory, and intercalated.

Secretory ducts. One kind of secretory duct is lined by the glandular cells that produce the secretion. (See Figs. 11-1, *C* to *E*, and 12-7.) In the salivary glands another type of secretory duct is found, and it contains glandular cells supplying additional substances to the secretion produced at some distance from the main gland cells. Special

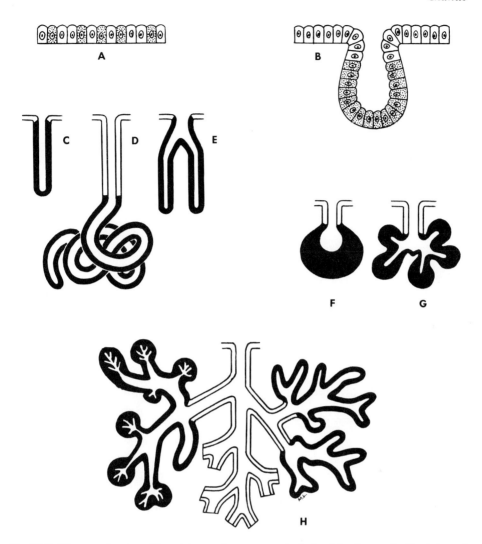

Fig. 11-1. Diagram showing different types of arrangement of glandular tissue. **A,** Glandular cells (granular) scattered among common epithelium cells (clear); **B,** glandular cells forming saclike invagination into underlying tissue; **C,** simple tubular gland; **D,** simple tubular gland coiled; **E,** simple branched tubular gland; **F,** simple alveolar gland; **G,** simple branched alveolar gland; **H,** compound gland. (Redrawn from Maximow and Bloom.)

techniques demonstrate the presence of basal striations in these cells, hence they are frequently called *striated ducts.*

Excretory ducts. Excretory ducts, formed of simple epithelium, presumably conduct secretions without taking part in the elaboration of major secretory components. (See Figs. 11-1, *D* and *F* to *H,* and 15-1.)

Intercalated ducts. Intercalated ducts are interposed between the glandular units and their conducting portions (for example, stri-ated or excretory ducts). (See Fig. 15-1.) The intercalated ducts are lined with flattened cells, which presumably do not produce a secretion. The latter are found only in the larger glands (for example, pancreas and salivary glands).

Classification

The simplest glandular unit is the unicellular gland, which consists of a cell that forms part of a lining epithelium and also elaborates a secretion. The goblet cells scattered along the lining of the intestine and respiratory tract are of this type.

The next simplest type is the intraepithelial gland, which consists of a strip of consecutive glandular cells forming a slight thickening or pocket entirely within the limits of the epithelium. The lining epithelium of the gut contains fingerlike or tubular projections of glandular cells, which are below the level of the epithelium in the underlying connective tissue and which maintain their connection to the surface by means of a duct. (See Figs. 11-1, *B*, *C*, and *E*, and 14-5 to 14-24).

Another means of classifying glands is by the manner and degree to which branching of the excretory or striated ducts occurs. If the ducts are absent (Fig. 11-1, *C* and *E*) or unbranched (Fig. 11-1, *D*, *E*, and *G*), the glands are termed *simple*. If the ducts branch (Fig. 11-1, *H*), the glands are called *compound*.

Simple and compound glands are subdivided according to whether the shapes of the secreting portions are tubular, alveolar (acinar), or tubuloalveolar. The name tubular is self-explanatory; an alveolar gland has secreting portions, which are spherical or flask shaped, whereas the tubuloalveolar variety may exhibit glandular portions intermediate between the two types already mentioned (Fig. 11-1, *H*, left side). Another variety of tubuloalveolar gland consists of tubular units and alveolar units attached to the same excretory duct. The simple tubular gland is further differentiated into tubular, coiled tubular, or branching tubular (Fig. 11-1, *C* to *E*). Also illustrated in Fig. 11-1, *G*, is the branching alveolar (compare Figs. 12-7 and 12-11, sebaceous glands). Other kinds of glands have been described such as those in the eyelid, but because of their highly specialized function and limited distribution, they will not be discussed here. Other classifications depend on the mode of secretion (holocrine, merocrine, apocrine) and on the product of secretion (mucous, serous, mixed, zymogenic).

Secretions

The secretions of exocrine glands are varied. Mucigen, for example, is an inadequately characterized mixture of carbohydrate and protein; zymogen (a precursor of enzymes) is in part protein and forms an important component of many serous secretions; sebum and cerumen contain protein, carbohydrate, and much lipid; in addition, secretions produced by the sweat, lacrimal, and lactating glands are extremely varied and complex. Glands such as the testes and ovaries and lymphoid and myeloid tissues are usually classed as *cytogenous*, since their chief activity is the production of living cells.

As indicated previously, the modes of secretion are utilized in classifying certain glands. In the case of *holocrine* secretion, the secretory product is stored in the gland cell, and the entire gland cell is extruded and destroyed in the process of secretion. The sebaceous glands are of this type. In *apocrine* secretion, the secretion accumulates in one or more large vacuoles below the free surface of the cell. During secretion a thin film of surface cytoplasm is removed with the secretory globules; the cell itself, however, is not usually destroyed in the process. In *merocrine* secretion, there is a cyclic increase and decrease of the secretory product, which is more or less continually released into the lumen of the gland without, however, destroying the cell or depleting the cytoplasm. Typical of this variety are the glands of the oral cavity and digestive tract.

Unicellular glands

The simplest glands are composed of one cell, and the most common representative of this group is the mucous or *goblet cell*. These cells are found in profusion in the digestive tract and in parts of the respiratory system. They are initially observed as tall columnar cells with elongate elliptical nuclei, distinguishable from their neighbors only by the absence of cilia or striated border. In the supranuclear position, minute granules appear, then droplets of mucigen, which migrate and accumulate at the free border of the cell. As more mucigen droplets accumulate in the cell the nucleus is forced toward the base, with concomitant changes in form from elliptical to a round and deeply staining conical form, until finally it appears as a flattened disk near the base of the cell. In addition, the apex of the cell expands laterally and distorts the neighboring epithelial cells. At this stage the cell looks like a goblet, with a narrow stem containing the nucleus and an expanded goblet-bell containing the nonstaining mucigen droplets in what appears to be a large cavity. In many instances the mucigen droplets nearest the surface are gradually released and dispersed in modified tissue fluid to form the viscid fluid known as *mucus.* In other instances the mucigen globules are released en masse; the goblet then collapses and appears as an irregularly outlined, tall columnar cell consisting of a narrow strip of cytoplasm containing a deeply staining, incredibly thin nucleus. The process of secretion is cyclic and may be repeated a number of times before the cell is replaced.

The presence of a large mass of nonstaining mucigen in hematoxylin and eosin preparations gives the impression of a large vacuole in cells filled with secretion. The principal ingredient of mucigen is a polysaccharide-containing protein called *mucin.* Aside from its adhesive properties, it has the ability to combine with and coagulate in the presence of acids to form a protective coating on surfaces. The PAS reaction demonstrates the polysaccharide moiety as a region that stains a red to purplish red. Certain aluminum-containing stain mixtures (mucicarmine, mucihematin) stain mucigen droplets a vivid red or blue.

Multicellular glands

The usual example employed to illustrate the multicellular variety of glands is the salivary glands. In these and similar glands the cells are grouped into *secretory units* of three types: mucous, serous, and seromucous (mixed) units (Fig. 11-2). They are usually arranged in alveoli (acini) and branched or straight tubules.

Mucous units are composed of a type of cuboidal epithelium, which is so disposed about a small lumen that the cells take on the form of truncated pyramids and are accordingly called pyramidal cells. At the beginning of a secretory cycle the nuclei tend to be round or ovoid and occupy a position nearer to the base of the cell rather than the center. As the mucigen globules accumulate near the lumen of the gland, the nuclei are displaced toward the base and are compressed to such an extent that they appear as flattened, darkly staining rods in contact with the cell boundary. Since the mucigen takes up so much of the volume of the cytoplasm and does not stain with hematoxylin and eosin, the cytoplasm of these cells does not appear eosinophilic and may on occasion even exhibit a pale bluish color. In certain of the salivary glands, the mucous units are easily detected under low power of the microscope as pale areas. With PAS the mucigen stains such a deep purplish red that all cellular detail may be obscured. Although these cells exhibit cyclic activity, the release of secretion is gradual and typical of the merocrine type of secretion.

Serous units are also composed of pyramidal cells but differ in that their nuclei are always centrally disposed in the cell. Their secretion granules are either slightly or extremely acidophilic and are primarily protein in character. Since these cells frequently elaborate enzymes (which are all partly protein), the secretion droplets within the cell all called *zymogen granules.* In many in-

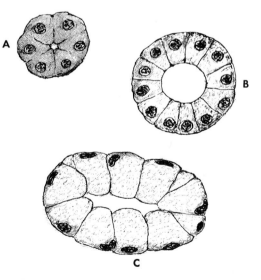

Fig. 11-2. Types of serous and mucus-secreting epithelium. **A,** Serous alveolus; **B,** alveolus secreting thick mucus; **C,** alveolus secreting thin mucus.

stances the granules are so small and so widely dispersed that the entire apex of the cell appears intensely acidophilic, whereas in other situations the granules are quite large and evenly distributed throughout the entire cell (Paneth cells). These cells produce an inactive precursor of the enzyme (zymogen). Zymogens are sometimes transported for a considerable distance before being activated. Since these cells are actively engaged in protein synthesis, the presence of large amounts of RNA or basophil substance in the perinuclear and subnuclear positions correlates well with their function. The serous cells of the pancreatic acini in well-stained hematoxylin and eosin preparations exhibit acidophilic apices and basophilic bases. The serous units of the salivary glands may be distinguished from the mucous units by the more central position of their nuclei and much greater affinity for dyes.

Mixed units are composed of both mucous and serous cells. The most easily demonstrated mixed units are found in the submaxillary glands of humans. In one type of mixed unit the mucous cells form a tubular portion joining the duct, and the terminal portion consists of the more deeply staining serous cells. On occasion the mucous cells are so numerous that they crowd the serous cells away from the lumen and form a crescentic cap of deeply staining cells or *demilune*. Occasionally, a mucous cell is also extruded into the *demilune* complex. In section it is not always possible to distinguish between a "pure" mucous unit and the tubular portion of a mixed unit. A "pure" serous unit exhibits a small but distinct lumen in its center. In favorable sections through the terminal part of a mixed unit the serous cells are separated from the lumen by mucous cells. In tangential sections of a demilune one may observe serous cells only; a central lumen is usually lacking, however. The student should be careful to distinguish between the mixed unit and the *mixed gland,* the latter being composed of both mucous and serous glands, and sometimes mixed units as well. Mixed glands of the type discussed here are also known as mucoserous or seromucous glands. The term *mixed gland* is also applied to glands that perform both an endocrine and exocrine function. (Compare pancreas, ovary, and so on.)

Occasionally certain stellate contractile cells may be found between the secretory unit and its basement membrane. These cells are called basket or myoepithelial cells and contain thin, prominent, dark-staining cresentic nuclei. They are said to propel secretions into gland ducts as a result of their contraction.

A number of serous or albuminous cells of certain oral glands are slightly PAS-positive and from a histochemical point of view are termed mucoserous cells. They are not, however, morphologically distinguishable from serous cells and are accordingly classed with them.

Glands that are neither serous nor mucous do not, as a matter of fact, form a group united by similarities of function or morphology. They are mentioned here merely to point out that many glandular organs exist which are not to be classified as serous or mucous. They are so varied that no general statement regarding them can be made, and they will be discussed individually in later chapters.

12

Integument

The skin consists of an epidermal and a dermal layer (corium) and rests upon the subdermal connective tissue. The epidermis is a stratified squamous epithelium, modified in some portions of the body by the addition of a thick cuticular layer and in others by the development of the hair and nails. The corium is a layer of dense connective tissue in which are located the various glands of the skin and the hair follicles. The subdermal or subcutaneous tissue is also fibrous, but it is more loosely arranged than the corium and generally contains adipose tissue.

HAIRLESS SKIN

No hair grows on the palms of the hands or the soles of the feet. They are covered with thick skin consisting of epidermis and dermis or corium (Fig. 12-1).

Epidermis

Stratum corneum. The outer layer of the epidermis, the stratum corneum, is thick in the palms and soles and consists of clear scalelike cells that become increasingly flattened as the surface is approached (Fig. 12-2). Nuclei are absent, and the cytoplasm is replaced by keratin proteins that are derived from tonofibrils of the deep layers of the epidermis. This keratin is soft keratin low in sulfur, in contrast to hard keratin occurring in nails. The peripheral surface of the stratum corneum undergoes constant desquamation and is known as the *stratum disjunctum.* There is a continual renewal of the desqua-

mated cells in the germinative layers, which move to the surface during the process of keratinization.

Stratum lucidum. Beneath the stratum corneum is the stratum lucidum, which consists of several rows of flattened nonnucleated cells that contain keratohyalin. They form a hyaline, highly refractile band that appears homogeneous and stains deeply with eosin. This layer is only present in the skin of the palms and the soles.

Stratum granulosum. Stratum granulosum consists of two to five rows of rhombic- or discoid-shaped cells arranged with their long axis parallel to the surface of the skin. The cytoplasm contains keratohyalin granules that stain intensely with hematoxylin. These granules are the precursors of soft keratin. There are from two to five layers of cells in which the cytoplasm is full of granules that stain deeply with hematoxylin. These layers make up the stratum granulosum, which is prominent because of its dark blue color. On closer examination it may be seen that the stratum granulosum differs from other epithelia in the arrangement of its cells. Rather than being closely applied to each other, they are separated by narrow spaces so that each is surrounded by a light line (in section). This is demonstrable in ordinary preparations. In exceptionally good preparations and under high magnification, it may be seen that the polygonal cells below the stratum granulosum are also separated by clefts and that the spaces are traversed by minute cytoplas-

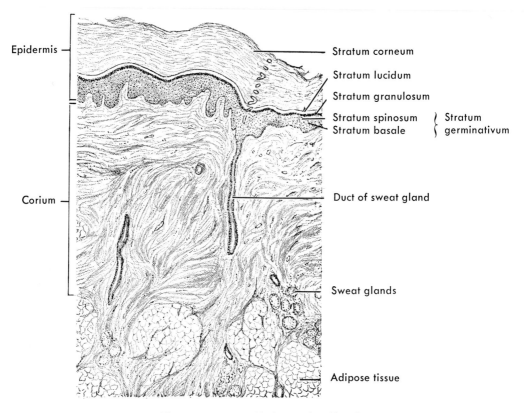

Epidermis

Stratum corneum

Stratum lucidum

Stratum granulosum

Stratum spinosum
Stratum basale } Stratum germinativum

Corium

Duct of sweat gland

Sweat glands

Adipose tissue

Fig. 12-1. Hairless skin from palm of hand.

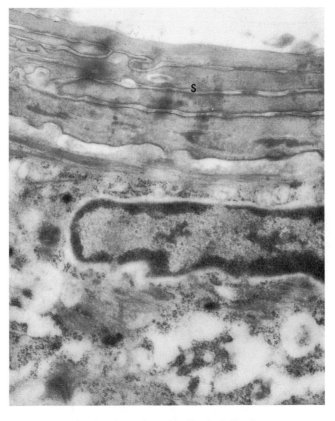

Fig. 12-2. Electron micrograph of surface of monkey lip. *S*, Cells of stratum corneum. (×29,000.)

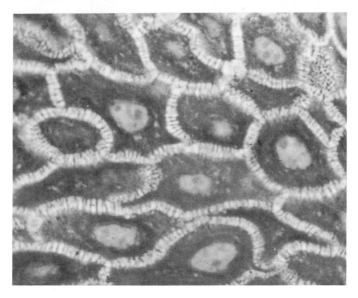

Fig. 12-3. Photomicrograph of part of stratum spinosum of human gingival epithelium showing intercellular bridges. (×1,200.)

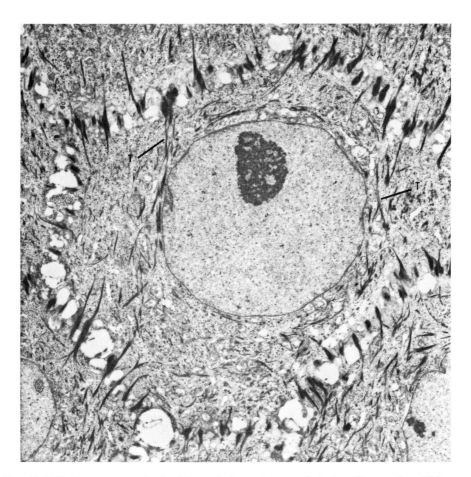

Fig. 12-4. Electron micrograph of cell from stratum spinosum of gingiva. These cells exhibit many tonofibrils, *T* (the intercellular bridges of light microscopy). Fibrils terminate in desmosomes on cell surface and do not, as was formerly supposed, extend to adjacent cells. (×6,000.)

mic bridges, uniting each cell to its neighbors. The name "prickle" cells is sometimes given to these polygonal cells and those of the stratum spinosum because of these protoplasmic strands (Figs. 12-3 and 12-4).

Stratum spinosum. The stratum spinosum layer of the epidermis (Fig. 12-5) is several cells in thickness and is composed of polyhedral cells, which are irregular in shape and noticeably separated from each other. In the surface layers the cells tend to flatten. The surface of these cells exhibits protoplasmic processes (Fig. 12-4), which appear to meet with similar processes from adjacent cells to form "intercellular bridges." These processes do not indicate protoplasmic continuity between these cells, which are sometimes referred to as prickle cells. Electron microscope studies have shown that the processes

contain tonofibrils and make intimate contact at a desmosome; accordingly, the cells are independent structures. The cytoplasm is intensely basophilic, which is associated with protein synthesis utilized in cell division and growth. This layer together with the basal layer is also known as the *stratum Malpighii* or *stratum germinativum*. It is the region in which cell proliferation and initiation of keratinization occurs. At the base of this zone are melanocytes containing colored pigment (melanin). Some of these granules are picked up by adjoining epithelial cells.

Stratum basale. The stratum basale, the most basal layer, is a region of active cell mitosis. It consists of a single layer of cuboidal cells that rest on a basement membrane (basal lamina and lamina reticularis). The cytoplasm stains intensely with hema-

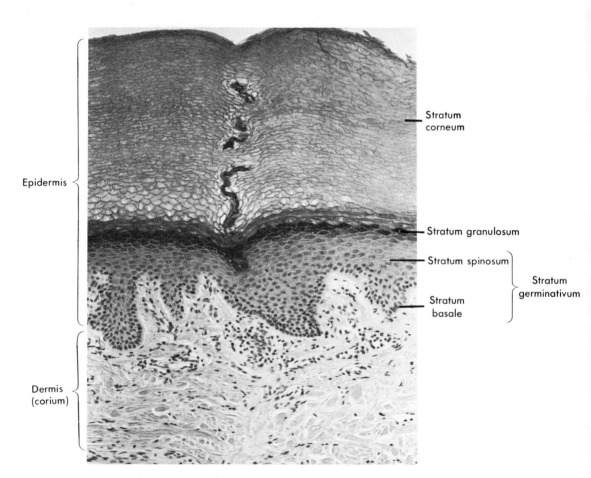

Fig. 12-5. Section of thick skin of human showing duct of sweat gland in epidermis. (×160.)

toxylin. Each cell exhibits short protoplasmic processes on the basal surface that fit into indentations of the basal lamina. Electron micrographs show that the border of the cell and the underlying basement membrane have an irregular arrangement, with strands of connective tissue occupying spaces between infoldings of the cell membrane. Hemidesmosomes occur at the base of these cells.

Corium (dermis)

The corium or dermis is a compact layer of connective tissue containing numerous collagenous, reticular, and elastic fibers. It varies in thickness from less than 0.5 mm on the eyelid and prepuce to 3 mm or more on the palms and soles. The upper surface in contact with the epidermis is usually thrown into nipplelike extensions called papillae that project into corresponding grooves at the base of the epidermis. The connective tissue within these papillae is richly vascular and contains delicate, loosely woven collagenous bundles, in addition to a rich network of sensory nerve endings. The dermis is divided into two strata that blend imperceptibly into one another. The subepithelial or *papillary layer* includes the papilla and ridges that extend into the epidermis. It is made up of fine collagenous, elastic, and reticular fibers. The deep or *reticular layer* is more extensive and is characterized by the presence of coarse collagen fibers and bundles of fibers that form a meshwork. Most of these fibers are arranged parallel to the surface of the skin.

The secretory coils of the sweat glands and the bases of the hair follicles (to be described later) are embedded in the dermis. Elastic fibers occurring in the reticular layer entwine around the sweat glands and the hair follicles, both of which are originally derived from downward extensions of the epidermis. The basal portion of the reticular layer sometimes contains networks of smooth muscle fibers that may cause the surface to be thrown into folds (for example, in the areolae of the nipples, the perineum, the scrotum, and the penis). Bundles of smooth

(erector pili) muscles are also attached to the hair follicles. In the skin of the face, bands of skeletal muscle (the facial musculature) are present in the dermis.

The subcutaneous layer *(hypodermis)* which is a looser variety of the dermis, lies beneath the reticular layer. Where the skin is firmly attached to underlying muscle or bone, this layer is composed of tightly woven collagenous fibers continuous with those of the dermis. In areas where the skin is more loosely attached to underlying structures, the fibers of the hypodermis are accordingly more loosely arranged. Frequently sheets of fat cells occur in the subcutaneous layer, for example, in the heel and in breast tissue. The subcutaneous layer is richly supplied with blood vessels and nerves.

HAIRY SKIN

In the skin of the greater part of the body, the basal layers of the epidermis extend into the corium to form hair follicles (Figs. 12-6 to 12-8). These are most extensively developed in the scalp, which may be used as an example of hairy skin (Fig. 12-7). In this locality protection is afforded by the hair, and the cornified layer is much thinner than it is on the hands and feet. In some cases it is reduced to less than one half the thickness of the basal and spinosum layers; the stratum lucidum is much reduced or entirely lacking, and there are few granular cells.

Hair

Hair consists of horny threads that are derived from the epidermis. They are located in pits that extend to various depths in the dermis. Hair consists of a *shaft*, the portion that projects above the surface, and a *root*, which is embedded in the skin. The root exhibits a bulbous extension, the undersurface of which is indented. The space within the indentation is occupied by connective tissue known as the *papilla* (Fig. 12-6). The root of the hair is enveloped by the *hair follicle* derived from an epidermal (epithelial) and a dermal (connective tissue) origin.

Hair is made up of three layers of epitheli-

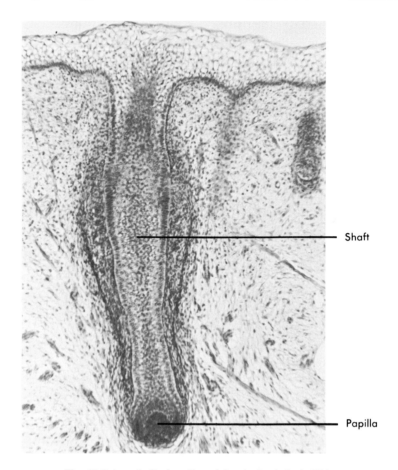

Shaft

Papilla

Fig. 12-6. Longitudinal section of developing hair. (×60.)

al cells. The *medulla* or central axis measures 16 to 20 μm in diameter and consists of two or three layers of cells. In the lower part they are cuboidal, whereas in the shaft they are cornified. The nuclei are either shrunken or absent. The *cortex* makes up the main bulk of the hair and consists of several layers of cells. In the deeper regions of the follicle the cells are cuboidal; at higher levels they become progressively flattened and cornified. Between the cells, pigment granules and air occur, which gives rise to color in the hair. The *cuticle* is a single layer of thin, clear cells that overlap each other like shingles on a roof.

Hair follicle

The hair follicle consists of (1) an inner and (2) an outer *epithelial root sheath* derived from the epidermis and (3) a connective tissue sheath derived from the dermis (Fig. 12-8).

1. The *inner epithelial root sheath* is made up of three layers: (a) a cuticle, (b) Huxley's layer, and (c) Henle's layer. The *cuticle* of the sheath, which lies adjacent to the cuticle of the hair, consists of thin scalelike overlapping cells that are nucleated in the deeper and nonnucleated in the upper regions. The two cuticles overlap in a linkage of cells to help hold the hair shaft in place. Huxley's layer, located outside the cuticle of the root sheath, appears as several rows of elongated cells that contain eleidin-like (*trichohyalin*) granules that give to the sheath of cells a glassy appearance due to keratinization. These cells are also nucleated in the deeper but nonnucleated in the upper regions of the

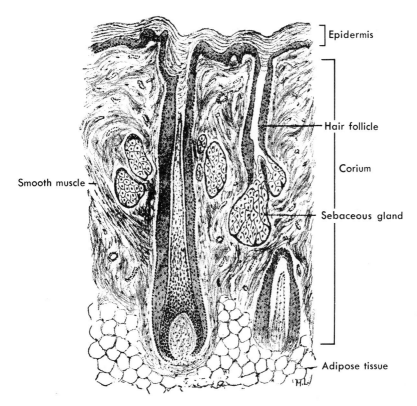

Epidermis

Hair follicle

Corium

Smooth muscle

Sebaceous gland

Adipose tissue

Fig. 12-7. Human scalp.

follicle. Henle's layer is made up of a row of clear flattened rectangular cells containing fibrils in the cytoplasm. Nuclei occur only in cells of the deeper portions. Also, there are short wedgelike processes between the cells. Both these layers (Huxley's and Henle's) consist of keratinized epithelium and represent an invagination of the epidermal surface.

2. The *outer epithelial root sheath* is a continuation of the Malpighian layer (stratum basale and *stratum spinosum*) and corresponds to it in structure. The outermost cells adjacent to the connective tissue are the tall cylindrical variety. The innermost cells are for the most part polygonal in shape and exhibit spinous processes, as do the prickle cells of the skin.

3. The *connective tissue sheath* may be divided into three parts: (a) an inner sheath, (b) a middle portion, (c) an outer division. The *inner sheath* is a homogeneous, nar-

row hyaline membrane applied to the base of the cylindrical cells of the outer sheath. The *middle portion* consists of a bundle of fine connective tissue fibers circularly arranged. The *outer division* is rather poorly defined and consists of coarse bundles of white fibers, longitudinally arranged, that serve to hold the hair down in the dermis.

All the layers of the hair follicle described are only visible a short distance above the bulb. Above and below this part of the shaft the different layers are less clearly defined or lacking.

GLANDS OF THE SKIN

The glands of the skin are of two kinds: the sweat glands and the sebaceous glands.

Sweat glands

Sweat glands are distributed over most of the surface of the body. They are simple tubular glands with convoluted secreting por-

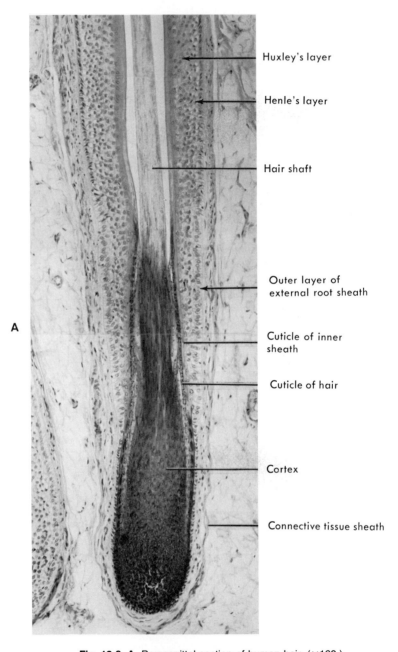

Huxley's layer

Henle's layer

Hair shaft

Outer layer of
external root sheath

Cuticle of inner
sheath

Cuticle of hair

Cortex

Connective tissue sheath

A

Fig. 12-8. A, Parasagittal section of human hair. (×160.)

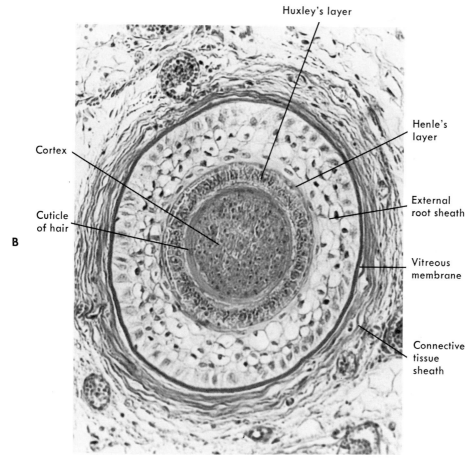

Huxley's layer

Henle's layer

External root sheath

Vitreous membrane

Connective tissue sheath

Cortex

Cuticle of hair

B

Fig. 12-8, cont'd. B, Transverse section through root of hair and follicle. (×1,000.) (Courtesy Ward's Natural Science Establishment, Inc.)

tions. The latter may lie in the subcutaneous tissue or in the deeper portion of the corium and are lined with cuboidal or columnar epithelium. The cytoplasm contains secretory granules or droplets (Fig. 12-9).

The ducts of the sweat glands are lined with a double layer of stratified cuboidal cells resting on a thin basement membrane (Fig. 12-10). The inner layer exhibits a homogeneous dark-staining cytoplasm, and the surface of the cells is refractile. In the epidermis the cellular constituents disappear and the duct consists of a noncellular channel.

In some regions of the body such as the axilla, the mammary areolae, and the circumanal region, the sweat glands are much larger than those located in the palms and other areas. These glands are of the apocrine type, producing thicker secretions than do the sweat formed by the smaller (merocrine) glands. Also included in this group of larger glands are the wax-secreting *ceruminous* glands located in the external auditory canal and the margin of the eyelid. The secretion of the glands is carried to the lower border of the epidermis, where it passes into a coiled channel through the tissues to emerge on the surface by way of a minute pore.

Sebaceous glands

A sebaceous gland and a strand of smooth muscle are associated with the hair follicle. The axis of the latter is never exactly perpendicular to the surface of the scalp, and the

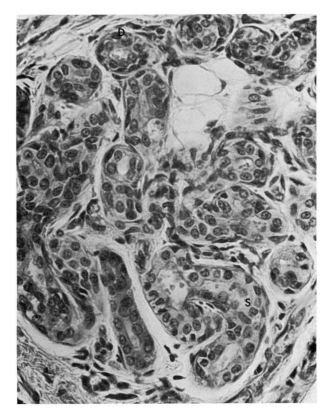

Fig. 12-9. Section of part of human sweat gland. *D,* Duct; *S,* secretory tubule. (×400.)

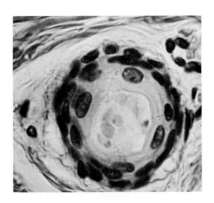

Fig. 12-10. Transverse section of duct of sweat gland of an infant. Note two layers of cells. (×400.)

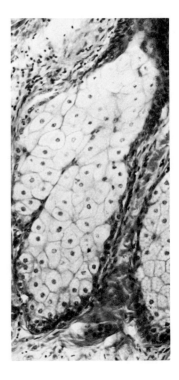

Fig. 12-11. Section of part of human sebaceous gland. (×160.)

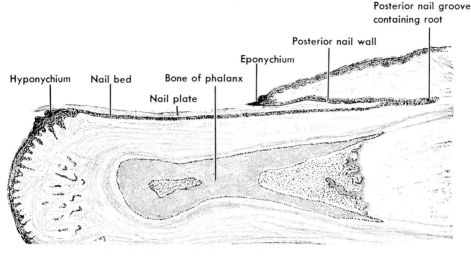

Fig. 12-12. Longitudinal section of finger of newborn child.

muscle and gland lie in the wider angle of the two that the follicle makes with the surface.

Sebaceous glands open through ducts into the spaces between the follicles and the hair shafts. Structurally they are different from any other glands thus far described. Their secreting portions are not composed of a single layer of cells grouped around a lumen but are rounded masses of cells. At the periphery of each mass the cells are cuboidal; in the center they are polygonal. The central cells are filled with vacuoles (Fig. 12-11) so that their appearance is somewhat similar to that of developing adipose tissue cells. The secretion of the sebaceous glands is accompanied by the breaking down of the central cells, remains of which are poured out with the oily accumulation into the hair follicle. The cells thus destroyed are replaced from the peripheral layer.

NAILS

The nails (Fig. 12-12), which are modifications of the epidermis, are composed of the (1) body, (2) wall, and (3) bed.

1. The *nail body* with its free edge is composed of several layers of clear, flattened cells, which differ from the stratum corium of the skin in that they are harder and also possess shrunken nuclei. The proximal part of the nail body lying under the fold of skin is called the root.

2. The *nail wall* is the fold around the proximal and lateral borders of the nail, marked off from the latter by the nail groove. The wall consists of skin that has all the layers of other parts of the skin except, sometimes, the stratum lucidum. The stratum corneum of the wall at the proximal part of the fold extends out over the body of the nail (eponychium).

3. The *nail bed* is the epidermis under the body of the nail. It lacks the stratum granulosum and stratum lucidum and consists of the deeper epidermal layers only. Under the proximal part of the nail, in the region called the lunula, the nail bed thickens to include all epidermal layers. It is from this region, the matrix, that growth of the nail takes place, the superficial cells of the matrix being transformed into nail cells. The corium of the nail bed has its connective tissue fibers arranged in two groups: (a) a group running in the long axis of the nail and (b) a group running vertically to the periosteum of the underlying bone. The dermal papillae of the nail bed form ridges, which run in the long axis of the nail.

13

Oral cavity

LIPS

The lips are muscular organs covered on the outside by skin and on the inside by the mucous membrane of the mouth. The muscles of the lips are striated and consist of the orbicularis oris, the compressor labii, and the mimetic. The lip is usually sectioned vertically in preparation for microscopic study and when so cut contains a core consisting of the cross sections of the orbicularis oris, with a relatively small number of strands of the mimetic and compressor labii muscles cut longitudinally (Fig. 13-1).

The skin covering the outside of the lip is like that of the greater part of the body. It consists of stratified squamous epithelium, which is cornified at the surface and rests on a layer of connective tissue. In the latter are sweat glands, sebaceous glands, and the bases of hair follicles. In the region transitional between skin and oral mucosa, hair follicles and glands disappear, and the epithelium is somewhat modified. Its basal layer follows an irregular course so that tall projections of the underlying connective tissue extend toward the surface of the lip. These cells are not pigmented but are well supplied with blood vessels, giving this part of the lip a brighter color than that of the surrounding skin.

On the oral surface the epithelium changes again. The height of the connective tissue papillae gradually diminishes, as does the cornification of the surface, and at the base of the lip on the inside, the mucous membrane

is similar to that lining other soft parts of the oral cavity. In this region there are seromucous glands lying in the connective tissue between the epithelium and the muscle.

LINING OF THE ORAL CAVITY

The epithelium lining the oral cavity is of the stratified squamous variety. It rests on a tunica propria of reticular or fine areolar tissue, which blends in most parts of the cavity with a submucosal layer of areolar tissue. Beneath the submucosa lie tissues that vary in different parts of the mouth. In the cheeks and lips, for example, the mucosa and submucosa lie against muscle, making a soft and somewhat elastic wall of the oral cavity (Fig. 13-2). In the hard palate and the gingivae, on the other hand, the layers in question lie directly against bone. Modifications of the mucous membrane are correlated with these differences in the tissue it covers.

Lips and cheeks

The inner surface of the lip is a good example of conditions in parts of the mouth that are bounded by muscle. The epithelium is not cornified. It has a surface layer of flattened cells that slough off in patches. Connective tissue papillae are low; the tunica propria blends without demarcation with the submucosa. The latter is fairly thick and in some regions contains glands, the ducts of which penetrate the mucosa and open into the oral cavity.

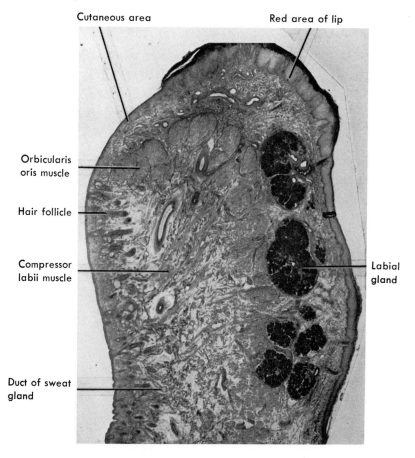

Cutaneous area   Red area of lip

Orbicularis
oris muscle

Hair follicle

Compressor
labii muscle   Labial
                                                gland

Duct of sweat
gland

Fig. 13-1. Parasagittal section of human lip in newborn infant. (×14.) (Courtesy Dr. S. Bernick.)

Gingivae and hard palate

Where the mucosa and submucosa lie over bony tissue, as in the gingivae and hard palate (Figs. 13-3 and 13-4), modifications of arrangement are to be observed. In the gingival region the connective tissue papillae of the tunica propria are long and slender and close together. The submucosa blends with the periosteum of the underlying bone. In the region immediately surrounding each tooth, fibers are present, which are specialized as part of the apparatus by which the tooth is held in its socket. No glands exist in this portion of the oral mucosa.

In the hard palate the papillae of the tunica propria are well developed, and there is a layer of elastic fibers, which forms a line of demarcation between the mucosa and sub-

mucosa. The latter coat blends here, as in the gingivae, with the periosteum of the underlying bone. There are glands in the submucosa of the palatal region.

TEETH

The human dentition consists of twenty deciduous and thirty-two permanent teeth. The teeth vary among themselves as to size, shape, and number of cusps and roots; each particular tooth, however, has its own unique morphological characteristics.

The hard tissues of the teeth are divided into two parts: (1) the crown, covered by enamel, is the part of the tooth that is ordinarily visible and extends beyond the margin of the gingivae; (2) the root is the part of the tooth that lies deep to the gingivae

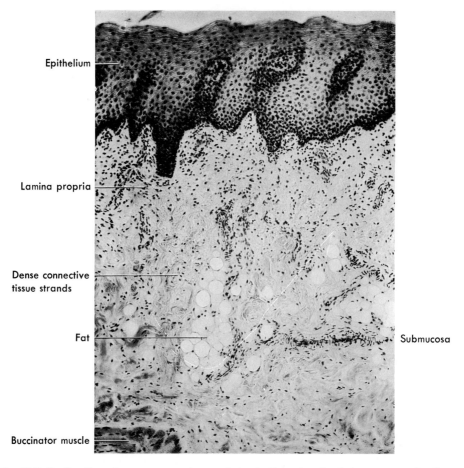

Fig. 13-2. Section through mucous membrane of cheek. Note strands of dense connective tissue attaching mucous membrane to buccinator muscle. (From Sicher, H., and S. N. Bhaskar [eds.] 1972. Orban's oral histology and embryology, 7th ed. The C. V. Mosby Co., St. Louis.)

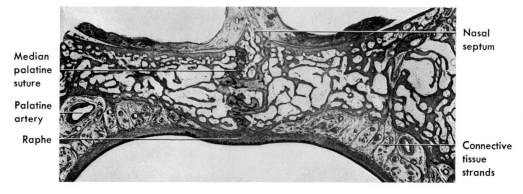

Fig. 13-3. Transverse section through hard palate. Palatine raphe; fibrous strands connecting mucosa and periosteum; palatine vessels. (From Pendleton.)

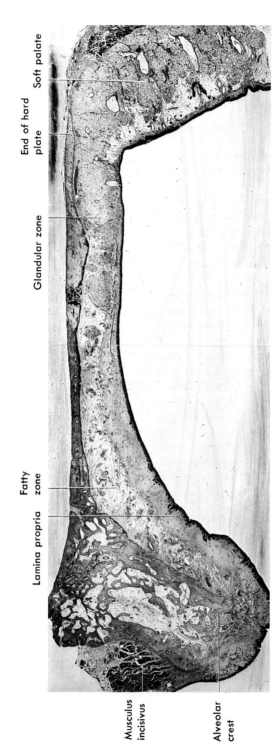

Fig. 13-4. Longitudinal section through hard and soft palates lateral to midline. Fatty and glandular zones of hard palate. (From Sicher, H., and S. N. Bhaskar [eds.] 1972. Orban's oral histology and embryology, 7th ed. The C. V. Mosby Co., St. Louis.)

and is implanted within the socket. The term *cervix*, or neck, is sometimes used to designate a slight constriction at the junction of the crown and root.

The tooth consists of enamel, dentin, and cementum, which are calcified tissues. In addition, each tooth has a vascular connective tissue component, the pulp, located within the pulp cavity.

Early development

The teeth are derived from two embryonic tissues: (1) ectoderm, which gives rise to the enamel, and (2) mesoderm, which gives rise to the dentin, cementum, and pulp and also the supporting tissues.

The dental lamina appears in the human embryo at approximately the sixth week of the gestation period. This lamina is derived from the oral epithelium. It consists of a band

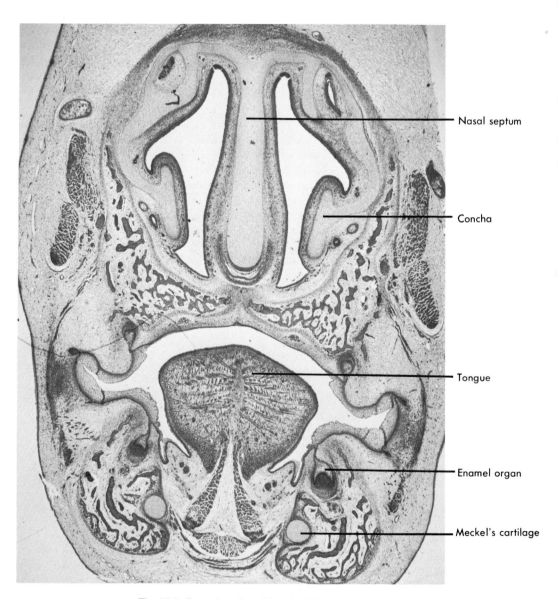

Fig. 13-5. Frontal section of head of 70 mm embryo. (×20.)

of cells that proliferate from the epithelium and extends into the underlying mesenchyme. Taken as a whole, the lamina is U-shaped, following the shape of the jaw and foreshadowing the shape of the dental arch. There is one labiodental lamina in each jaw (Fig. 13-5).

Soon after the dental lamina is differentiated, one can observe that it is made up of two parts; one part consists of the original lamina, the other of an outgrowth that is inclined away from the tongue and is known as the gingival lamina. Later this lamina hollows out from the oral surface. The tissue located labially gives rise to the inside of the lip, and the tissue located lingually gives rise to the epithelium of the gums; the cavity between the two becomes the vestibule (Fig. 13-5).

Development of enamel organ

In each of the two dental laminae localized proliferations of tissue occur in the region where the future teeth are to form. There are ten of these outgrowths in each jaw; they are known as tooth buds or germs. These buds lie some distance removed from the oral epithelium and are connected with it by a narrow strand of the dental lamina. The tooth buds are at first rounded and solid. They gradually become invaginated on their distal surface by the invasion of the subjacent mesenchyme. The mesenchyme continues to proliferate; eventually this leads to a rearrangement of the epithelial part of the tooth germ from a solid organ to one that is hollow and goblet shaped. While the change in the external configuration takes place, a differentiation of the tissues in this structure now known as the enamel organ also occurs. The rearrangement and differentiation result in the reestablishment of four distinct parts of the enamel organ: the outer enamel epithelium, the stellate reticulum, the stratum intermedium, and the inner enamel epithelium (Fig. 13-6).

In this stage of development in the human

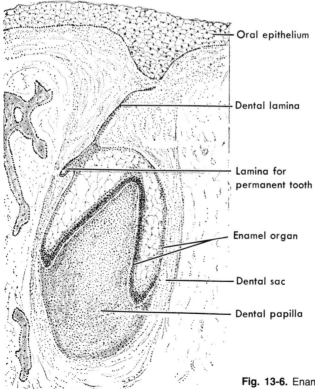

Oral epithelium

Dental lamina

Lamina for permanent tooth

Enamel organ

Dental sac

Dental papilla

Fig. 13-6. Enamel organ and dental papilla of pig embryo before formation of dentin.

being (about 12 weeks), the portion of the dental lamina connecting the enamel organ and the oral epithelium becomes reduced in size and begins to disintegrate. Its distal portion, however, now appears as a small projection on the lingual aspect of the enamel organ and later develops into the anlage for the permanent tooth. Enamel organs of permanent teeth that do not have deciduous predecessors are derived from the original dental lamina in the same manner as are the deciduous enamel organs, but at a later time.

Enamel formation. In the fifth to sixth month of intrauterine life, shortly after dentin has begun to form on the crown of the developing tooth, enamel formation begins (Figs. 13-7 and 13-8). Before this occurs, the several layers of cells that comprise the enamel organ come together to form the combined enamel epithelium, which is closely applied to the tip of the crown. The cells that compose the innermost layer, the inner enamel epithelium, have by this time differentiated into tall columnar cells with prominent nuclei, which are located peripheral to the surface that is in contact with the dentin. These cells, known as ameloblasts, elaborate a rather wide protoplasmic process from the free surface of the cell, Tomes' enamel process, which comes in contact with the dentin. This is the region of

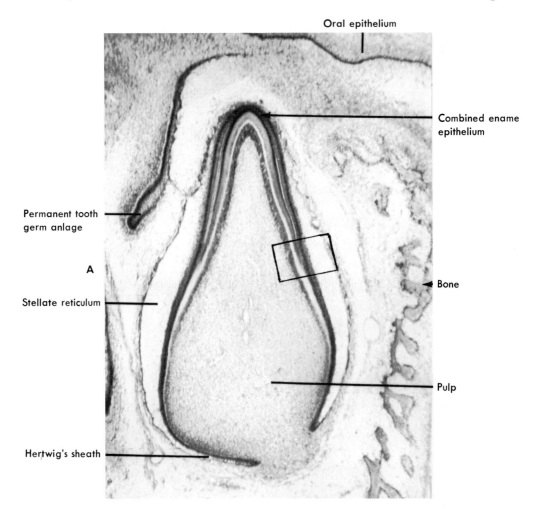

Oral epithelium

Combined enamel epithelium

Permanent tooth germ anlage

A

Stellate reticulum

Bone

Pulp

Hertwig's sheath

Fig. 13-7. A, Developing canine showing initial stages of mineralization. **B,** Part of developing tooth indicated by box in **A,** showing early stages of dentin formation. (×160.)

the future dentinoenamel junction. In the process of enamel formation this tissue is first laid down at the periphery of dentin; as more enamel is deposited, the ameloblasts move outward, away from the odontoblasts.

The space formerly occupied by Tomes' processes gradually become impregnated with mineral salts; this eventually leads to the production of the fully calcified enamel rod (Fig. 13-9). Between the rods are fine interstices, which also contain calcified material and are known as the interprismatic areas. The process of enamel formation continues until the crown is completely formed. By the time the tooth erupts, the ameloblasts and the other enamel epithelia in the coronal

region degenerate, leaving only the enamel cuticle covering the crown.

Mature enamel. Enamel is the hardest tissue in the body. It is approximately 98% calcified. It also contains small amounts of enamel protein and moisture. Enamel covers the crown of the tooth and is whitish in color. It is in contact with dentin, cementum, and the gingiva.

Enamel consists of highly calcified rods or prisms, which are separated by minute amounts of interprismatic substance (Figs. 13-9 and 13-10). The enamel rods extend from the periphery of the dentin to the free surface of the crown. Their direction generally is radial in the region of the tip or the

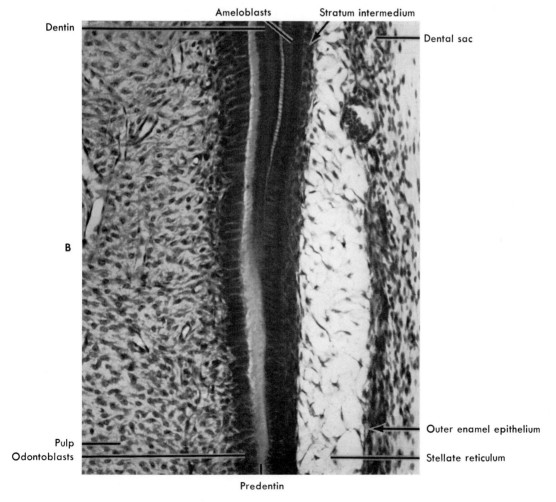

Fig. 13-7, cont'd. For legend see opposite page.

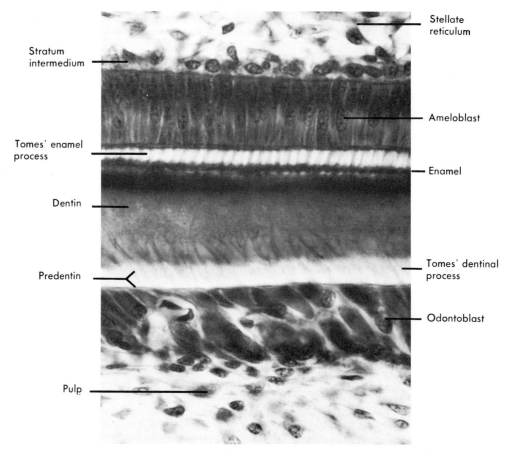

Stellate
reticulum

Stratum
intermedium

Ameloblast

Tomes' enamel
process

Enamel

Dentin

Tomes' dentinal
process

Predentin

Odontoblast

Pulp

Fig. 13-8. Section of developing tooth showing formation of dentin and enamel. (×420.)

cusp; toward the cervix of the crown they sometimes form a slight angle with reference to the dentinal tubules. In certain parts of the crown the rods frequently intertwine. When viewed in longitudinal section, this enamel appears gnarled. The shape of the enamel rod in cross section varies. It is sometimes hexagonal.

Recent studies have shown that in transverse section the enamel rods have a typical keyhole appearance (Fig. 13-10).

Contour (imbrication) lines, known as the striae of Retzius, are frequently observed in sections of enamel. They represent modification or change in the degree or rate of mineralization occurring during the formative period of the tooth. These striae originate at the dentinoenamel junction and extend to the free surface of the crown in an arc paralleling

the surface of the dentin. In transverse sections of the crown the striae appear concentrically arranged.

Organic material in the form of enamel protein appears in enamel of most teeth as strands or tufts that originate at the dentinoenamel junction. This organic component is most readily observed in transverse sections of the crown.

Development of dentin. Dentin is laid down in the developing deciduous tooth just before the appearance of enamel.

The first step in the development of this tissue consists of the formation of reticular fibers, which radiate from the pulp to the distal surface of the inner enamel epithelium. This tissue and other elements incorporated into dentin are derived from the mesenchyme or the primitive pulp. The reticular

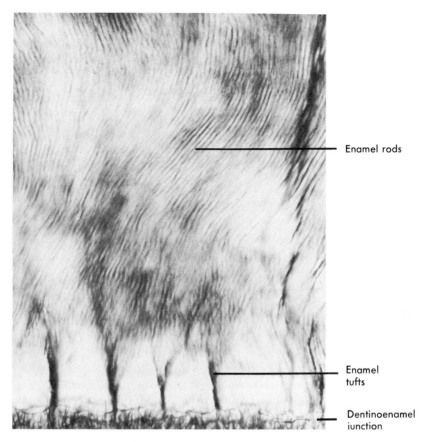

Enamel rods

Enamel
tufts

Dentinoenamel
iunction

Fig. 13-9. Ground section of part of crown of human tooth showing enamel rods. (×420.)

fibers become arranged radially, first at the tip of the crown and later toward the apex of the developing tooth.

These radially arranged reticular fibers undergo two important changes during the development of dentin: (1) they come to lie within the calcified tissue more or less parallel to the contour lines of the tooth and (2) they change from reticular to collagenous fibers.

Dentin is first differentiated at the tip of the crown; then it gradually envelops the entire pulp cavity. When dentin is first formed, certain cells, which align themselves along the periphery of the pulp cavity, gradually differentiate into special columnar cells known as odontoblasts. The odontoblasts have a dark-staining, rounded basal nucleus and relatively clear cytoplasm, which stains intensely with eosin. A protoplasmic extension known as Tomes' dentinal process, which comes to occupy a space in the dentin, is elaborated at the free surface of the cell. The basal surface of these cells frequently ends in a blunt, tapering projection. In the tip of the crown the layer of odontoblasts is several cells deep. Approaching the apex, the cells thin out until eventually they are arranged in a single epithelioid layer. It is in such an area that they may be most advantageously studied in sections of the developing tooth (Figs. 13-7 and 13-8).

The first dentin, which can be observed in hematoxylin and eosin preparations, appears as a relatively narrow zone of tissue peripheral to the pulp cavity in the coronal region of the tooth. It takes the eosin stain, and one may observe that Tomes' dentinal

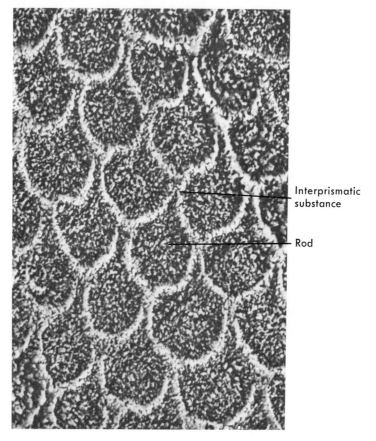

Interprismatic substance

Rod

Fig. 13-10. Scanning electron micrograph of transverse section of human enamel rods (prisms). Note typical keyhole shape of rods. (×3,500.) (Courtesy Dr. H. Nakahara.)

fibrils occupy a radial position within this tissue. In this, the uncalcified state, it is known as predentin.

After the initial zone of predentin has been established, examination of a slightly later stage in tooth development reveals that a new zone of predentin has formed on the pulpal side of the first increment. During this process the odontoblasts retreat pulpward, retaining meanwhile their connection with the dentin by means of the dentinal processes, which lie embedded in the dentin.

While the second zone of predentin forms, the initial (peripheral) zone undergoes partial calcification. In this process small droplets of bluish staining material appear, which come together to form calcoglobules. This gives a fairly characteristic globular appearance to calcifying dentin. In the later stages of development the globules usually coalesce to form a tissue that is fairly uniform in appearance.

The dentinal processes meanwhile do not calcify. They occupy spaces within the calcified tissue that are known as dentinal tubules (Fig. 13-11).

In comparing the development of enamel with that of dentin, it should be emphasized that enamel is a solid, nontubular tissue, which grows peripherally with reference to the dentin. Unlike dentin, which retains vital connections by means of Tomes' dentinal processes, enamel loses all contact with vital tissues when the tooth erupts. This has an important bearing on the metabolism of these tissues in the erupted tooth.

Peritubular dentin   Matrix   Dentinal tubule

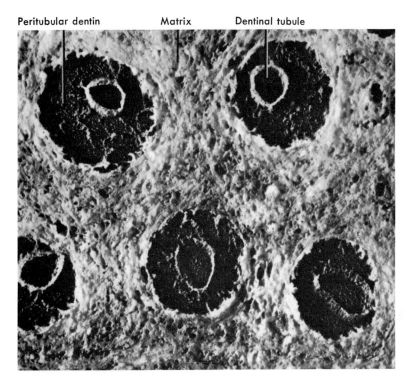

Fig. 13-11. Electron photomicrograph of demineralized section of dentin. (×5,000.) (Courtesy Dr. D. Scott.)

Mature dentin. Mature dentin is a translucent, compressible tissue consisting of a calcified component (apatite) and an organic component, which is chiefly collagen. It also contains moisture. Examination of a ground section of this tissue reveals a relatively homogeneous translucent calcified tissue (Fig. 13-12). The collagenous fibers that are embedded within this calcified tissue are not visible except in specially prepared sections. Dentin is traversed by numerous tubules, which extend from the pulp to the periphery of the dentin. In the living state these tubules contain Tomes' dentinal processes and tissue fluid. Each tubule is arranged in the form of the letter S in the crown. In the root they are relatively straight. Before they terminate, the tubules divide dichotomously into from two to four branches. As the tubules traverse the dentin, they also give off many lateral side branches known as tubiculi; some of these later connect with other tubiculi or adjacent tubules. The tubiculi are best shown in ground sections stained with silver nitrate. In decalcified sections stained with hematoxylin and eosin, a dark zone called Neumann's sheath surrounds the dentinal tubules.

Variations of dentin. On the periphery of the root one may observe in ground sections of a tooth an imperfectly calcified zone of dentin, which, because of its characteristic appearance, is known as Tomes' granular layer. In addition, imbrication lines, also known as the lines of Owen, are frequently observed in dentin. They are rather wide bands of dentin that follow the contour of the tooth and have a less dense appearance in section. They probably indicate disturbances in metabolism during the formation of dentin.

More extensive variations in the appearance of dentin may also be observed in many teeth that have developed under conditions of faulty mineral metabolism. These areas in the dentin are readily seen in ground sections of teeth and are most commonly ob-

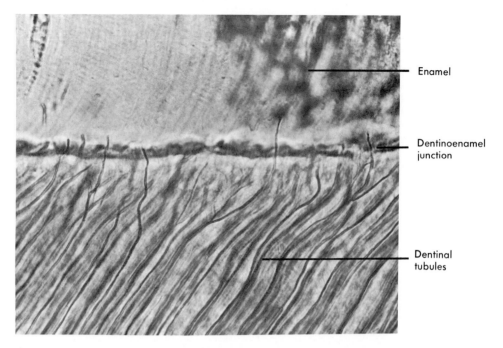

Enamel

Dentinoenamel junction

Dentinal tubules

Fig. 13-12. Ground section of human dentin. (×640.)

served in the crown just below the dentino-enamel junction. This tissue is known as interglobular dentin and represents areas practically devoid of calcified materials. The scallop-edged areas appear black in ground section.

Abrasion of tooth surfaces and caries also produce variations in the histological appearance of dentin. In the former situation the dentin in contact with an abraded area usually becomes nonvital or sclerosed, and in both these situations an irregular variety of the tissue known as secondary dentin may be deposited on the margin of the pulp cavity in an apparent attempt to protect pulp tissues from the oral environment.

Cementum

Cementum is a calcified tissue that forms a thin shell around the periphery of the root. In origin, appearance, and composition it closely resembles bone. It is first formed in the cervical part of the tooth; gradually it encloses the entire root.

There are two varieties of cementum: (1) primary or cell free, which appears hyaline in ground sections and usually occurs on the coronal part of the root (Fig. 13-13) and (2) secondary or cellular, which is deposited later than primary cementum and occupies a position on the periphery of the apical third of the root. In ground sections of the tooth one observes a hyaline calcified tissue in which scattered cells, cementoblasts, occupy a space within lacunae—much as in sections of bone. The fibers of the peridental membrane, which suspend the tooth in the socket, are firmly anchored to the root of the tooth by means of cementum.

Pulp

Pulp is essentially a connective tissue organ. In ordinary sections the pulp in the young tooth is extremely cellular. The appearance of the pulp cells is similar to that of fibroblasts. Histiocytes also have been described as being present in the pulp. As the tooth increases in age, the character of the pulp changes: the relative number of cells decreases, and the fibers increase.

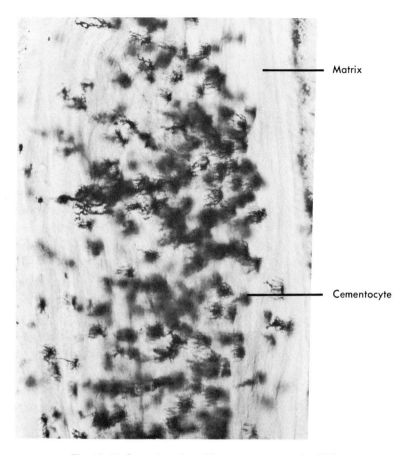

Matrix

Cementocyte

Fig. 13-13. Ground section of human cementum. (×420.)

The odontoblasts previously referred to occupy a position on the periphery of the pulp. These cells constantly retreat pulpward as dentin is slowly deposited throughout the life of the tooth. In the mature tooth the region just below the odontoblasts may have fewer cells than do other parts of the pulp, and it is known as the cell-poor zone of Weil.

The pulp tissue contains an abundant nerve, vascular, and lymph supply.

Gingiva

The gingiva is the modified part of the oral mucous membrane that covers the surface of the alveolus (Fig. 13-14). It is attached to the tooth at the level at which the tooth is inserted into the oral cavity. It consists of two parts: (1) dense connective tissue, the lamina propria, and (2) a covering of stratified squamous epithelium.

The tissues that make up the gingivae are normally attached to the alveolus and to the tooth surfaces. The undersurface of the epithelium is frequently thrown into folds or pegs. The outer surface usually shows a slight degree of cornification. The chief function of this tissue is protective. The following parts of the gingivae are usually recognizable in sections: (1) the outer border of the gingiva, known as the gingival margin; (2) the gingival crevice, a space of variable size between the tooth surface and the gingiva; (3) the epithelial attachment, a strip of stratified squamous epithelium, which originates at the approximate level of the cementoenamel junction. It is attached to the tooth at this level by means of desmosomes and continues up to the free margin of the gingiva. For some considerable distance it is in intimate contact with the cervical part of the crown.

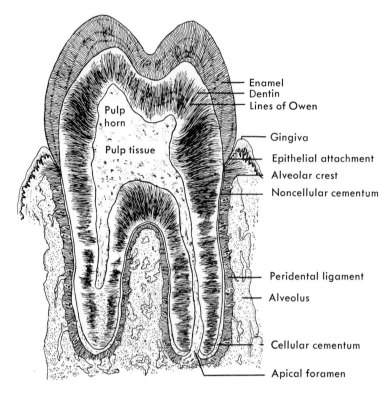

Fig. 13-14. Section of human maxillary molar cut buccolingually to show general relationships of tooth and surrounding tissues.

With advancing age this tissue migrates rootward.

PERIDENTAL LIGAMENT

Peridental ligament is a term used to designate a group of collagenous fibers that suspend the tooth in the socket and support the gingivae. The fibers occupy a space between the bony socket or alveolus, on the one hand, and the periphery of the root, on the other. Above the level of the alveolus the fibers run up to the gingiva. They also connect the cervical parts of adjacent teeth.

The fibers concerned with the suspension of the tooth and support of the gingivae are known as principal fibers. They are relatively short fibers that, in the region of the root, are arranged horizontally or obliquely with reference to the long axis of the tooth.

Other fibers, known as interstitial fibers, occur in the peridental space as isolated is-

lands of connective tissue in which one may observe in section the vessels and nerves that supply this tissue. Clusters of dark-staining cells, the epithelial rests, may frequently be seen in the peridental ligament. They are remnants of the enamel epithelium.

ALVEOLUS

The alveolus, or socket, is the bony crypt in which the tooth is suspended (Fig. 13-14). The alveolus proper consists of a thin lamina of bone, which surrounds the root just peripheral to the peridental ligament. This plate is made up of compact bone. The distal ends of the fibers of the peridental ligament are firmly cemented into this tissue. Between the compact bone making up the alveolus and the external parts of the jaw are numerous trabeculae of supporting bone, which are advantageously arranged to take up the stresses that the teeth transmit to the bone surrounding them.

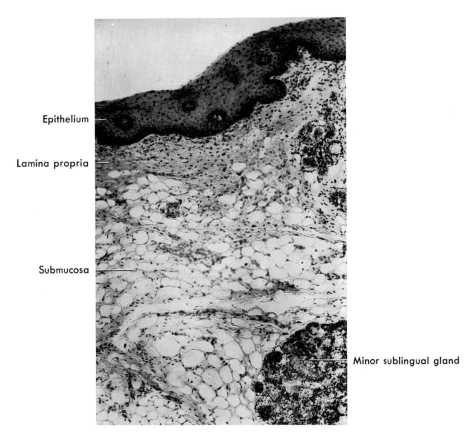

Epithelium

Lamina propria

Submucosa

Minor sublingual gland

Fig. 13-15. Mucous membrane from floor of mouth. (From Sicher, H., and S. N. Bhaskar [eds.] 1972. Orban's oral histology and embryology, 7th ed. The C. V. Mosby Co., St. Louis.)

TONGUE

The tongue is primarily a muscular organ. It is covered with a mucous membrane (Fig. 13-15), parts of which are modified to conform to its function as an organ of mastication and of taste.

The muscles of the tongue are in three main groups: longitudinal, transverse, and sagittal fibers. They are arranged in interlacing groups and embedded in areolar and adipose tissue.

The mucosa covering the dorsal surface of the tongue is modified to form a great number of elevations or papillae. It should be noted that these papillae are different from the projections of connective tissue of the epithelium, which have been mentioned in descriptions of the parts of the oral mucosa. The papillae of the tongue are elevations of both connective tissue and epithelium. Within each of them there also may be projections of the tunica propria into the epithelium, which are termed secondary papillae. The distribution and characteristic forms of the papillae of the tongue are filiform, fungiform, foliate, and vallate.

Filiform papillae

Filiform papillae are the most numerous of the papillae and are distributed over the entire dorsal surface of the tongue. Each consists of a conical elevation of the tunica propria and stratified squamous epithelium. The whole papilla is inclined in an anteroposterior direction. Its surface epithelium is cornified, the cornification extending in strands, which gives this type of papilla its name (threadlike) (Fig. 13-16).

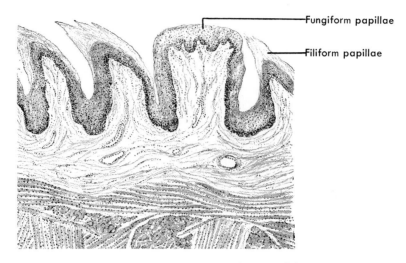

Fig. 13-16. Dorsal surface of tongue of dog.

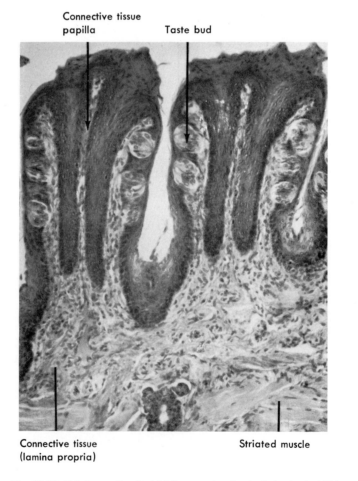

Fig. 13-17. Foliate papilla of rabbit tongue showing taste buds. (×160.)

Fungiform papillae

Fungiform papillae are distributed unevenly among the filiform papillae on the dorsal surface of the tongue, being most numerous near the margin of the organ but never as numerous as the filiform variety. They are club shaped, with flattened free surfaces, and have a diameter somewhat greater than that of the basal portion of a filiform papilla. The epithelium covering them shows little, if any, cornification and is relatively thin. This, combined with the fact that they have a rich blood supply, gives them a red color in the living state. Their secondary papillae are a characteristic feature of these structures (Fig. 13-16). Taste buds are sometimes visible on the free surfaces of fungiform papillae but are small and not always noticeable.

Foliate papillae

Foliate papillae are well developed on the tongues of certain rodents but are rudimentary in man. When fully developed they have some features in common with fungiform papillae, being club shaped with flat tops. The types are readily distinguishable, however, by the following facts: (1) the foliate papillae occur in groups along the lateral margins of the tongue and are not intermingled with filiform papillae; (2) they have numerous prominent taste buds set close together along their sides; and (3) they are characterized by the presence of the secondary connective tissue papillae, which occupy approximately three fourths of the depth of the primary papilla. Lingual glands occur in the same part of the tongue as do the foliate papillae (Figs. 13-17 and 13-18).

Vallate (circumvallate) papillae

Vallate (circumvallate) papillae are the largest papillae of the tongue and the least numerous. There are only twenty to thirty of them, arranged along the sulcus terminalis, and they are so large that they are macroscopically visible. Each projects only a short distance above the surface of the tongue but is, as the name implies, surrounded by a deep groove (Fig. 13-19). Their

Stratified squamous epithelium

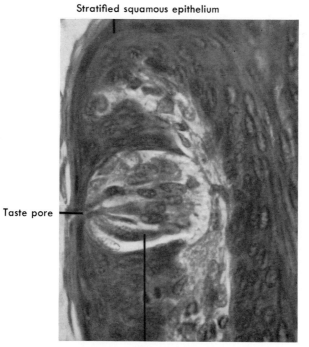

Taste pore

Cell in taste bud

Fig. 13-18. Taste bud showing pore. (×640.)

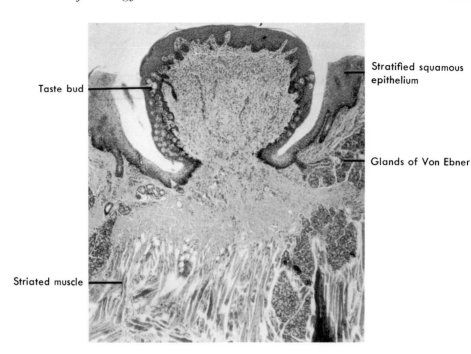

Taste bud

Stratified squamous epithelium

Glands of Von Ebner

Striated muscle

Fig. 13-19. Section through circumvallate papilla. (×40.)

secondary papillae are short and usually occur only on the surface. The outstanding characteristics, aside from their size and positions, are (1) the walls of the grooves surrounding them are beset with large taste buds and (2) the grooves serve as the point of exit for the ducts of conspicuous serous glands, which are present in this part of the tongue (Ebner's glands).

The taste buds are composed of two kinds of cells: the specialized taste cells and the supporting cells. In ordinary sections the two kinds may be distinguished by their nuclei, those of the taste cells being dark and spindle shaped and those of the supporting cells pale and round or oval. The taste bud as a whole is a flask-shaped structure lying in the epithelium and opening onto the surface through a minute circular pore (Fig. 13-18). In specimens treated with silver nitrate, nerve fibers may be traced into the center of the buds.

The ventral surface of the tongue is covered by mucous membrane not unlike that lining the lips and cheeks (Fig. 13-15). In all parts of the organ the interlacing bands of striated muscle are a characteristic feature.

In regions where glands occur, their secreting portions lie in the connective tissue, which forms a stroma around the muscles, producing an arrangement of glandular and muscular tissue not often seen in other organs. It may be said that the tongue has no submucosa, this layer being replaced by a mixture of connective tissue, muscle, and glands.

GLANDS OF THE ORAL CAVITY

Saliva, the fluid in the oral cavity, is secreted principally by three large glands—the parotid, the submaxillary, and the sublingual—which lie outside the lining of the cavity and communicate with it by means of large ducts.

Contributions to the saliva are also made by numerous smaller glands that are situated in the submucosa of some parts of the wall of the oral cavity and among the muscles of the tongue. They are of three kinds: (1) serous, (2) mucous, and (3) seromucous—and are located as follows:

1. The serous glands are located in the tongue, in the region of the vallate papillae (Ebner's).

Epithelium   Lamina propria

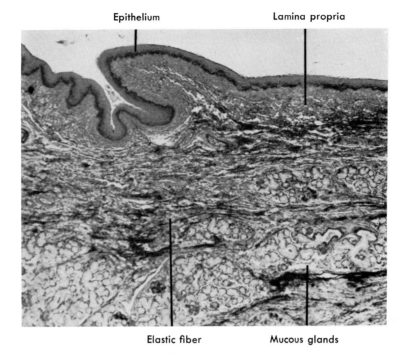

Elastic fiber   Mucous glands

Fig. 13-20. Longitudinal section of laryngeal portion of pharynx of dog. (×16.)

2. The mucous glands are located on the anterior surface of the soft palate (palatine), on the hard palate, on the borders near the foliate papillae (lingual) of the tongue, and on the root of the tongue.

3. The seromucous glands are located on the anterior portion (anterior lingual) of the tongue and on the lips (labial).

Posterior to the sulcus terminalis there are no papillae on the dorsal surface of the tongue. It is covered by stratified squamous epithelium similar to that lining the remainder of the cavity at this point. The tunica propria consists of reticular tissue and contains condensations of lymphoid tissue, as well as the palatine and lingual tonsils described in Chapter 8. Mucous glands are present in the submucosa of the fauces.

PHARYNX

The oral cavity opens through the *fauces* into the oropharynx. This region is only partly separated from the upper respiratory region or *nasopharynx* by the soft palate and the uvula. The latter abuts on the *pharyngeal tonsils* (adenoids). At the level of the hyoid

bone the oropharynx merges into the *laryngeal pharynx*, which in turn leads to the epiglottis of the respiratory system and the esophagus of the digestive system.

The pharynx is thus the meeting place for nasal passages, oral cavity, larynx, and esophagus. Histologically the pharynx takes on the mixed characteristics of all these structures (Fig. 13-20).

The nasopharynx has a lining characteristic of the respiratory tract, that is, a pseudostratified epithelium and a tunica propria that is separated from the submucosa by an elastic membrane. This region will be described in Chapter 16.

The oropharynx and laryngopharynx are intermediate in composition, as they are in position between the oral cavity and the esophagus. They are lined with nonkeratinized stratified squamous epithelium and have a lamina propria containing numerous elastic fibers, some of which form an incomplete membrane at the border of the mucosa. Branches of this elastic lamina also extend between groups of muscle bundles (Fig. 13-20).

In the superior lateral regions of the pharynx the submucosa may be of considerable extent and may contain the secreting portions of mucous glands. In some parts of the pharynx, however, the elastic membrane of the mucosa rests immediately on the muscular layer, in which situation the glands occupy a position between the strands of muscle, similar to the pattern found in the tongue. The arrangement described has given rise to the statement that the pharynx has no submucosa. It is obvious, however, that in a transitional region such as the pharynx, different conditions obtain at different levels of the organ. Sections of the laryngopharynx are, in fact, difficult to distinguish from those of the upper part of the esophagus, especially since the elastic lamina is thoroughly dispersed in this region.

The muscular layer of the pharyngeal wall consists of bundles of striated muscle obliquely arranged to form a constrictor. The bundles interlace and form irregular layers.

14

Digestive tract

The digestive tract is a hollow tube running from the oral cavity to the anus, modified in its various parts but consisting throughout of four coats or layers: mucosa, submucosa, muscularis, and adventitia or serosa (Fig. 14-1).

The coats of the digestive tract are summarized as follows:

1. Mucosa
   a. Epithelium
   b. Lamina propria containing:
      *Glands**
      Lymphoid tissue
      Scattered muscle fibers
      Capillaries and small lymphatics
      Muscularis mucosae
2. Submucosa
   a. Areolar tissue containing:
      Heller's plexus of blood vessels
      Meissner's plexus of nerves
      Lymphatics
      Glands
      Lymphoid tissue
3. Muscularis
   a. *Oblique layer*
   b. Circular layer
   c. Connective tissue containing Auerbach's plexus of nerves
   d. Longitudinal layer
4. Adventitia or serosa
   a. Areolar tissue containing:
      Adipose tissue
      Blood vessels
      Mesothelial covering

---

*Italics indicate the structures present in some but not all divisions of the digestive tract.

Mucosa. The mucosa is made up of (1) an epithelial lining that borders on the lumen of the tract and rests on (2) a lamina propria of reticular or fine areolar tissue. The lamina propria may contain glands, scattered fibers of smooth muscle, and lymph nodules. The nodules are often large, extending below the mucosa into the adjacent coat of the tract. They are a response to frequent invasions of microorganisms across the gut lining and represent a defense against infection. Fine capillaries and lymphatics are present in the lamina propria. In the greater part of the digestive tube the mucosa includes a third layer, (3) the muscularis mucosae, which is a thin coat of smooth muscle fibers. This muscle layer directly beneath the surface lining probably helps throw the surface into folds to facilitate movement of material past the secreting and absorbing cells of the epithelium.

Submucosa. The second coat of the wall is the submucosa. This is composed of areolar tissue, which contains a plexus of small blood vessels known as Heller's plexus. It also includes numerous lymphatics and a plexus of nerves (Meissner's plexus). In the esophagus and the duodenum the submucosa contains the end pieces of mucous galnds. In other parts of the tube, lymphoid tissue extends from the mucosa into the submucosa.

Muscularis. The muscularis is usually composed of two layers of muscle. The fibers of the inner coat are arranged circularly about the tube, whereas those of the outer coat lie in its long axis. This arrangement is followed

207

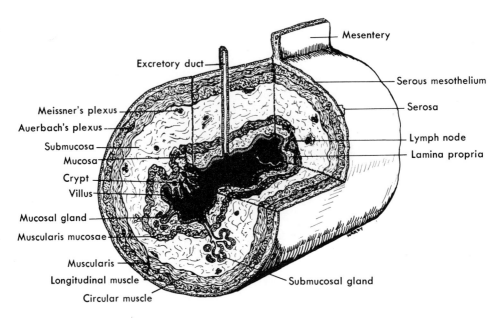

Fig. 14-1. Stereogram of general plan of gastrointestinal tract.

throughout the tract, but in the stomach there is a third oblique layer, next to the submucosa. Thickenings of the circular layer form sphincters at various points of the tract. In the upper end of the esophagus and the lower end of the rectum the muscle is striated; elsewhere it is smooth. The two layers of muscle are separated by a thin layer of connective tissue in which is seen the myenteric (Auerbach's) plexus of nerves.

Adventitia or serosa. The adventitia or serosa, the fourth layer of the tract, is composed of loose areolar tissue frequently containing adipose tissue. Where the tract borders on the body cavity the areolar tissue is covered by the mesothelium and is called the serosa. Elsewhere it blends with the surrounding fascia and is called the adventitia.

ESOPHAGUS

Mucosa. The esophageal region of the mucosa of the digestive tract is distinguished from the remainder by the fact that it is lined with stratified squamous epithelium, which rests on a fairly thick lamina propria (Figs. 14-2 and 14-3). Particular attention is called to the wide lumina of the ducts, which lead from the glands of the submucosa to the

surface. In many mammals the epithelium is cornified at its surface. Two narrow zones of glands are present in the mucosa of the esophagus, one at its junction with the stomach and the other at the level of the cricoid cartilage. These glands, called superficial glands *(cardiac)*, are shallow branching tubules that secrete mucus into the lumen of the organ. The mucosa also contains small lymph nodules and scattered lymphoid tissue.

The muscularis mucosae is absent in the upper part of the esophagus, its place being taken by a rather indefinite elastic membrane, which separates the mucosa from the submocosa (Fig. 14-2). Smooth muscle first appears about one fourth of the way down the tube in the form of scattered bundles longitudinally arranged. Farther down the tract these are consolidated in a complete layer. Unique features of the muscularis mucosa of the esophagus are that it is thicker than in any other part of the digestive tract and that the fibers run in only one direction.

Submucosa. The submucosa of the esophagus is generally described as a layer of areolar tissue containing throughout its length blood vessels, nerves, and the secreting portion of mucous glands. The ducts of the

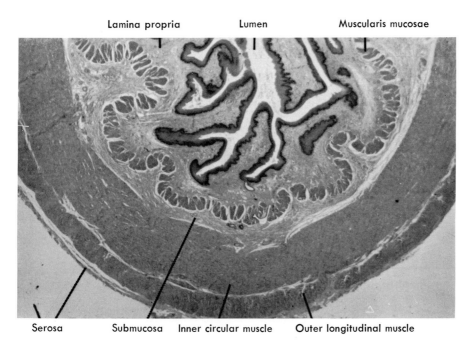

Lamina propria Lumen Muscularis mucosae

Serosa Submucosa Inner circular muscle Outer longitudinal muscle

Fig. 14-2. Transverse section of esophagus of dog. (×16.)

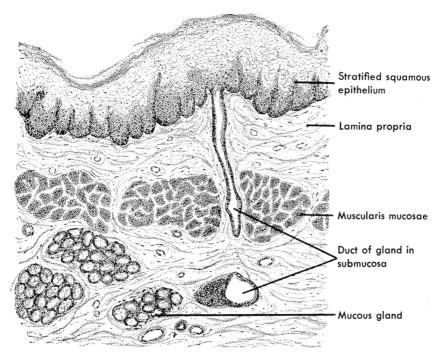

Stratified squamous epithelium

Lamina propria

Muscularis mucosae

Duct of gland in submucosa

Mucous gland

Fig. 14-3. Mucosa and submucosa of human esophagus.

glands run through the mucosa to open onto the epithelial surface. As a matter of fact, the glands are not constant in their distribution, and some animals (for example, the monkey) have only a few in this layer.

Muscularis. In the upper half of the esophagus the muscle is striated like that of the tongue. It is not, however, under voluntary control. In the lower half of the esophagus the muscle changes to the smooth variety; in the middle portion the two kinds may be found intermingled. The arrangement of the muscular coats of the esophagus is less regular than that of other parts of the digestive tract. Two coats are present, but both may have the fibers obliquely placed so that the typical orientation in any inner circular and outer longitudinal layer may not be apparent. This is particularly true in the esophagus of the dog.

STOMACH

Mucosa. At the junction of the esophagus and stomach the lining epithelium changes abruptly from stratified squamous to simple columnar (Fig. 14-4), the cells of which secrete mucus. The epithelium of the stomach, unlike that of the small intestine, does not have a cuticular border. The surface of the mucosa is thrown into folds *(rugae)*, the height and number of which depend on the degree of distention of the organ. In addition to the rugae, the surface of the mucosa is marked by closely set pits, which are lined with the same type of epithelium (Fig. 14-5). Beneath the epithelium is a lamina propria of reticular or fine areolar tissue, and below the level of the pits this layer contains glands. The shape and proportionate depth of the pits and the characteristics of the glands are different in different parts of the stomach. At the junction of the esophagus and stomach the pits are shallow, and the glands, which are lined with a simple cuboidal epithelium, have wide lumina and secrete thin mucus (Fig. 14-6).

In the fundic region (Fig. 14-7) the mucosa is much deeper than in the zone immediately below the esophagus, and it contains a greater number of glands. The lamina propria is reduced to a fine interglandular stroma in its deeper portion, and the pits extend only about one fourth of the distance from the surface to the muscularis mucosae. The glands are called fundic glands, or, since they are found in all parts of the organ ex-

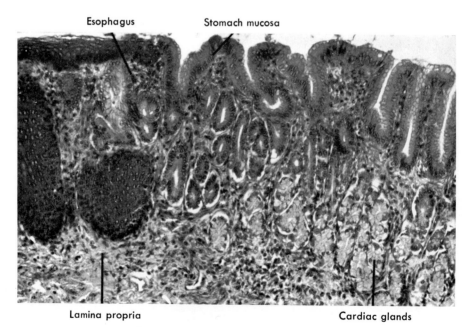

Esophagus   Stomach mucosa

Lamina propria   Cardiac glands

Fig. 14-4. Gastroesophageal junction in dog. (×160.)

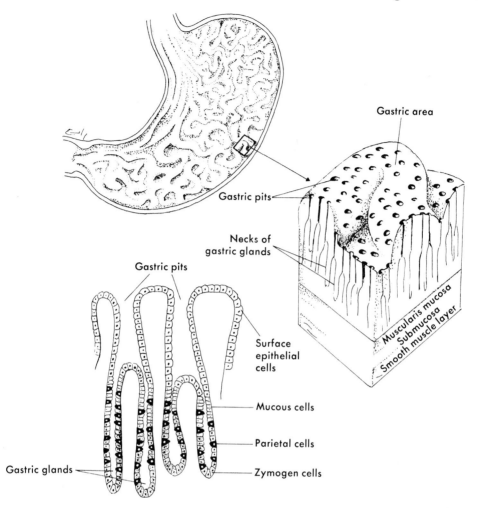

Fig. 14-5. Diagram showing folding of stomach mucosa and detail of a gastric area and gastric pits. A section through a gastric gland is shown on the lower left. (Drawing by Emily Craig.)

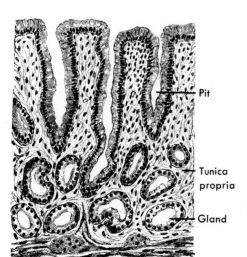

Fig. 14-6. Mucosa of cardiac region of stomach of monkey.

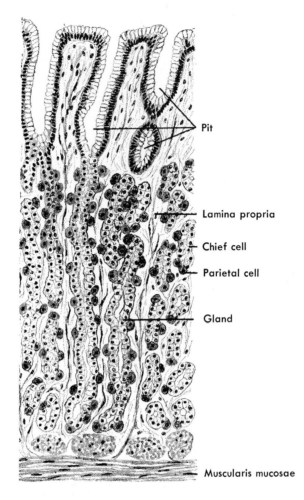

Pit

Lamina propria

Chief cell

Parietal cell

Gland

Muscularis mucosae

Fig. 14-7. Mucosa from fundus of stomach of monkey.

cept the cardiac and pyloric zones, they may be called gastric glands.

The surface mucous cells cover the entire surface and line the pits. They are columnar cells with nuclei located in the basal region. With routine preparations the apical cytoplasm stains faintly and has a foamy appearance. The electron microscope shows dense elliptical secretory granules in the apical part of the cell (Fig. 14-8). Each gastric gland is composed of four kinds of cells: (1) chief (peptic) cells, (2) parietal or oxyntic cells, (3) neck mucous cells, and (4) argentaffin cells.

1. The *chief cells* (Fig. 14-9) line the lower part of the gastric glands. They are low columnar and have the appearance of typi-

cal serous cells. These cells contain abundant striated basophilic material corresponding to the cisternae of the endoplasmic reticulum, which supports the synthesis of a large amount of protein for export. The chief cells also exhibit numerous mitochondria and secretory granules containing the precursor of pepsin.

2. The *parietal cells* are relatively large and intensely acidophilic. They are most numerous at the neck of the gland. They do not border directly on the lumen but are crowded away from it by the chief cells. The parietal cells appear somewhat oval, with the narrow end directed toward the lumen. These cells elaborate the antecedent of hydrochloric acid and are believed to elaborate the *intrinsic*

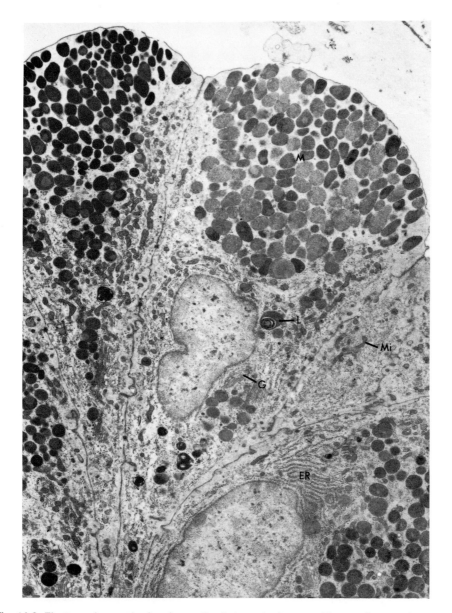

Fig. 14-8. Electron micrograph of surface cells of stomach of mouse. These cells are columnar and contain numerous mucinogen granules, *M,* at the distal surface. *ER,* Endoplasmic reticulum; *G,* Golgi apparatus; *L,* lysosome; *Mi,* mitochondrion. (×9,000.)

factor in humans, needed for the absorption of vitamin B_{12}. At the electron microscope level it has been shown that the cytoplasm contains numerous mitochondria and surface indentations, the secretory canaliculi (Fig. 14-10). The surfaces of the canaliculi are lined with microvilli. These specializations of the cell surface greatly enhance its surface area and represent the means by which the cell can secrete a strong acid. The details of this process are unclear but are believed to involve the elaborate canaliculi system.

3. The *neck mucous cells* are relatively few in number, have a wide base, and taper in the apical region. They are smaller than the surface cells and exhibit a considerable amount of basophilia. The mucous droplets in these cells, as shown by the electron mi-

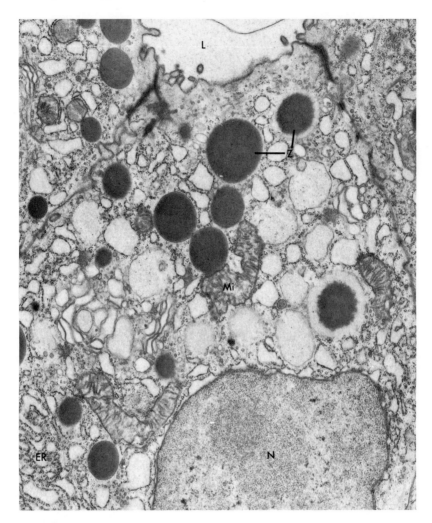

Fig. 14-9. Electron micrograph of apical part of a chief (zymogen) cell of gastric gland of mouse. *ER*, Rough endoplasmic reticulum; *L*, lumen; *Mi*, mitochondrion; *N*, nucleus; *Z*, zymogen granule. (×16,000.)

croscope, are larger and less dense than those of the surface cells, and they are distributed deep in the cell as well as in the apical region.

4. The *argentaffin cells* stain strongly with bichromatic salts. They are few and are scattered between the basement membrane and the chief cells. They contain characteristic granules, which are clearly shown in electron micrographs (Fig. 14-11). The granules are believed to contain monoamines such as serotonin, a vasoconstrictor that stimulates the contraction of smooth muscle. The nucleus is markedly infolded.

Argentaffin cells belong to a widespread group of cells, derived from neuroectoderm embryologically and having certain biochemical features in common. They are referred to as the APUD cell line, based on their capacity to synthesize monoamines *(Amine Precursor Uptake and Decarboxylation).* In the gut they can be found (here and there in the mucosal lining) all the way from the stomach to the colon. This far-flung distribution ensures that their secretion will represent an integrated response to the composition and consistency of the luminal contents. As a group they regulate the composition of

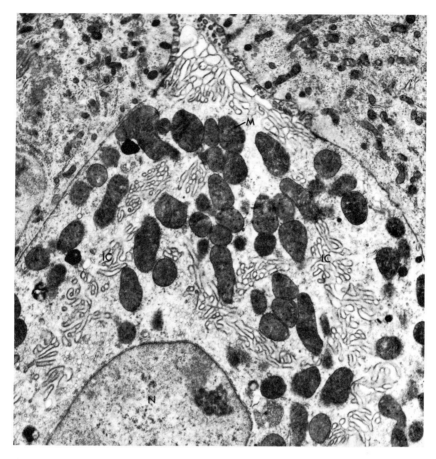

Fig. 14-10. Electron micrograph of a parietal cell of mouse gastric mucosa. The extensive intracellular secretory canaliculae, *IC,* within the cell exhibit numerous irregularly oriented microvilli. *N,* Nucleus; *M,* mitochondrion. (×15,000.) (Courtesy Dr. S. Luse.)

gastric secretions (water, enzyme, and electrolyte content), the motility of the gut wall, and the processes of absorption and utilization of nutrients. Among the hormones that have been localized immunocytochemically are secretin (which can be found in granular cells between the crypts and villi of the small intestine), cholecystokinin, and gastrin (in the antrum of the stomach).

In the pyloric region the pits are relatively deep, extending at least halfway to the muscularis mucosae (Fig. 14-12). They are V shaped, tapering off into the glands that open into them. The glands in this portion of the stomach are composed of large mucus-secreting cells and have wide lumina. No parietal cells exist in the pyloric glands except in the transition zone, where they merge with glands of the gastric type.

The muscularis mucosae of all parts of the stomach is a complete layer of smooth muscle, which includes both circular and longitudinal fibers.

Submucosa. The submucosa is composed of areolar tissue and does not contain glands in any part of the stomach. In a section of the junction of the esophagus and stomach some of the end pieces of deep mucous glands may extend into the submucosa of the stomach, but, since their ducts open into the esophagus, they should be considered as part of the wall of the latter organ. Small arteries, veins, and lymphatics may easily be seen in the submucosa. Meissner's plexus

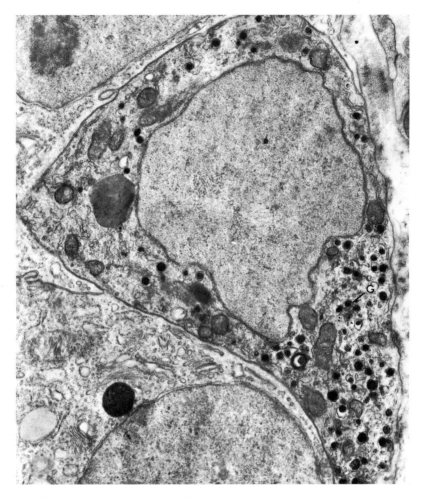

Fig. 14-11. Electron micrograph of argentaffin cell from gastric gland of mouse's intestine. The argentaffin cell contains numerous dense spherical granules, *G,* enclosed by a membrane. (×15,000.) (Courtesy Dr. S. Luse.)

of nerves and ganglia is less conspicuous.

Muscularis. In the stomach the muscular coat consists of two complete layers (inner circular and outer longitudinal), with an incomplete layer of obliquely arranged fibers between the circular layer and the submucosa. The circular layer is by far the thickest of the three coats. The arrangement of fibers is somewhat irregular, and it may be difficult to distinguish the three coats of the muscularis in a microscopic section of this region. Auerbach's plexus is present between the circular and longitudinal fibers.

The woven arrangement of muscle fibers in this sack-like organ permits the mixing and kneading action required to mix gastric

secretions with ingested food. This mechanical, grinding action reduces food to small particles in a slurry called chyme, which is then discharged at intervals into the duodenum.

In addition to more gentle mixing actions in the body of the stomach, the stomach displays intense peristaltic waves in the antrum, which squeeze the chyme and cause it to reflux back up into the body for further mixing. The body of the stomach has relatively little muscle tone and can bulge outward to store food as it enters the stomach from the esophagus.

The mesenteric (Auerbach's) plexus between the muscle sheets is needed to coordi-

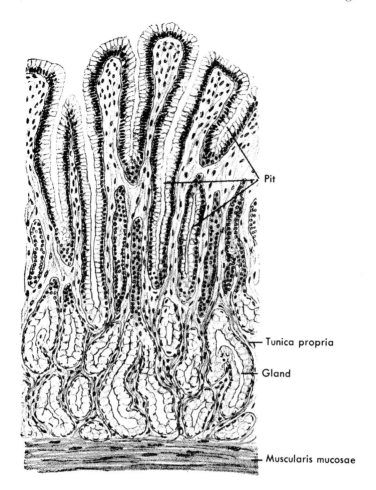

Fig. 14-12. Mucosa from pyloric region of stomach of monkey.

nate the otherwise weak and ineffectual intrinsic contractions of the smooth muscle. Parasympathetic discharges into the muscle sheet ensure that the cells contract en masse rather than individually.

Serosa. The greater part of the stomach is covered with a layer of mesothelium located outside the loose connective tissue that invests the muscle layers. This is, however, usually destroyed in the preparation of the piece of tissue for sectioning; all that is seen of the serosa is a coating of areolar tissue containing blood vessels, adipose tissue, and occasional nerve trunks.

SMALL INTESTINE

The small intestine extends from the pyloric part of the stomach to the large intestine. Its inner surface may be seen, on gross examination, to be marked by the presence of ridges that are circularly disposed and that extend into the lumen throughout this part of the tract. These ridges are the *plicae circulares* (Fig. 14-13). Each consists of a projection of the connective tissue of the submucosa covered by the mucosa. The plicae circulares provide a greater surface for the absorption of food.

Mucosa. The mucosal surface available for absorption is still further increased by the presence of minute fingerlike projections, of epithelium and lamina propria, which cover the surface of each plica. These villi are hardly visible to the naked eye (Fig. 14-13 to 14-15).

Villi. Under the microscope each villus is

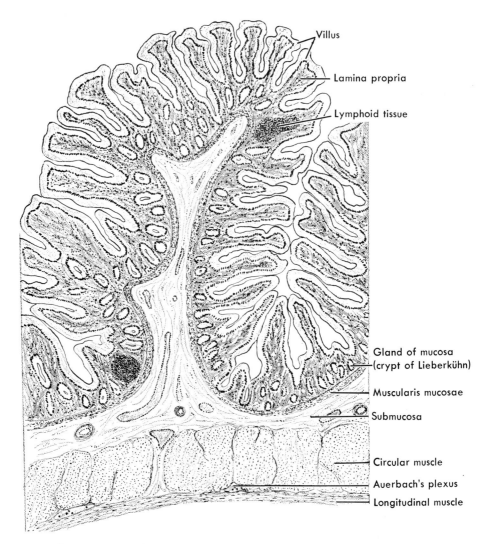

Fig. 14-13. Longitudinal section of jejunum of monkey showing a plica circularis.

seen to consist of a projection of the lamina propria covered by simple columnar epithelium and scattered goblet cells. The lamina propria is reticular tissue and contains capillaries, lymphatics, and scattered muscle fibers (Fig. 14-16). In an injected specimen, it is apparent that the vessels have a definite plan of distribution. In each villus is a central lymphatic called a lacteal (Fig. 14-14), available for absorption, into which certain lipids from the tract are absorbed. An arteriole enters the villus at one side and breaks up into capillaries at the distal end. Blood is collected from the capillaries by a venule, which

passes out along the side opposite that occupied by the arteriole. Villi occur in all parts of the small intestine and are its most characteristic feature. In the duodenum they are leafshaped; in the jejunum, tall and somewhat enlarged or forked at their distal ends. The ileum has shorter, club-shaped villi. Other parts of the tract have projections that at first sight might be mistaken for villi. In the stomach, for instance, the tissue between two pits has somewhat the same form as a villus and consists of a mass of reticular tissue covered by columnar epithelium. Closer examination reveals, however, that

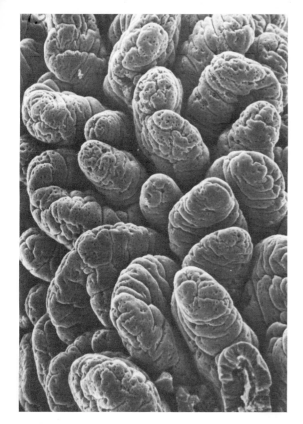

Fig. 14-14. Scanning electron micrograph of inner surface of small intestine of crab-eating monkey showing three-dimensional aspect of villi. (×65.) (Courtesy Dr. H. Nakahara.)

Fig. 14-15. Scanning electron micrograph of freeze-fracture preparation of section of jejunum of crab-eating monkey showing several villi. (×150.) (Courtesy Dr. H. Nakahara.)

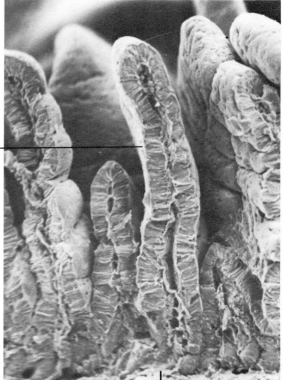
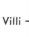

Villi

Lamina propria

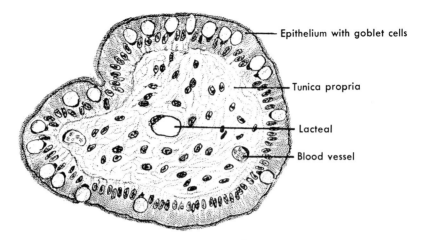

Epithelium with goblet cells

Tunica propria

Lacteal

Blood vessel

Fig. 14-16. Transverse section of villus.

the organization of vessels which is characteristic of a villus is lacking in the stomach.

The epithelium lining the villi rests on a delicate basement membrane (basal lamina plus the lamina reticularis) and consists of two distinct varieties: (1) the columnar absorbing cells and (2) goblet cells.

1. The *absorbing cells* are usually of the tall columnar variety, although they vary in shape as an adaptation to intestinal movements. The cytoplasm is finely granular and may contain lipid droplets. The nucleus is oval and located in the lower third of the cells.

A striking and distinguishing feature of the absorbing cells is the presence of a *striated* (brush) border. At the optical microscope level this border appears as a homogeneous refractive layer covering the surface of the cell. At the electron microscope level it is apparent that the striated border consists of numerous closely packed microvilli (Fig. 14-17). The surface of the microvillus is coated with branching filaments (fuzz) that stain positively for mucopolysaccharide (Fig 14-18). The center of the microvillus contains fine filaments longitudinally oriented, which terminate in the subjacent cytoplasm in a group of filaments known as the *terminal web*. Taken together, the folds of the intestinal lining, ranging from the large plicae circulares to the minute microvilli, increase

the surface area over 600 times what would be available if the gut lining were a simple smooth tube of the same diameter.

In addition to these features, the microvilli contain several enzymes such as alkaline phosphatase, ATPase, maltase, and amino peptidase. Accordingly, the striated border not only provides a tremendous increase in the luminal surface to carry on absorption but also contains several enzymes that participate in the digestive process.

Mitochondria, the Golgi complex, and endoplasmic reticulum do not exhibit unusual characteristics. The smooth variety however, is most prevalent in the apical region. Intercellular junctions at the adluminal surface are numerous and typical of junctional complexes previously described (Chapter 2).

2. The *goblet cells* are scattered among the columnar absorbing cells. During the elaboration of mucous, the apical part of the cell becomes distended into a typical goblet shape, and the nucleus and cytoplasm are displaced into the narrow basal region of the cell. During routine preparation of tissues, the mucigen droplets are dissolved and the upper part of the cell appears empty. Special staining methods show that the mucigen droplets are basophilic, periodic acid-Schiff positive, and metachromatic. These cells exhibit a few attenuated microvilli.

Glands. Between the bases of the villi,

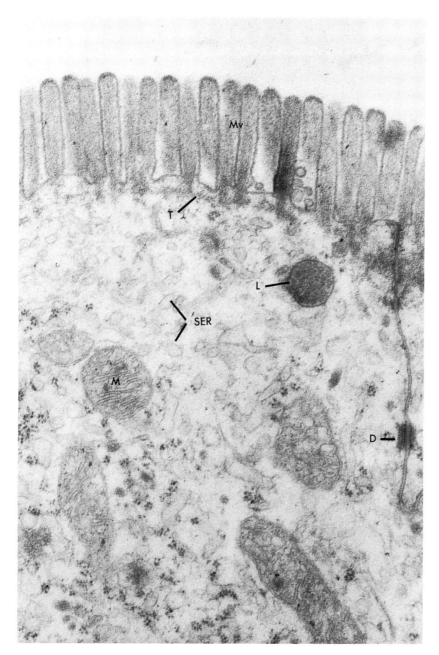

Fig. 14-17. Electron micrograph of portion of epithelial cell from small intestine of mouse. *D,* Desmosome; *L,* lysosome; *M,* mitochondrion; *Mv,* microvilli; *SER,* smooth endoplasmic reticulum; *T,* terminal web. (×48,000.)

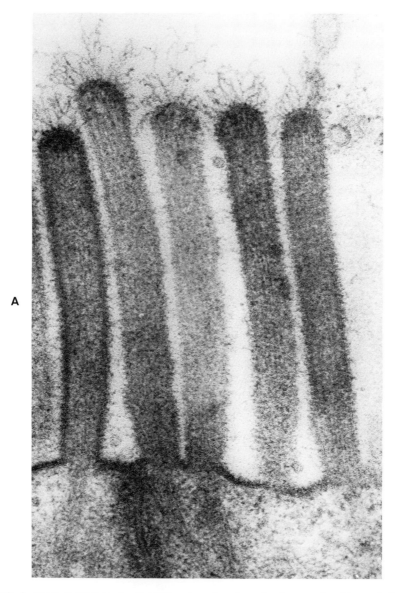

Fig. 14-18. A, Electron micrograph of apical region of portion of columnar absorbing cell shown at higher magnification than in Fig. 14-17. Note microvilli, terminal web region, and prominent fuzzy coat covering surface of microvilli. **B,** Electron micrograph of transverse section of several microvilli showing plasmalemma and core of filaments in each microvillus. (**A** ×150,000; **B** ×100,000.) (Courtesy Dr. H. Nakahara.)

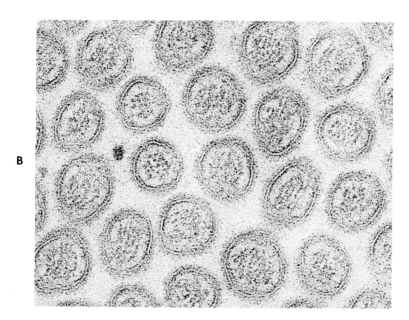

B

Fig. 14-18, cont'd. For legend see opposite page.

glands extend into the lower part of the mucosa (Fig. 14-19). These are the intestinal glands (crypts of Lieberkühn). At the base of each gland is a group of cells, the cells of Paneth, which are somewhat larger than the surrounding cells and have paler nuclei (Figs. 14-20 and 14-21). Their cytoplasm is sometimes darker, sometimes lighter, than that of the surrounding cells. Cells similar to the Paneth cells have been found in other parts of the digestive tract, but it is in the small intestine that they are most numerous and therefore most easily found.

It has long been assumed that Paneth cells secrete lysozyme. It appears that cell secretion is related in some way to amino acid and protein metabolism, since in children with severe protein malnutrition (kwashiorkor), Paneth cells are markedly reduced or absent. These cells reappear when nutrition is restored to normal. There is at present no evidence that Paneth cells do secrete digestive enzymes, and in fact the burden of information suggests that the cells may be involved in some other aspect of digestion. They are more numerous in the ileum than in the upper parts of the small intestine.

The rest of the crypt is lined with columnar epithelium somewhat resembling that which covers the villi. Its cells, however, are not quite as tall as those covering the villi, and fewer of them are goblet cells. Special stains bring out the fact that some of the lining cells have an affinity for silver stains, but this type (argentaffin cells) is not distinguishable when stained with hematoxylin and eosin. Like the cells of Paneth, argentaffin cells occur in other parts of the gut as well as in the small intestine. The cells of the crypts provide new cells for the villi surfaces to replace those shed into the lumen. It has been estimated that the villus surface is renewed every few days in humans.

Lymphoid tissue. Lymphoid tissue is widely distributed throughout the mucosa of the small intestine. In the ileum the nodules are gathered into groups (Peyer's patches) and fill not only the mucosa but also the submucosa. These groups of nodules will be further described later in this discussion.

Muscularis mucosae. The muscularis mucosae consists of two thin layers of smooth muscle, an inner circular and an outer longi-

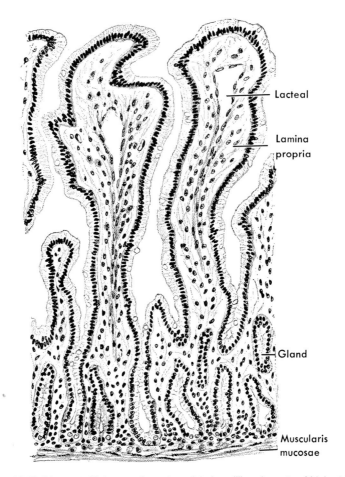

Fig. 14-19. Mucosa of jejunum of monkey showing villi and crypts of Lieberkühn.

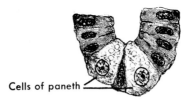

Fig. 14-20. Epithelium at base of crypt of Lieberkühn.

tudinal layer. It thus repeats in miniature the arrangement of the muscularis coat.

Submucosa. The submucosa of the intestinal wall is different in the three divisions of the small intestine. Its basis is the same throughout: a layer of areolar tissue containing the vessels and nerves of Heller's and Meissner's plexuses, respectively. In the duodenum the layer contains, in addition,

groups of mucous glands. These are duodenal glands of Brunner (Fig. 14-22). Their secretion, which is mucus similar to that formed in the cardiac glands of the stomach, enters the duodenum through ducts, which open on the surface between the crypts of Lieberkühn or into the crypts themselves. These glands are thought to secrete a fluid that aids in protecting the duodenal surface from the

Fig. 14-21. Electron micrograph of several cells at base of intestinal gland of mouse. Cell with prominent dark granules. *P,* Paneth cell; *ER,* endoplasmic reticulum. (×6,700.)

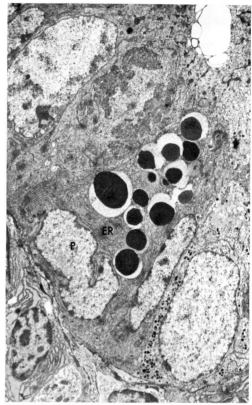

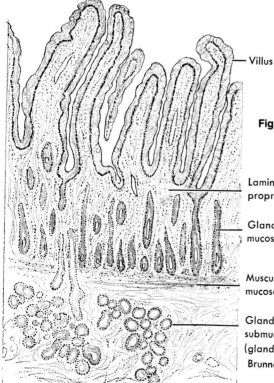

Villus

Fig. 14-22. Mucosa and submucosa of duodenum of monkey.

Lamina propria

Gland of mucosa

Muscularis mucosae

Glands of submucosa (glands of Brunner)

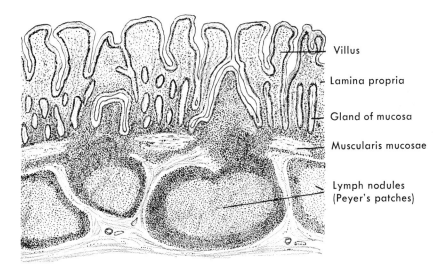

Villus

Lamina propria

Gland of mucosa

Muscularis mucosae

Lymph nodules
(Peyer's patches)

Fig. 14-23. Mucosa and submucosa of ileum showing Peyer's patches.

acidic contents of the stomach as they enter the duodenum. In adults these glands do not extend much beyond the mouth of the duct of Wirsung, through which the pancreas empties its buffered secretions into the duodenum. In the ileum, groups of lymph nodules occupy both mucosa and submucosa (Fig. 14-23). Each group consists of from ten to sixty nodules with germinal centers, and the groups are so large that they are visible to the naked eye. They not only fill the submucosa and the mucosa but also extend a little into the lumen of the intestine, obliterating the villi. They are called Peyer's patches or the aggregate lymph nodules of the intestine. Similar aggregates may be present in the lower part of the jejunum, but the majority of the sections from this part of the tract have only a small amount of lymphoid tissue. Glands are never found in the submucosa of the jejunum. It is characterized by its exceptionally high branching plicae circulares and its long villi.

Muscularis. The muscularis of the small intestine consists, throughout its length, of an inner circular and an outer longitudinal layer of smooth muscle. Between these, as in other parts of the tract, lies Auerbach's plexus of nerves.

Serosa. As in the stomach, the serosa is a layer of connective tissue covered by meso-

thelium. This arrangement of muscle supports the mixing and propulsive contractions of the gut tube. These movements are dependent mainly on the myenteric plexus of the gut, although very weak contractions can occur even if the plexus is blocked by atropine. The intensity of contraction is increased by parasympathetic stimulation and diminished by sympathetic stimulation.

LARGE INTESTINE

In the large intestine the plicae circulares are replaced by the semilunar folds. These folds include not only the mucosa and submucosa but also the inner layer of the muscularis and are grossly visible on the outside, as well as on the inside, of the gut. As the name implies, they are crescentic in shape, each one extending about one third of the way around the wall of the large intestine. A description of the characteristics of the four coats of this region follows.

Mucosa (Fig. 14-24). Water and electrolytes are absorbed from the large intestine, and its lining is well supplied with mucus-secreting cells. It has no villi. In the embryo, villi are present in the large intestine but disappear during late fetal life. The epithelium consists of simple columnar absorbing cells and numerous goblet cells. The lamina propria contains many glands. These are sim-

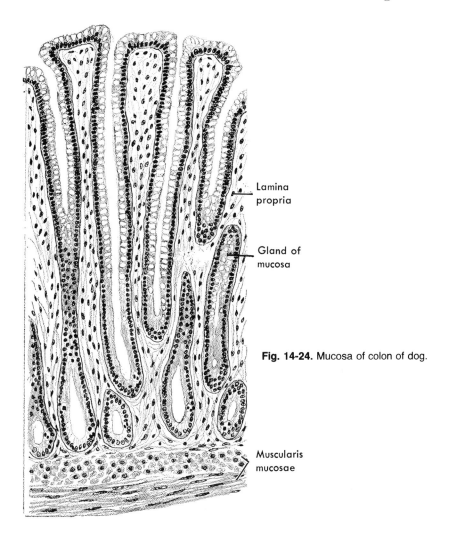

Lamina
propria

Gland of
mucosa

Fig. 14-24. Mucosa of colon of dog.

Muscularis
mucosae

ple tubular glands, closely set, lined with epithelium similar to that covering the surface of the mucosa. They have few cells of Paneth. The lamina propria contains blood and lymph capillaries, but these are not organized in definite units, as are those of the small intestine. Solitary lymph nodules are present and are often so large that they break through into the submucosa. The muscularis mucosae is composed of an inner circular and an outer longitudinal layer (Figs. 14-24 and 14-25), as in the small intestine.

Submucosa. The submucosa of the colon has no glands. Besides the areolar tissue with vessels and nerves, it contains only the solitary lymph nodules, mentioned previously.

Muscularis. The inner circular layer of the muscularis is continuous around the wall and is thrown into folds with the mucosa and submucosa. The longitudinal layer is in the form of three bands, which run through the length of the large intestine. These are called the taeniae coli. When dissected away from the rest of the wall, they are found to be considerably shorter than the wall, and this difference in length produces the semilunar fold in the longer parts. The effect of the taeniae is like that of a drawstring run through a piece of cloth.

Serosa. The serosa contains large deposits of adipose tissues, which protrude on the outer surface of the tube and are macroscopically visible as the appendices epiploicae.

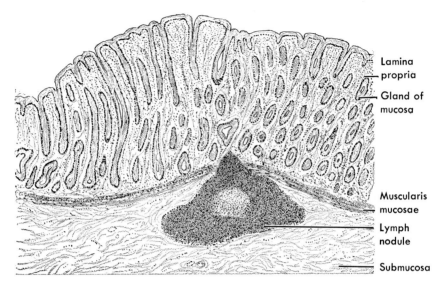

Fig. 14-25. Mucosa and submucosa of colon of dog showing a solitary lymph nodule.

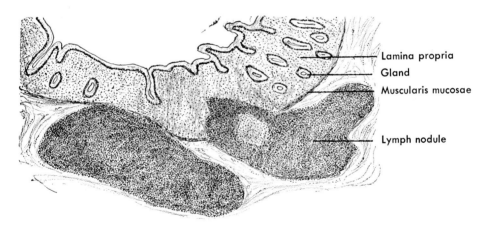

Fig. 14-26. Mucosa and submucosa of human appendix.

VERMIFORM APPENDIX

The wall of the vermiform appendix resembles that of the colon but is thickened by accumulations of lymphoid tissue (Fig. 14-26).

Mucosa. The epithelium of the mucosa is simple columnar and in the normal appendix is highly folded. Extending from the surface are simple tubular glands containing numerous mucus-secreting and occasional Paneth cells. Argentaffin cells are a frequent occurrence in the middle third of the wall of the crypts. The lamina propria contains an accumulation of lymphoid follicles resembling those of the pharyngeal tonsils and, like the latter, may show inflammatory changes. In a condition of subacute inflammation of the appendix, the lumen may be narrowed or obliterated and the mucosa replaced in part by fibrous scar tissue and confluent nodules of lymphoid tissue. This condition is seen rather frequently. The muscularis mucosae is interrupted by the lymph nodules and in places is reduced to only a few strands of muscle. The mucosa of the appendix is basically arranged like that of the

Table 3. Peculiarities in parts of digestive tract

	Mucosa	Submucosa	Muscularis
Esophagus	Stratified squamous epithelium Glands confined to two narrow zones Muscularis mucosae lacking in upper part	Mucous glands	Striated in upper part

Stomach	Cardiac—Shallow pits
	    Mucous glands
	Fundus—Pits elongated
	    Fundic (gastric)
	    Glands prominent
	Pylorus—Pits relatively deep
	    Glands mucous type
			Oblique layer of muscle
			    inside circular layer

Duodenum	Villi; leaflike	Mucous glands; plicae are low	
Jejunum	Villi; tall	Tall branching plicae	
Ileum	Villi; club-shaped	Large groups of lymphoid nodules	
Colon	No pits or villi Many goblet cells in epithelium		Longitudinal muscle ar- ranged in three bands
Appendix	No pits or villi; much lymphoid tissue	Much lymphoid tissue	
Rectum	Like colon; stratified squamous		
Anus	Noncornified, stratified squamous epithelium		Internal circular muscle forms internal sphincter

colon except that the glands are less numerous and the lymph nodules more prevalent in the appendix.

Submucosa. The submucosa is composed of areolar tissue with vessels, nerves, and lymphoid tissue.

Muscularis. The muscularis is composed of two complete layers, as in other parts of the tract.

Serosa. The serosa presents no exceptional features.

• • •

The peculiarities of the different parts of the digestive tract that may be used as diagnostic features in identifying sections are presented in Table 3.

RECTUM AND ANUS

The rectum is divided into an upper and a lower part. The upper part extends from the third sacral vertebra to the diaphragm of the pelvis. The mucosa of this part is similar to that of the colon. The crypts of Lieberkühn however, are, longer and contain many goblet cells. The muscularis mucosa,

submucosa, and circularly arranged smooth muscle are also similar to those of the colon. The taeniae coli, however, spread out and form a continuous layer, which is much thickened in the dorsal and ventral surface of the gut wall.

The surface of the lower part of the rectum (anal canal) is thrown into several longitudinal folds known as the rectal columns (of Morgagni). At the lower termination these folds unite with one another to form the anal valves. At the level of the anal valves the epithelium becomes stratified squamous of a noncornified variety. The noncornified epithelium extends nearly to the anal orifice, where it changes to stratified squamous, characteristic of the epidermis. At the level of the anal orifice, hairs, sweat glands, and sebaceous glands occur. The sweat glands are of two types. One type has the structure characteristic of glands found in various parts of the body; the second type (circumanal) is large and resembles the axillary sweat glands.

At the approximate level of the anal valves, the muscularis mucosae becomes much diminished and eventually is lacking entirely. The submucosa contains an abundant supply of arteries and veins. The inner circular layer of the muscularis of the anal canal is composed of smooth muscle, is relatively thick, and serves as the internal anal sphincter. The outer longitudinal layer of smooth muscle continues over the internal sphincter and attaches to connective tissue. Also present is an external sphincter composed of striated muscle lying internal to a third sphincter, the levator ani.

BLOOD SUPPLY OF THE STOMACH AND INTESTINES

The arteries that supply the gut pass through the mesentery to reach the serosa where they branch into smaller vessels. The latter continue through the two coats of the muscularis to the submucosa, where they form an extensive (Heller's) plexus. From the plexus of the submucosa, blood passes to the mucosa and to the muscular coat of the gut (Fig. 14-27).

NERVE SUPPLY OF THE STOMACH AND INTESTINES

The nerve supply of the stomach and intestines consists chiefly of nonmyelinated and myelinated (preganglionic) fibers of the autonomic system. When the nerves reach the connective tissue between the two layers of the muscularis coat, they are associated with ganglion cells to form the plexus of Auerbach. From the plexus, fibers pass to the submucosa where they form another plexus, Meissner's plexus.

LYMPHOID TISSUE IN THE GUT MUCOSA

Few tissues have such a dense or diverse accumulation of lymphoid cells as the gut. These cell groups can be divided into three categories: lymphoid follicles, accumulations of plasma cells, and epithelial lymphoid cells (the theliolymphocytes). The lymphoid follicles occur in the mucosa or submucosa throughout the entire extent of the gut. They are most prominent, however, in the lower

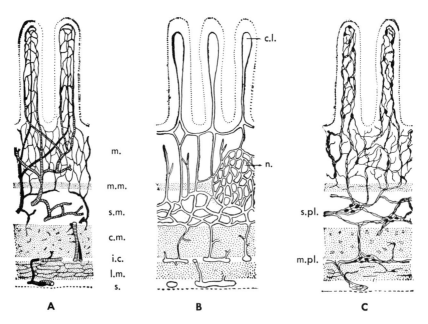

Fig. 14-27. A, Diagram of blood vessels of small intestine; arteries appear as coarse black lines; capillaries as fine ones; and veins are shaded. **B,** Diagram of lymphatic vessels. **C,** Diagram of nerves based on Golgi preparations. Layers of intestine: *m,* mucosa; *mm,* muscularis mucosae, *sm,* submucosa; *cm,* circular muscle; *ic,* intermuscular connective tissue; *lm,* longitudinal muscle; *s,* serosa; *cl,* central lymphatic; *n,* nodule; *spl,* submucous plexus; *mpl,* myenteric plexus. (**A** and **B** after Mall; **C** after Cajal; from Bremer, F., and H. Weatherford. 1948. Text-book of histology. The Blakiston Co., Philadelphia.)

ileum (Peyer's patches), the appendix, and the nasopharyngeal adenoid tissue. The theliolymphocytes can be observed between the epithelial cells in the basal third of the lining of the gut, especially in the small intestine. The lymphoid follicles and the theliolymphocytes (which are thought to be young lymphocytes returning to the lamina propria by way of the bloodstream), are said to be the equivalent of the bursa of Fabricius, a hindgut lymphoid organ present in birds that appears to be involved in the development of the immunoglobulin-producing system *(humoral immunity)*. In contrast, the thymus is held responsible for controlling development of *cell-mediated immunity*. (Chapter 10). Plasma cells are uniformly scattered in the lamina propria of the villi and between glandular crypts as well, especially in the duodenum, jejunum, and colon. Most of the plasma cells produce immunoglobulin A (IgA) in contrast to cells of the lymph nodes and spleen, which produce mostly immunoglobulin G (IgG). It has been suggested that these plasma cells respond to local antigenic stimulation, since IgA production is scant or lacking in germfree animals, a situation that is reversed when animals are placed on a septic diet. IgA is secreted onto the luminal surface in the mucus. These molecules may be bactericidal and may help tie up foreign protein before it can cross the gut wall and enter the bloodstream or interact with tissue mast cells to elicit histamine release and an allergic response. A similar protective mechanism operates in the respiratory tract.

15

Glands associated with the digestive tract

In addition to the glands situated in the wall of the digestive tract, large masses of glandular tissue lie outside the limits of the tube and pour their secretions into it through ducts. These are the salivary glands, the ducts of which open into the oral cavity, and the pancreas and liver, secretions of which go to the intestine. The pancreas resembles the salivary glands and is most conveniently studied in connection with them. The gallbladder will also be included in this discussion.

SALIVARY GLANDS AND PANCREAS

Because microscopically the tissues of the salivary glands closely resemble those of the pancreas, they are discussed in the same section of this chapter. Differentiation between the two is discussed on p. 249 and in Figs. 15-1 and 15-2.

Salivary glands

The salivary glands consist of several glandular structures that secrete a fluid known as *saliva*. Numerous small glands are located in the oral mucous membrane. The secretions of these glands serve to moisten and lubricate the membrane. In addition, three pairs of large glands are situated some distance from the oral cavity. These structures, usually known as the salivary glands proper, are the parotid, submaxillary (submandibular), and sublingual glands. In the human, the parotid gland has only serous alveoli; the submaxillary and sublingual

glands have both serous and mucous alveoli. Accordingly, the parotid glands are classified as serous, the palatine glands as mucous, and the submaxillary and sublingual glands as mixed.

Saliva assists in the process of chewing by dissolving readily soluble components of the food, initiating digestion of starch (by salivary amylase), softening the food mass, and coating the mass with a lubricant film. Saliva also contains substances (such as IgA) that discourage bacterial growth and thus may help to suppress tooth decay. Although the amount of antibodies in saliva is small, from 600 to 800 ml of saliva is secreted per day, containing a total of about 200 mg of immunoglobulin. During sleep little saliva is secreted by the major salivary glands. A small amount of saliva is continuously secreted by the minor salivary glands. Circadian rhythms are evident in daily saliva output as well.

The salivary glands consist of the glandular tissue proper, also known as the *parenchyma*, and a supporting interstitial connective tissue framework, the *stroma*. The connective tissue septum divides the glands into units known as lobes and lobules. Collecting ducts and vascular and nerve elements are located in the septum.

Parotid glands

The parotids, the largest major salivary glands, are located below and somewhat anterior to the ears. In man as well as the dog,

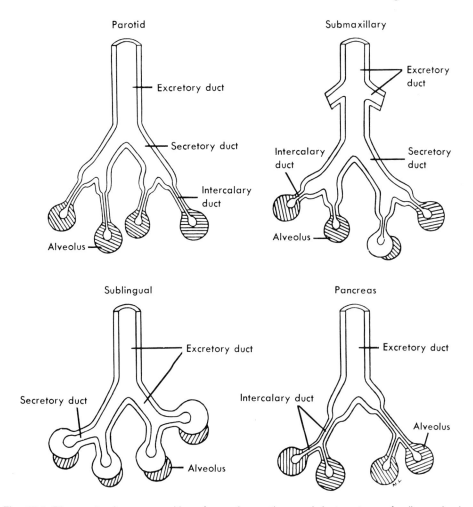

Fig. 15-1. Diagram to show composition of secreting portions and duct systems of salivary glands and pancreas. Alveoli and crescents that are shaded are serous cells; those unshaded are mucous cells.

cat, and rabbit it is entirely serous. The main excretory (Stensen's) duct opens into the oral cavity opposite the second molar tooth.

As will be seen from Figs. 15-1 to 15-3, the parotid has excretory, secretory, and intercalary (intercalated) ducts, which lead out from serous alveoli. The arrangement of these elements in sequence is not as clear in sections as it is in Fig. 15-1. Numerous alveoli with intercalary and secretory ducts are crowded together to form a lobule. A fine connective tissue stroma, often containing fat cells, surrounds the alveoli, and a heavier sheath of the same tissue separates adjacent lobules. A group of lobules forms a lobe, covered in turn with a connective tissue sheath that mingles at the outer borders of the gland with the surrounding fascia. Within the lobule the alveoli and ducts are cut in various directions, and their connections are not always clear. One may, however, find a group of alveoli through which the plane of section passes vertically, and in such a case the arrangement is visible.

Several alveoli open together into a fine duct called the intercalary duct. This tubule is composed of flattened cells. Several intercalary ducts open into a tubule lined with columnar epithelium, the secretory (striated) duct. The cells of this duct have a centrally located, spheroidal nucleus and a cytoplasm

Secretory duct

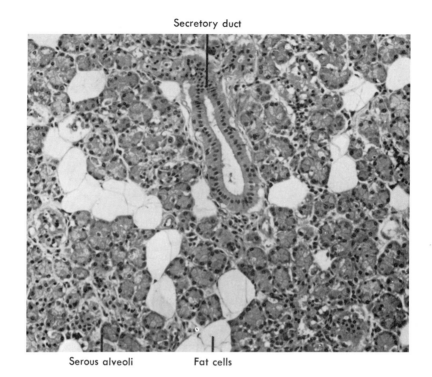

Serous alveoli   Fat cells

Fig. 15-2. Section of human parotid gland. (×160.)

Serous alveolus

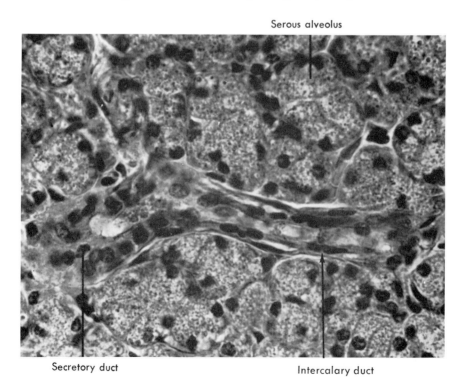

Secretory duct   Intercalary duct

Fig. 15-3. Human parotid. (×640.)

that is finely granular and acidophilic. The basal part of the cell exhibits a marked striated appearance. The numerous rod-shaped mitochondria located in this part of the cell are perpendicular to the base of the cell. Also present are basal infoldings of the plasma membrane extending into the cytoplasm. The arrangement of mitochondria and plasma membrane infoldings in these cells is similar to the configuration observed in the cells of the proximal convoluted tubules of the kidney and, as in the kidney cells, is concerned with actively transporting ions and regulation of fluids. These ducts open, in turn, into excretory ducts, which are lined with tall columnar epithelium. As one traces these ducts toward the opening into the oral cavity, the epithelium is seen to change from columnar (in the secretory ducts) to pseudostratified,

then stratified columnar, and finally stratified squamous.

The end pieces or alveoli are composed entirely of serous cells, which are wedge shaped and are grouped about a small lumen. The cell boundaries are usually indistinct. The appearance of the cells varies considerably, depending on the state of activity. In the resting condition numerous granules appear in the distal portion of the cell. After secretion the number of granules is reduced, whereas the number of vacuoles is increased. The fate of these vacuoles is uncertain, since the membrane material does not appear to be recycled for use in new secretory granules. The granules, which are refractile, are known as *zymogen granules* and are concerned with the elaboration of the enzyme produced by the cell (Fig. 15-4).

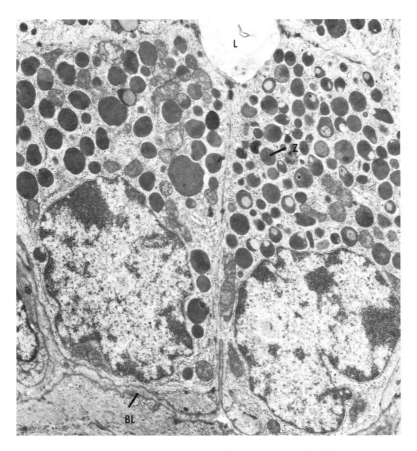

Fig. 15-4. Electron micrograph of two acinar cells of rhesus parotid. *BL,* Basement lamina; *Z,* zymogen granules; *L,* lumen of acinus. (×9,400.)

In addition to mitochondria and a Golgi apparatus, which are common to secreting cells, the rough endoplasmic reticulum, appearing as a group of membranes adjacent to the nuclei, is also an important cytologic component of the serous cells. The granules associated with the endoplasmic reticulum are strongly basophilic, are composed of ribonucleoprotein, and are associated with the synthesis of proteins within the cell, such as zymogen granules.

With the aid of special techniques, delicate *intercellular secretory canaliculi* may be demonstrated in serous alveoli. These canaliculi appear to penetrate the cells themselves and are then known as the *intracellular secretory canaliculi*. They are common to serous alveoli. An additional element, is a peculiar stellate-shaped cell occupying a position between the secreting cells and the basement membrane (Fig. 15-13). Closely associated with the secreting cells, their processes form a basketlike structure around the alveolus. They are known as *basket* or *myoepithelial cells.*

Myoepithelial cells (Fig. 15-9) receive sympathetic fibers, and the stimulation of these fibers contracts the cells. The function of myoepithelial cells in the secretion of saliva is speculative. Besides assisting in moving the acinar fluid along the ducts, the myoepithelial cells may also take part in changing the composition of saliva by controlling the contact time of the passing fluid with the duct cells. Myoepithelial cells have been shown to possess strong alkaline phosphatase activity as well. Saliva is quickly expelled into the mouth by myoepithelial contraction, and it has been suggested that this action would aid in expelling highly viscous saliva.

Fine structure of acinar cells. The parotid is a serous type of gland and the pyramid-shaped cells rest on a well-defined basement lamina. The nucleus is prominent, irregularly shaped, and basally located. In favorable sections a cytocentrum is observed in a supranuclear position and close to the Golgi apparatus. Profiles of rough endoplasmic

Serous alveolus   Secretory duct

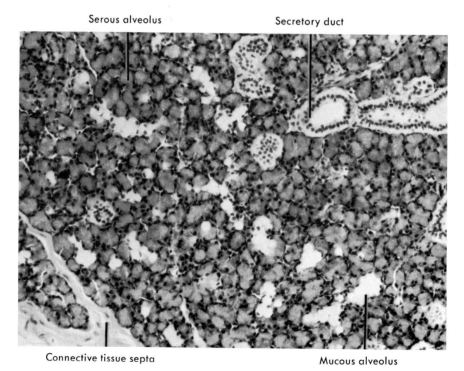

Connective tissue septa   Mucous alveolus

Fig. 15-5. Mixed salivary gland (submaxillary) of cat, serous type. (×40.)

reticulum cisternae are numerous and are scattered throughout the cytoplasm. Mitochondria are few and are usually located in the distal part of the cell. The most prominent feature of the cytoplasm is the presence of numerous, large, spherical secretory granules containing the precursor of amylase, which is concerned with the digestion of carbohydrates. The cells lie in close apposition to one another, and desmosomes occasionally occur where the cells appose each other. The distal surface that forms the border of the lumen of the acinus subtends small microvilli (Fig. 15-4).

Submaxillary (submandibular) glands

The submaxillary gland is a mixed gland, but the proportion of mucous and serous alveoli varies in different species. In humans

it is mostly serous. The secretion is conveyed chiefly by Wharton's duct, which opens in the oral cavity beneath the tongue. This duct is lined with pseudostratified columnar epithelium, plus a stroma of longitudinally arranged smooth muscle cells.

As in the parotid glands, there are excretory, secretory, and intercalary ducts in the submaxillary glands (Figs. 15-1 and 15-5), but the last named are short and difficult to find. The alveoli are of two kinds. Many are pure serous, like those of the parotid; others are mixed serous and mucous (Figs. 15-6 and 15-7). The mucous cells of a mixed alveolus are grouped around the lumen and are distinguished from the serous cells by their paler cytoplasm and their basal, flattened nuclei. The serous cells are arranged in the form of a cap outside the mucous cells. They

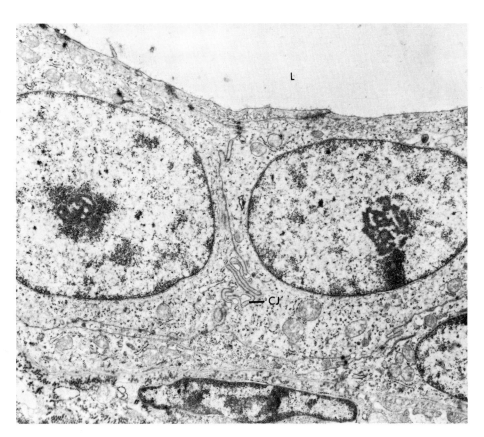

Fig. 15-6. Electron micrograph of part of epithelium of intercalated duct of submaxillary gland of the cat. These cells are low cuboidal type, having large centrally placed nuclei and prominent cell junctions, *CJ;* lumen, *L.* (×12,000.)

Serous alveolus

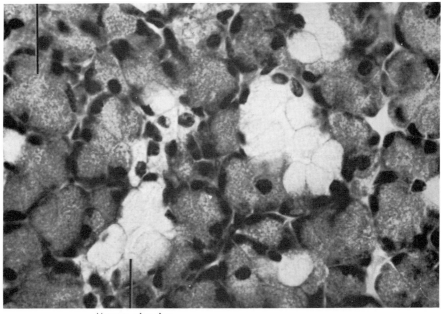

Mucous alveolus

Fig. 15-7. Mixed salivary gland (submaxillary) of cat, chiefly serous alveoli. (×640.)

Lumen

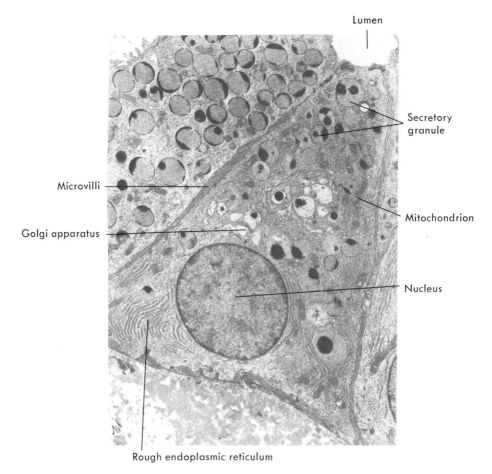

Secretory
granule

Microvilli

Mitochondrion

Golgi apparatus

Nucleus

Rough endoplasmic reticulum

Fig. 15-8. Electron micrograph of serous cell from human submandibular gland. (×6,500.) (Courtesy Dr. H. Nakahara.)

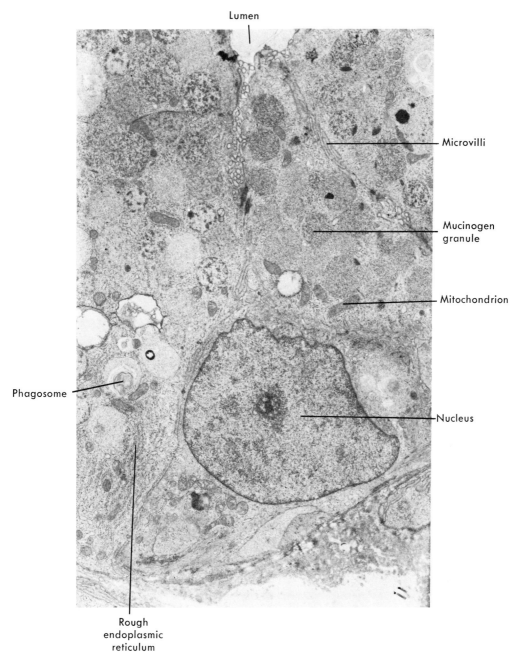

Lumen

Microvilli

Mucinogen granule

Mitochondrion

Nucleus

Phagosome

Rough endoplasmic reticulum

Fig. 15-9. Electron micrograph of mucous cells from human submandibular gland. (×9,000.) (Courtesy Dr. H. Nakahara.)

do not border on the lumen of the alveolus, but pour their secretion into it through minute channels between the mucous cells. Such groups of serous cells are often crescent shaped in sections and are called demilunes of Heidenhain. In the submaxillary gland, which has many purely serous alveoli, the demilunes of the mixed alveoli are small. The serous cells, when viewed at higher magnifications, reveal the presence of a prominent rough endoplasmic reticulum, Golgi complex, and many Golgi-derived secretory granules (Fig. 15-8).

The mucous cells occurring in either the mixed or pure mucous alveoli are modified cuboidal or low columnar cells. When stained with hematoxylin and eosin, they ap-pear as follows: the cells rest on a fine reticular basement membrane, and in this resting condition their nuclei appear flattened and occupy a position near the base of the cell. The cytoplasm appears pale blue in contrast to the deeper blue or purple coloration of the serous cells. The cytoplasm contains a basephilic network and numerous granules. In the active condition, the granules enlarge and become droplets, which may occupy a considerable portion of the cell (Fig. 15-9). During secretion the droplets of mucin are discharged, and the cell returns to the resting state. Mitochondria and the Golgi apparatus are not prominent features of these cells, and intracellular canaliculi are lacking.

Secretory duct

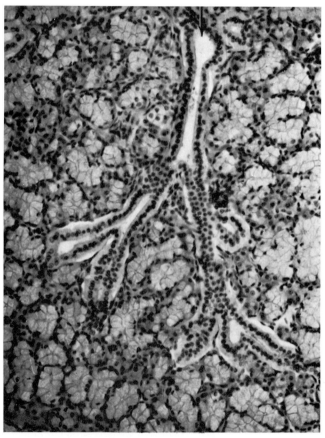

Fig. 15-10. Mixed salivary gland, sublingual, of dog, chiefly of mucous alveoli together with ducts in septa. (×200.)

Sublingual glands

The sublingual glands are mixed glands in man as well as the dog, cat, and sheep and are the smallest of the chief salivary glands. They consist of a group of glands that lie beneath the mucous membrane of the floor of the mouth. Several ducts empty into the mouth at the side of the frenulum of the tongue near the opening of Wharton's duct.

The duct system of the sublingual gland differs from that of the other salivary glands in that the intercalary ducts are usually lacking entirely and the striated or salivary ducts are few in number. The larger ducts are lined by pseudostratified epithelium, which is replaced by simple columnar epithelium in the smaller ducts (Figs. 15-10 and 15-11). The overall appearance of a section of this gland shows it to be a mixed gland, predominantly mucous in character (Figs. 15-11 and 15-12). The terminal alveoli are usually mucous. Pure serous alveoli are infrequently present. However, large serous cells, in the form of demilunes surrounding mucous alveoli, are numerous. This gland does not have a distinct capsule. Myoepithelial cells are also present (Fig. 15-13).

Blood and nerve supply

The salivary glands have a relatively rich blood supply consisting of arteries, veins, and lymphatics, which run in the connective tissue septa along with the ducts. The arteries branch into capillary networks where they eventually surround the alveoli. The innervation of the salivary glands is complicated and involves fibers of the sympathetic and parasympathetic systems.

Physiology of salivation

The flow of saliva is regulated by nerves of the autonomic nervous system. Both sets of nerves, parasympathetic and sympathetic, are able to affect the secretory process, which occurs reflexly.

Beta-adrenergic receptor stimulation is accompanied by an increase in cyclic AMP, causing secretion of amylase. During sympathetic stimulation cyclic AMP thus provides a link in the coupling between stimulation and secretion. Since saliva can be secreted at pressures higher than capillary pressure, it is agreed that saliva formation and secretion is not due to hydrostatic filtration, as is urine formation.

Fig. 15-11. Mixed sublingual gland in dog. (×640.)

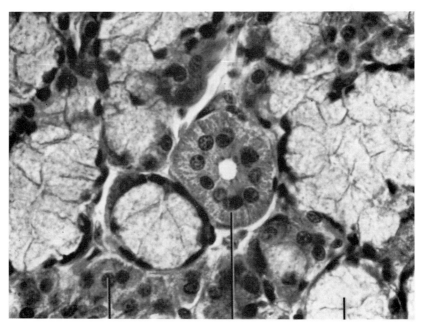

Serous cells   Striated duct   Mucous cells

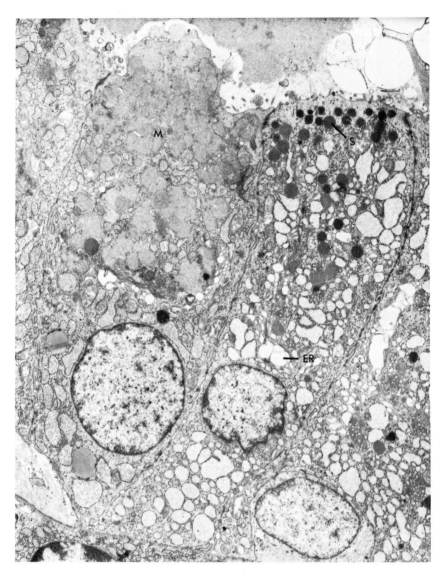

Fig. 15-12. Electron micrograph of part of acinus of sublingual gland of cat. Left, mucous cell with droplets of mucinogen, *M;* right, serous cell exhibiting numerous dilated cisternae of endoplasmic reticulum, *ER,* and distally, secretory granules, *S.* (×7,200.)

The energy for salivary secretion is provided by metabolism of the acinar cells, which produce the secretion and are responsible for the secretory pressure also. Adjustments in electrolyte content of the secretion are made by the duct cells, which can reabsorb salt across the duct wall.

In spite of this difference in the formation of precursor fluid, there are important parallels between saliva and urine formation. Evidence from micropuncture and microperfusion studies indicate that the salivary gland, like the kidney, elaborates in its proximal segment a fluid that is isotonic to plasma and is high in sodium ions and low in potassium ions. Resorption of sodium ions and secretion of potassium ions occur in the more distal segments of the gland. Sodium resorption by the salivary ducts is dependent on the presence of aldosterone in a manner not unlike

Acinar (serous) cells   Lumen

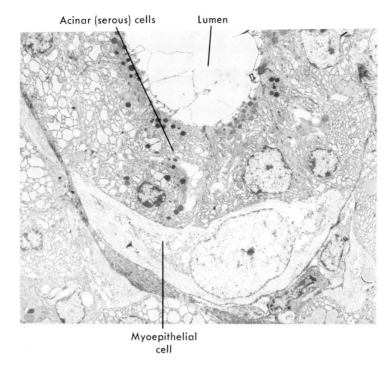

Myoepithelial
cell

Fig. 15-13. Electron micrograph of sublingual gland of cat. (×4,800.) (Courtesy Dr. H. Nakahara.)

its action on the kidney tubule, where aldosterone stimulates a net sodium retention in body fluids and potassium excretion in the urine.

The acinar and intercalary duct region is the only site for the net movement of water in saliva. Bicarbonate is actively secreted by the main excretory duct. Localization of secretory and resorptive functions in specific cell types of the salivary unit has not been determined.

Pancreas

The pancreas is really a union of two organs having entirely different functions. These are the pancreatic tissue proper and the islands of Langerhans. The former tissue elaborates the pancreatic juice, containing several digestive enzymes that are conveyed to the duodenum. The islands of Langerhans, the endocrine portion, produces hormones that play an important role in the regulation of carbohydrate metabolism.

The pancreas has long intercalary ducts,

which lead directly into excretory ducts without the intervention of a secretory portion (Fig. 15-1). The alveoli are shorter and rounder than are those of the parotid and are composed of pyramidal cells resting on a basement membrane. The basal portion of the cells appears basophilic, the apical portion is characterized by the appearance of *zymogen granules*, their number depending on the functional state of the cell (Fig. 15-14).

A peculiar feature of the pancreatic alveoli is the presence of one or more small epithelial cells lying in contact with the apices of the secreting cells. These are the *centroalveolar cells*. Although the function of these cells was previously unknown, it has now been established that they are a continuation of the epithelium of the intercalary duct, which is carried over into the acinus as a projection rather than directly into the lumen (Fig. 15-15).

Fine structure of the acinar cells

The basal portion of the cell (Fig. 15-16) contains an extensive endoplasmic reticular

Zymogen granules

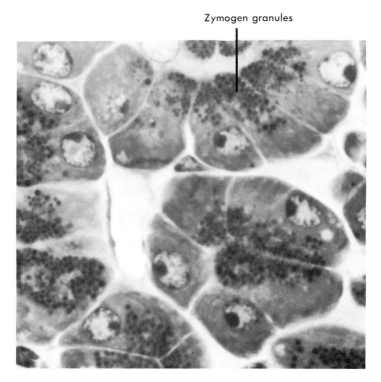

Fig. 15-14. Photomicrograph of acinar cells of pancreas showing zymogen granules. (×800.)

Acinar cells   Intercalary duct

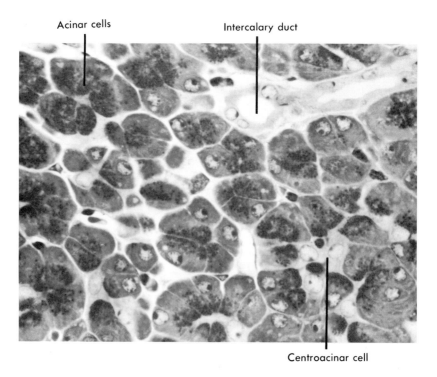

Centroacinar cell

Fig. 15-15. Photomicrograph of section of pancreas of monkey. Note dark secretory granules in apical parts of acinar cells. (×400.)

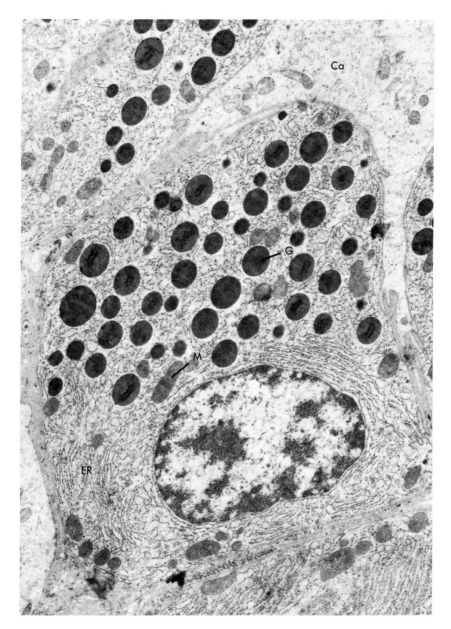

Fig. 15-16. Electron micrograph of pancreatic acinar cell of monkey. Characteristic of cytoplasm is prominent endoplasmic reticulum, *ER,* and numerous dense zymogen granules, *G. M,* Mitochondrion; *Ca,* centroacinar cell.

system exhibiting parallel cisternae studded with ribosomes. Ribosomes are also present in great numbers in the cytoplasm. The endoplasmic reticulum and free ribosomes correspond to the basophilic substance (ergastoplasm) observed in the basal part of the cell at the optic level. The mitochondria, although not numerous, are well defined and contain granules distributed in the matrix between the cristae. A prominent Golgi apparatus located in a supranuclear position consists of parallel arrays of membranes, vacuoles, and sinuses. Many of the vacuoles contain a dense homogeneous material representing the precursor of zymogen. The zymogen granules located in the distal region of the cell appear dense and are enclosed by a membrane.

Islands of Langerhans

The islands of Langerhans are collections of cells that arise as outgrowths from the walls of the ducts of the pancreas during embryonic life. Although they are thus connected developmentally with the ducts, they do not secrete into the tubules. They may become entirely detached from them or retain a connection through a cord of cells that has no lumen. They consist of coiled anastomosing cords of cells penetrated by a network of capillaries into which they secrete (Fig. 15-17, A).

In hematoxylin and eosin preparations, the islands appear as spheroidal masses of pale-staining cells arranged in the form of anastomosing cords. Interspersed between the cords of cells are numerous blood capillaries. The walls of these blood vessels are in intimate contact with the cells making up the cords, an arrangement that facilitates exchange of secretion between the cells and the vessels, which are surrounded by a basement membrane thinner than that in the exocrine pancreas.

At least three cell types can be distinguished in the islets: (1) the alpha or A cell, (2) the beta or B cell, and (3) the delta or D cell. Some authors also recognize another cell type, the C cell that has a pale cytoplasm, few organelles, and no secretory granules.

1. The alpha (A) cells in man tend to be found in clusters at the edges of the islets but may also occur individually within the deeper parts of the cell mass. They cannot be readily distinguished from the beta or delta cells with routine hematoxylin and eosin staining, but special stains such as chrome hematoxylin-phloxine permit identification on the basis of the differential color reaction of the granules within the cells. With the chrome hematoxylin-phloxine stain, the granules of alpha cells appear as small, intensely red–staining bodies, whereas the granules of the more numerous beta cells are larger and stain dark blue. The most distinguishing ultrastructural feature of the alpha cells is the presence of dense spherical granules of uniform size, arranged

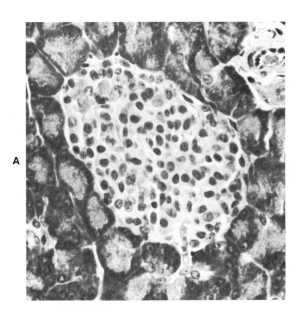

Fig. 15-17. A, Photomicrograph of island of Langerhans of squirrel monkey surrounded by acinar cells. (×400.)

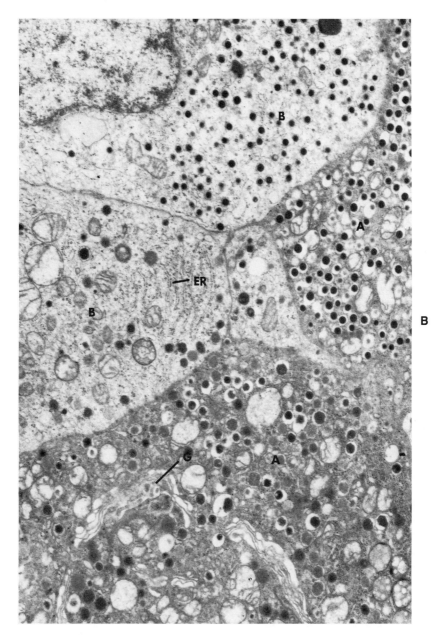

Fig. 15-17, cont'd. B, Electron micrograph of island cells of rhesus monkey pancreas. Character and size of granules are the most important distinguishing features of these cells. *A,* Alpha cell; *B,* beta cell; *ER,* endoplasmic reticulum; *G,* Golgi apparatus. (×11,500.)

primarily on the side of the cell facing the capillary bed (vascular pole). These granules are separated from a surrounding membrane by a clear space of low electron density. The cells contain mitochondria similar to those of beta cells although noticeably smaller, a Golgi complex smaller than that of the beta cells, and a few cisternal profiles of rough endoplasmic reticulum, as well as many free ribosomes. The nucleus is often indented or lobulated (Fig. 15-14, *B*). The alpha cells have been divided into two groups, one of which has an affinity for silver stains. The argyrophilic alpha$_1$ cells may secrete gastrin, a hormone that affects gastric secretion and the motility of gut muscle. The nonargyrophilic alpha$_2$ cells have been shown to produce glucagon, a hormone involved in maintaining body metabolism during fasting.

2. The beta (B) cells tend to occupy the middle of the islets (Figs. 15-17, *B*, and 15-18). They are responsible for the secretion of insulin, a hormone concerned with controlling the utilization of nutrients shortly after a meal. Beta cells are similar in appearance to alpha cells in both size and shape and can only be distinguished from alpha cells by special stains or by ultrastructural features. The beta cells show a wide species variation in the structure of the secretory granules. In humans the beta granules contain one or more elongate or polygonal crystals surrounded by a homogeneous matrix of relatively low density. The cells also contain another granule type that lacks a crystalline core. It has been suggested that these other granules are an immature form. Both granule types contain insulin. The beta cells have slightly larger mitochondria and a more extensive Golgi apparatus than do alpha cells. The endoplasmic reticulum is less prominent and the nucleus is of a fairly regular form.

3. The delta (D) cells have numerous membrane-bound granules of a somewhat larger size and lower density than alpha cell granules. The cell is often rounded in shape with a pale cytoplasm and a spherical or indented nucleus. Delta cells are usually found within alpha cell clusters. Delta cells have been shown by immunocytochemical

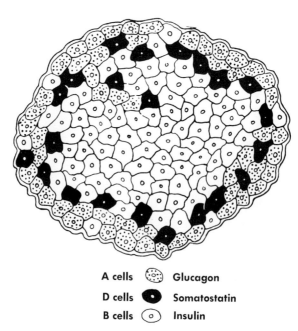

A cells — Glucagon
D cells — Somatostatin
B cells — Insulin

Fig. 15-18. Schematic representation of an island of Langerhans showing distribution of glucagon, somatostatin, and insulin-containing cells. Island cell types for which a function has not yet been positively established are omitted. (From Unger, R., and L. Orci. 1975. Lancet **2:**1243-1244.)

methods to contain somatostatin, a polypeptide that can regulate insulin and glucagon secretion (Fig. 15-18).

Functions of the pancreas

The pancreas represents a complex mixture of exocrine and endocrine glandular tissue. The exocrine glands secrete an alkaline fluid, the pancreatic juice. This fluid contains proteases such as trypsin, which splits proteins into amino acids; amylase, which converts starch to maltose; and lipase, which hydrolyzes neutral fats to glycerol and fatty acids. The secretion is regulated by two hormones released from the gut during the entry of partially digested food (chyme) into the duodenum. One of these hormones, secretin, regulates the amount of buffered fluid released by the pancreatic exocrine tissue; the other, pancreozymin-cholecystokinin, regulates the enzyme content of the fluid. Pancreatic juice is released into the duodenum where it neutralizes the acidic chyme as it enters the small intestine from the stomach and continues the process of enzymatic digestion of the macromolecules contained in the chyme.

The other component of the pancreas is the accumulation of small islands of Langerhans, an endocrine tissue. The beta cells secrete insulin. Insulin stimulates glucose uptake by most cells and enables cells such as liver, kidney, and muscle to store glucose in the form of glycogen. It is basically a hormone that promotes storage of nutrients and the initiation of growth and repair processes. The alpha cells of the pancreas secrete glucagon, a hormone that works in a way opposite to (*antagonizes*) the actions of insulin. Glucagon stimulates the production of glucose by gluconeogenesis and glycolysis in the liver and is responsible for maintaining normal blood sugar levels during fasting. Both hormones also influence the storage and release of fats from adipose tissue. Insulin stimulates fat synthesis (lipogenesis) and glucagon stimulates fat breakdown (lipolysis). The two hormones act together to control the day-to-day storage and utilization of carbohydrates, proteins, and fats as energy sources, and the ratio between insulin and glucagon influences whether the body is in a fed or fasted energy economy. It is not surprising that they are positioned in the island so that they can interact (Fig. 15-18).

Blood and nerve supply

The blood supply to the pancreas is derived chiefly from the superior and inferior pancreaticoduodenal arteries and also from divisions of the splenic artery. As in the salivary glands, the arteries pass in the connective tissue septa to end in capillaries among the acini and islands of Langerhans. Corresponding veins return the blood to the superior mesenteric and portal veins. The nerves that supply the pancreas are derived from the splanchnic and the vagus nerves.

Summary

It is sometimes difficult for students to distinguish the four glands just described (parotid, submaxillary, sublingual, and the pancreas). The following facts may be emphasized. Of the four glands, two contain no mucous cells. These are the parotid and the pancreas, which are alike in that the cells of their alveoli are all serous. They are differentiated by the presence of islands of Langerhans and centroalveolar cells in the pancreas. In differentiating between the submaxillary and sublingual glands, one should look for purely serous alveoli in the former. It must be remembered, however, that the large serous crescents of the sublingual may be cut so that their relation to the mucous alveoli is not seen and they appear to be separate alveoli. Such instances are, however, isolated; if more than half the cells in a section are serous, it is certain that the section is from the submaxillary gland. Some specimens are difficult to identify, especially since the proportions of serous and mucous cells vary in different animals and even in different parts of the same gland.

LIVER

The liver develops as an outgrowth from the wall of the gut, lying in the pathway of the vitelline and umbilical veins. The space between the vessels becomes broken up into a multitude of small sinusoids having extremely permeable walls. The blood supply of the liver is complicated, and an understanding of its arrangement and distribution within the liver is essential for a proper appreciation of the manner in which the liver functions.

The two cells of special interest in regard to liver function are (1) the parenchymal cells (hepatocytes), which form thin plates or sheets separated by the sinusoids, and (2) the phagocytic reticuloendothelial cells, which form the lining of the sinusoids.

1. The hepatocytes are engaged in many functions. They are involved in synthesizing the secreting bile components; in the uptake and storage of nutrients; in the removal of drugs, toxins, and naturally produced compounds such as hormones; and in the synthesis and release of several blood proteins such as albumin, transport globulins, and blood-clotting proteins.

2. The phagocytic cells are involved in filtering the blood as it passes through the sinusoids. These cells play a key role in maintaining the normal defense responses of the body against infection. Although the role the liver plays in trapping bacteria that escape into the bloodstream from the intestinal tract remains controversial, decrease in phagocytic capacity due to liver disease may lead to a serious compromise of body defense against infection.

The liver is thus a complicated organ both structurally and functionally and is actually several organs in one. It is a compound tubular exocrine gland secreting bile, an organ in the reticuloendothelial system that filters and stores blood, and a massive collection of cells that synthesize and release many substances into the bloodstream.

The liver is located in the upper right portion of the abdominal cavity just below the diaphragm and is divided into four lobes. It is surrounded by a connective tissue capsule that contains a number of elastic fibers. This surface sheet of connective tissue, called *Glisson's capsule,* is covered by an incomplete tunica serosa derived from the peritoneum. At the point where the major af-

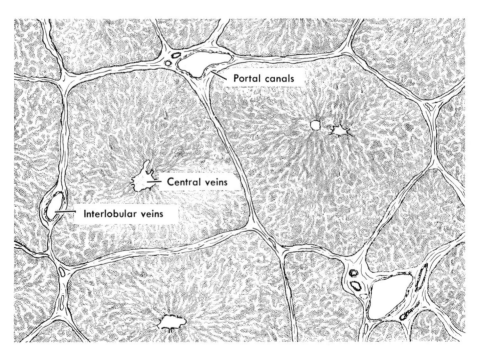

Fig. 15-19. Liver of pig, low magnification, showing relations of lobules to portal canals, central veins, and interlobular veins.

ferent and efferent vessels and the efferent bile duct enter and leave the liver (the *porta hepatis*), the capsule surrounds the vessels and follows them in to the organ, forming a connective tissue framework that divides the mass of hepatocytes into lobules. This framework is not obvious in the human liver, but in the pig liver (which is often used as an example of liver tissue in laboratory exercises) the connective tissue forms an easily identifiable sheath around each lobule (Fig. 15-19).

The lobules are cylindrical or roughly prismatic in shape (Fig. 15-19) and have two main constituents: (1) a parenchymal portion, consisting of the hepatocytes, and (2) a system of anastomosing vascular channels (sinusoids) (Fig. 15-20). The hepatocytes are arranged in irregular branching and anastomosing plates of cells that are disposed in a radiating fashion around the central vein of the lobule. At sites where three or more structural units (lobules) join, there is usually a more abundant accumulation of connective tissue, together with a bile duct, one or more branches of the portal vein, and hepatic arteries and lymph vessels. This triangular-shaped zone, the *portal canal*, helps to delineate the periphery of the lobules. The ducts and vessels contained within it are

referred to as the *portal triad*. Of the vessels present in this complex, the vein is by far the largest; the bile duct is readily recognized by the presence of its columnar epithelial lining (Fig. 15-21).

Blood flows from the rim of each lobule (called the *limiting plate*) through the sinusoids toward the center of the lobule where it drains into the central vein. At points within the sinusoid and along the periphery of the lobule, more highly oxygenated blood from the hepatic arteries is mixed with the nutrient-laden venous blood from the portal veins. Blood in the central veins passes into the sublobular veins and is conveyed to the inferior vena cava.

As a result of the unusual blood supply of the lobule, which is more richly oxygenated at the edges with only a minor infusion of oxygenated blood near the middle of the lobule, the cells in the hepatocyte mass are functionally different. Rappaport has described the functional unit (*acinus*) of the human liver in terms of blood supply. The acinus is an angular mass of parenchyma forming a pie-shaped wedge surrounding an axis consisting of the terminal branch of a portal vein, a hepatic artery, and a bile duct. The acinus extends inward to the central vein (Fig. 15-21). This definition of a functional unit takes into account the territory of drainage of a branch of a portal vein and is based on the portal canal as a boundary. The cells nearest the rim of the parenchymal mass (where the venous and arterial blood supply penetrates the sinusoids) would be expected to have the richest blood supply, whereas the cells around the central vein would be the most impoverished. The metabolic processes that occur in the hepatocytes nearest the edge of the acinus (zone 1 of Rappaport) are likely to involve oxidative metabolism, whereas the cells deepest in the acinus (zone 3) are most likely to be engaged in anaerobic metabolism. This is confirmed by differences in the distribution of enzymatic activity within the acinus.

Liver cells and sinusoids

Liver cells are arranged as a series of anastomosing perforated plates that are con-

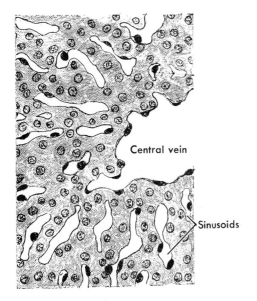

Fig. 15-20. Region of liver lobule immediately surrounding central vein.

Central vein

Sinusoids

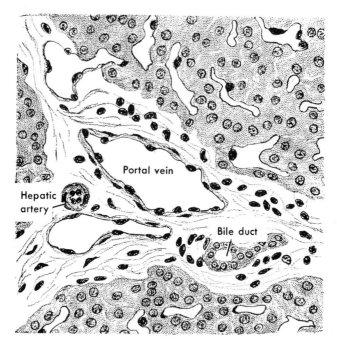

Fig. 15-21. Portal canal containing branch of portal vein. Upper left, small vein opening into sinusoid.

tiguous with the blood-filled sinusoids on all but one side (Fig. 15-22). They extend from the periphery of the lobule to the central vein in a radial manner. The hepatic cells form the secretory part of the liver. The excretory duct system of the liver consists of minutes channels that begin as grooves within the lateral surfaces of hepatocytes (Fig. 15-23). Two (or sometimes three) hepatocytes join their surfaces at these grooves by means of tight junctions and form spaces into which bile is secreted. The channels are called *bile canaliculi.*

The cell membrane facing the sinusoidal walls is thrown into numerous microvilli that project into the narrow perisinusoidal space, the *space of Disse,* which separates the hepatocytes from the vessel walls (Fig. 15-24). The liver sinusoids are highly permeable and contain pores measuring as much as a micrometer in diameter that permit large molecules of blood proteins to traverse the walls. The fluid in the space of Disse flows along the surfaces of the hepatocytes and then either reenters the sinusoidal bed or is drained into the lymphatics. The micro-

villi greatly enhance the absorptive capacity of the hepatocytes. Along the lateral margins of the cells are numerous membrane projections and indentations that serve to anchor the cells together. There are also many focal points of attachment (desmosomes).

The parenchyma of the liver is composed of large polyhedral-shaped cells supported by reticular fibers (Figs. 15-20 and 15-25). They usually exhibit visible cellular boundaries. The appearance of the cytoplasm varies, depending on its location and its physiological condition. The nuclei are centrally placed with a prominent nucleolus and as many as one fourth of the cells are binucleate. The mitochondria are fairly numerous, especially at the edge of the acinus nearest the portal canal where the oxygen supply is greater. The Golgi apparatus is situated adjacent to the bile canaliculus. The rough and smooth components of the endoplasmic reticulum are both abundant, and at the light microscope level the cell is seen to contain scattered basophilia corresponding to both the rough endoplasmic reticulum and numerous free ribosomes (Figs.

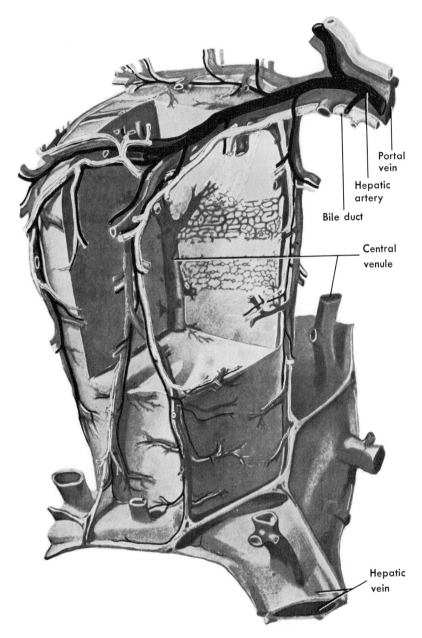

Portal
vein

Hepatic
artery

Bile duct

Central
venule

Hepatic
vein

Fig. 15-22. Reconstruction of liver lobule of pig showing relation of blood vessels and bile ducts to liver parenchyma. (Modified from Braus. 1924. Anatomie des Menschen. Julius Springer, Berlin. Vol. 2. from Nonidez, J., and W. Windle. 1953. Textbook of histology. McGraw-Hill Book Co., New York.)

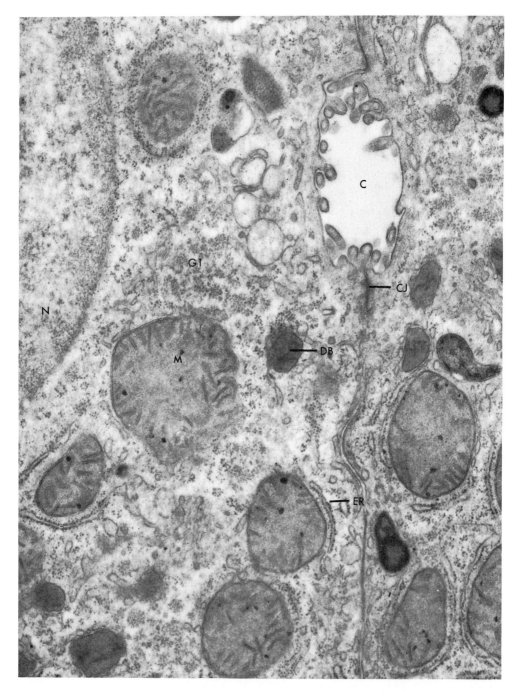

Fig. 15-23. Electron micrograph of parts of two adjacent cells of rat liver, showing bile canaliculus, *C. CJ,* Cell junction; *DB,* dense body; *ER,* rough endoplasmic reticulum; *Gl,* glycogen; *N,* nucleus; *M,* mitochondrion. (×15,000.) (Courtesy Dr. S. Luse.)

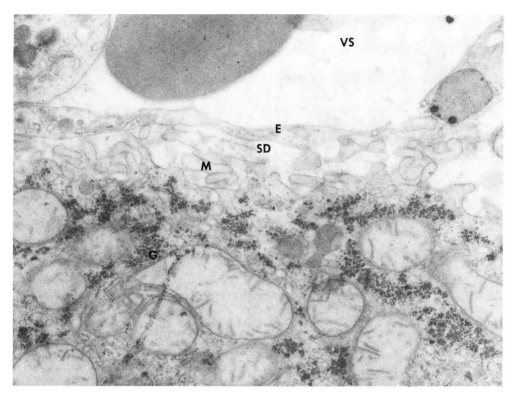

Fig. 15-24. Electron micrograph of sinusoidal surface of mouse liver cell showing relation of surface microvilli, *M;* space of Disse, *SD;* and endothelial cells, *E. G,* Glycogen; *VS,* vascular space.

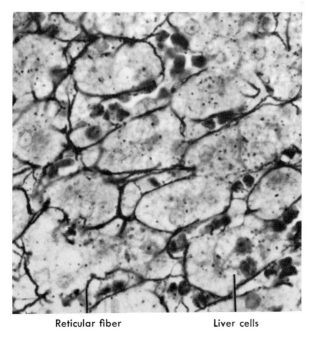

Reticular fiber   Liver cells

Fig. 15-25. Section of human liver showing reticular fibers. (Bielschowsky method; ×640.)

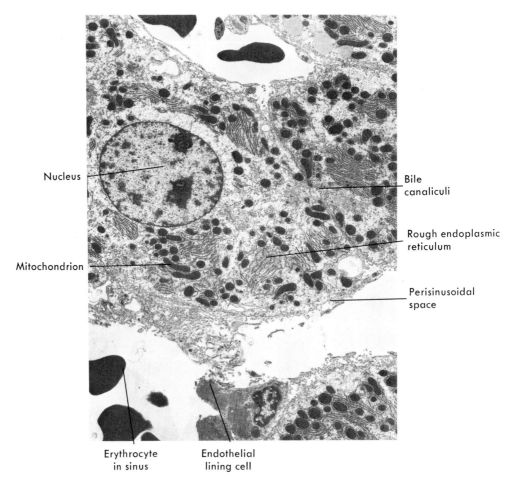

Nucleus

Mitochondrion

Bile
canaliculi

Rough endoplasmic
reticulum

Perisinusoidal
space

Erythrocyte
in sinus

Endothelial
lining cell

Fig. 15-26. Electron micrograph of liver cells of rat. (×4,500.) (Courtesy Dr. H. Nakahara.)

15-23 and 15-26). The cells contain numerous inclusions as a result of their multiple functions. The various kinds of observable granules are glycogen, lipids, lipofuscin, and bile pigment. At the ultrastructural level the cells exhibit numerous lysosomes and microbodies, the latter being electron-dense organelles containing oxidase systems with a high affinity for oxygen.

The cords consisting of hepatocytes anastomose freely, forming a spongy network that radiates from the central vein. The meshes of the network of hepatocytes border on the sinusoids, which are lined by three varieties of endothelial cells. About 25% of the lining cells protrude into the sinusoidal lumen as stellate phagocytic (Kupffer) cells,

50% are flat phagocytic cells, and the remainder are differentiated endothelial cells. In ordinary preparations stained with hematoxylin and eosin, the lining of the sinusoids appears to consist of cells that lie along the borders of the hepatocytes. The nuclei of these cells are small and dark, and their cytoplasm forms a thin film along the border of the sinusoids. With special methods the stellate Kupffer cells can be seen bulging into the lumen of the sinusoids. The reaction of the phagocytic cells lining the sinusoids (which represent about 60% of the total population of reticuloendothelial cells in the body) to vital stains is similar to that of other reticuloendothelial cells elsewhere in the body (Fig. 15-27).

Hepatic cell   Macrophage (Kupffer)   Red blood corpuscles in hepatic sinusoid

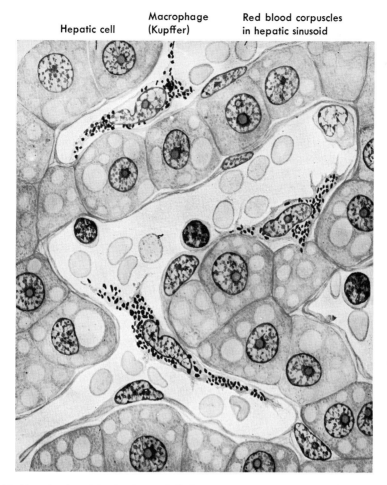

Fig. 15-27. Hepatic sinusoids showing endothelial cells and macrophages lining them. (×1,200.) (From Nonidez, J., and W. Windle. 1953. Textbook of histology. McGraw-Hill Book Co., New York.)

Circulation

As already indicated, the circulation of the liver is derived from two sources: about 75% from the portal vein (Fig. 15-22) and 25% from the hepatic arteries.

The portal vein carrying venous blood from the intestine and spleen, together with branches of the hepatic artery, enters the liver at the porta hepatis. These vessels divide and run through the connective tissue septa of the lobes as the interlobar vessels. The interlobar veins give off branches that run between the lobules and are known accordingly as interlobular veins. These vessels encircle the lobule, eventually penetrate it, and break up into fine vessels, the hepatic sinusoids. The sinusoids empty into the cen-

tral vein, which is considered to be the first part of the efferent system of the hepatic vessels. The central vein passes down through the lobule, collecting blood from many sinusoids, and eventually unites with other central veins that lead into the sublobular vein. Blood from these veins is eventually collected by the hepatic vein and is finally carried to the vena cava (Fig. 15-22).

Biliary tree

The biliary tree provides the exit channels for the secretion of bile, a fluid containing bile salts (important in emulsifying fats and in facilitating the absorption of lipids from the gut), and a number of compounds that represent excretory forms of the end-prod-

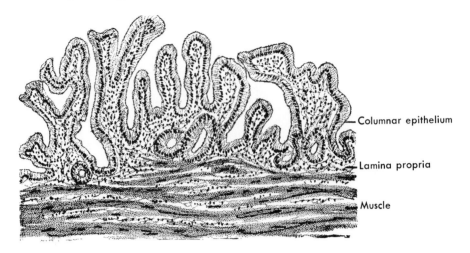

Columnar epithelium

Lamina propria

Muscle

Fig. 15-28. Gallbladder of monkey.

ucts of hemoglobin metabolism (bilirubin) and the inactivation of drugs and hormones (various glucuronides and sulfates). All the hepatocytes continuously form small amounts of bile, which are secreted into the bile canaliculi that lie between the hepatocytes in the hepatic plates (Fig. 15-23). The bile then flows peripherally toward the interlobular septa where canaliculi empty into terminal bile ducts, finally reaching the hepatic ducts and common bile duct, from which the bile empties directly into the duodenum or is diverted into the gallbladder.

Lymphatics

The liver sinusoids are extremely permeable, and large quantities of fluid pass through their walls into the space of Disse. Much of this is drained off into the lymphatics. Under resting conditions as much as half the lymph formed in the body is contributed by the liver. If the pressure in the venous system of the liver rises by only 3 mm Hg, excessive amounts of fluid begin to flow through the lymph channels, soon exceeding their capacity; fluid then diffuses through the capsule of the liver into the abdominal cavity. Because of the permeability of the sinusoids, this fluid is almost pure plasma. The manner in which the lymph is collected and formed has not as

yet been resolved. Lymphatics have not been found near the sinusoids or within the liver plates, although normal lymph channels may be observed in the connective tissue of the capsule, in the portal canals, and in the sparse sheath of connective tissue surrounding the hepatic veins.

Nerve supply

The nerves supplying the liver are chiefly nonmyelinated sympathetics. These nerves play a role in the storage and release of blood by the liver. Because the liver is an expandable and compressible organ, it can store large quantities of blood. Normally the liver holds about 500 ml of blood (equivalent to about 10% of the blood pumped by the heart each minute). About 1,500 ml of blood (counting both the portal blood and arterial blood) are pumped into the liver each minute. Much of the blood held in the liver as a reservoir is pooled in the veins, with a lesser amount in the sinusoids. When stimulated by sympathetic nerves, these vessels constrict and can expel as much as 350 ml into the general circulation within a few minutes.

GALLBLADDER

The gallbladder is a hollow, pear-shaped organ closely adherent to the posterior surface of the liver. It consists of a blind end

Epithelium

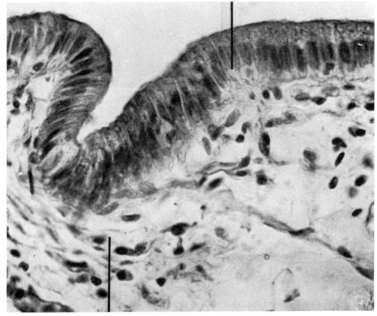

Lamina propria

Fig. 15-29. Mucosa of gallbladder. (×640.)

known as the fundus, a body, and a neck, which continues as the cystic duct.

The layers common to other parts of the digestive tract are poorly developed and are more or less intermingled in the gallbladder (Fig. 15-28). It is lined with a columnar epithelium in which the cell walls are distinct (Fig. 15-29). This epithelium rests on a connective tissue layer (lamina propria) that represents the lamina propria and submucosa of other parts of the tract. The connective tissue and epithelium are irregularly folded, forming numerous elevations and pockets. After the latter are tangentially cut, they appear as closed sacs, which look like glandular follicles. There is, however, no secretion in the gallbladder except that of a small group of mucous glands near its neck.

Outside the connective tissue is a layer of smooth muscle, which consists of intermingled groups of circular, longitudinal, and oblique fibers. The muscular coat is thick and has much connective tissue combined with the muscle fibers. There is a fairly thick serosa of loose connective tissue covered by the mesothelium.

Blood and nerve supply

The gallbladder is supplied by the cystic artery, and the venous blood is collected by veins that empty into the cystic branch of the portal vein. The gallbladder is richly supplied by lymphatics, and many plexuses occur in this organ. Branches of both the vagus and splanchnic nerves supply the gallbladder.

16

Respiratory tract

Functionally, the respiratory tract can be divided into a *conducting portion*, consisting of cavities and tubes that convey air from outside the body into all parts of the lungs, and a *respiratory portion*, consisting of those divisions within the lung where exchange of gases between the air and the blood occur. Anatomically, the conducting passageways consist of structures outside the lung (nose, nasopharynx, larynx, trachea, and main bronchi) and inside the lung (smaller bronchi, bronchioles, terminal bronchioles) (Fig. 16-1). Each terminal bronchiole terminates in several respiratory bronchioles that mark the entrance into the respiratory division of the lung. Each respiratory bronchiole branches into a system of alveolar ducts and alveoli in which gaseous exchange takes place (Fig. 16-4).

Embryologically, the primordium of the respiratory tract arises as a small bud from the ventral wall of the foregut. This bud gives rise to a tube, the trachea, which soon loses all connection with the foregut except at the opening of the larynx. The trachea then begins to branch and at the time of birth seventeen subdivisions of the original tube have occurred, during which the bronchi, bronchioles, and terminal bronchioles are formed. With the beginning of breathing at birth, the ends of the terminal bronchioles (the smallest passageways in the conducting system) expand into alveolar ducts and alveoli, and six more sets of branches are added. For the purpose of presentation, the respiratory tract will be divided into an upper part, including the passageways above the larynx, and a lower part, beginning with the first derivative of the embryonic bud from the foregut wall, the trachea. The problems of wall construction in these two parts of the respiratory system are solved in different ways. Since air is moved through these passages by negative pressure, the air passages must resist collapse in order to function. Without the reinforcement of bone, the large masses of cartilage and dense fibrous tissue of the upper respiratory passages would collapse. In the tubes making up the lower passageways, rings and plates of cartilage gradually give way to layers of muscle and elastic fibers braided around the air passageways (Fig. 16-4). Breathing stretches the lung and holds these slender passageways open; reinforcement of the walls is then no longer necessary. Instead, provision is made to permit greater elasticity and ability to adjust in both diameter and length with the changes in lung size. The muscle also participates in adjusting the volume of the airways or *respiratory dead space*. Muscle tone is controlled by the parasympathetic nervous system, and changes in tone during coughing or cold weather act as a protective device for the lung passageways.

Aside from its respiratory function (which involves the exchange of gases between the tissue fluids, plasma, and air spaces in the lung), the air in the respiratory system must be moistened, filtered, and warmed to per-

Fig. 16-1. Topographic representation of respiratory apparatus.

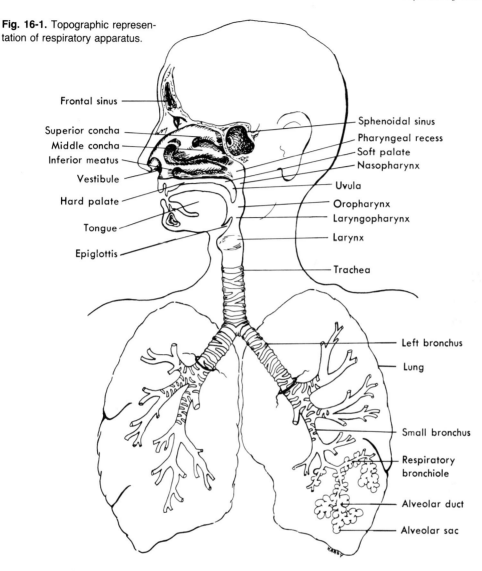

Frontal sinus

Superior concha

Middle concha

Inferior meatus

Vestibule

Hard palate

Tongue

Epiglottis

Sphenoidal sinus

Pharyngeal recess

Soft palate

Nasopharynx

Uvula

Oropharynx

Laryngopharynx

Larynx

Trachea

Left bronchus

Lung

Small bronchus

Respiratory
bronchiole

Alveolar duct

Alveolar sac

mit proper functioning of the component parts. The mucus supplied by goblet cells in pseudostratified columnar epithelium and by the submucosal glands serves to entrap dust particles and bacteria and also to supply enzymes that lyse certain bacteria. The same secretion serves to moisten the air and also dissolves certain molecules, which are perceived as odors, with the aid of the olfactory organ in the nasal passages. The coordinated beating of cilia on cell surfaces moves the secretions from the nasal passages through the nasopharynx to the oropharynx, while similar activity of ciliated cells located in the bronchioles, bronchi, and trachea propels mucus to the glottis. From this locus the secretions are either expectorated or pass into the esophagus. An abundant supply of venous blood vessels in the submucosal tissues of the nasal passages warms the air. Several of the functions mentioned are facilitated by an abundant surface area in each nasal passage occurring in (1) four accessory sinuses (frontal, ethmoidal, sphenoidal, and maxillary, named for the bones that enclose them) and (2) the presence of three conchae containing the tortuously twisted turbinate bones. Certain phagocytic cells called *dust cells* are located in the lung tissues. They remove and store foreign particles that enter the lungs. The olfactory organ serves to warn the organism of the presence of noxious substances in the air. The specialized respiratory epithelium of the lung alveoli is admirably suited for its function of gas exchange. The conducting tubules are constructed so that open passageways for gases are maintained under the widely fluctuating pressures produced in ventilation. These tubules gradually change in structure from thick-walled, rigid tubes to increasingly thinner and softer ones, and a similar change occurs in blood vessels that accompany them.

Upper parts of the respiratory tract

NASAL PASSAGES

The nose consists of two passageways separated by the cartilage-containing *nasal septum*. Each passageway begins at the *external nares* as an inflection of the keratinized stratified squamous epithelium of the wings (alae) of the nose. The inflected portion forms the *vestibule* of the nose and is covered by nu-

merous hairs (vibrissae). Large sebaceous glands and numerous sweat glands are also found in this region. The connective tissue papillae are deep, and scattered mixed serous and mucous glands may be observed. In the posterior region of the vestibule the epithelium becomes nonkeratinized, or forms only small patches of nonhairy keratinized epithelium. The latter indicates the beginning of the so-called *respiratory* part of the nasal passage, which, in turn, terminates in a small orifice called the *choana* leading into the nasopharynx.

The respiratory portion of each nasal passage includes the sinuses, olfactory organ, the three conchae, including the meati, and the upper surface of the hard palate. In general, the epithelium of this region is ciliated pseudostratified columnar, usually exhibits four to five rows of nuclei, and contains goblet cells. The underlying lamina propria, composed of both elastic and collagenous fibers, is adherent to a nearby periosteum or perichondrium (Fig. 16-2). A basement membrane containing elastic fibers occurs irregularly.

The sinuses indicated are located in cer-

Epithelium   Lamina propria

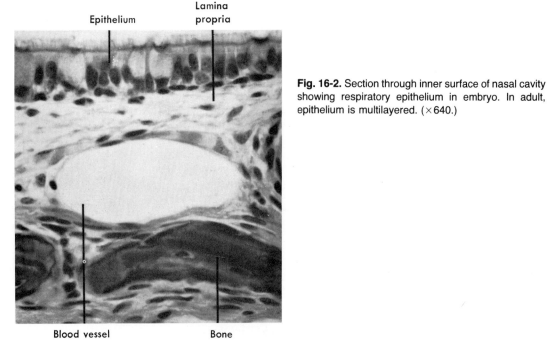

Blood vessel   Bone

Fig. 16-2. Section through inner surface of nasal cavity showing respiratory epithelium in embryo. In adult, epithelium is multilayered. (×640.)

tain bones of the head and are usually observed in decalcified sections of the head of an embryo or fetus. They are usually identified by their location rather than by histologic characteristics. The epithelium is ciliated pseudostratified columnar, of approximately half the thickness of other parts of the tract. The lining of sinuses exhibits two or three rows of nuclei and few goblet cells. The basement membrane is thin and rarely observed. The lamina propria, also thin, is mainly collagenous and is closely adherent to the periosteum. It has few glands but is frequently supplied with lymphoid aggregations and other leukocytic forms.

The superior, middle, and inferior conchae are usually observed in frontal sections through the head of the human fetus as coiled and recurved projections arising from the walls opposite the septa (paraseptally). In animals such as the pig, only parts of the conchae are visible because the head is prolonged into a snout. The space inferior to each concha is, in sequence, the superior, middle, and inferior meatus.

The middle and inferior conchae bear the usual thick type of pseudostratified columnar epithelium, containing many goblet cells. The basement membrane is thick and is readily demonstrated. The lamina propria exhibits both serous and mucous alveoli, as well as a large number of prominent venous passages. The latter may be engorged with blood or collapsed, and their walls exhibit both circular and longitudinal bands of smooth muscle. Each meatus bears a thin epithelium containing a few goblet cells, which rests on a thin basement membrane. The superior concha and parts of the roof of the nasal passage and adjacent septum form part of the olfactory organ. The epithelium of the organ is thick and, since the neural processes are almost impossible to trace in hematoxylin and eosin preparations, its appearance is similar to that of stratified columnar epithelia. The surface cells contain pigment granules when properly preserved, and the cilia present are covered by a coagulated secretion, which gives the impression that the tissue is covered by a cuticle.

NASOPHARYNX

In the parts of the nasopharynx that do not come into contact with surfaces of other tissues, the epithelium is ciliated pseudostratified columnar and the lamina propria contains mixed or seromucous glands. In certain transitional zones stratified columnar epithelium may occur but it is not easily distinguished from the pseudostratified variety. In the superior and posterior portions of the nasopharynx are many aggregations of lymphoid cells, which may be extensions of the pharyngeal tonsils or adenoids. Similar aggregations forming the tubal tonsils are found surrounding the entrance of the eustachian tubes into the nasopharynx. At about the lower level of the tonsils the posterior wall of the nasopharynx is covered by a nonkeratinized stratified squamous epithelium with numerous low papillae. The superior surface of the soft palate and uvula also bear a nonkeratinized stratified squamous epithelium.

LARYNX

The uppermost portion of the larynx is known as the epiglottis. The lingual or anterior surface of the epiglottis is covered by a nonkeratinized stratified squamous epithelium and bears many seromucous glands in the lamina propria, especially near its connection with the base of the tongue. The upper part of the posterior surface of the epiglottis is covered by a nonkeratinized stratified squamous epithelium, which merges into a transition zone and appears as irregularly ciliated stratified columnar epithelium. The lower part of the posterior surface bears ciliated pseudostratified columnar epithelium exhibiting goblet cells, and near the base one may observe scattered taste buds. The lamina propria includes some mucous and serous units. The zone between the two surfaces is occupied by a large area of cartilage containing serveral thick elastic fibers, the so-called elastic cartilage. In the epiglottis of some animals the cartilage may contain a central zone invaded by fat cells. No perichondrium, however, occurs in the invaded zone (Fig. 16-3).

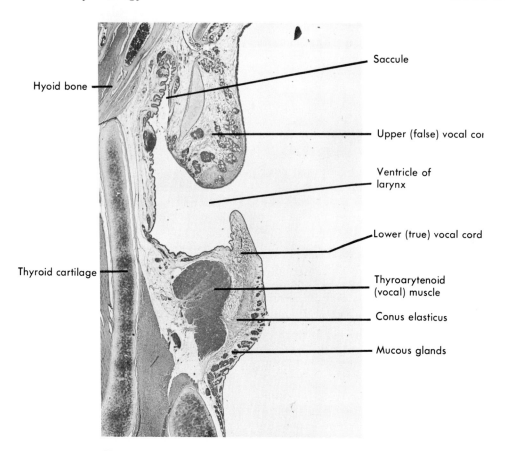

Hyoid bone

Thyroid cartilage

Saccule

Upper (false) vocal cor

Ventricle of larynx

Lower (true) vocal cord

Thyroarytenoid (vocal) muscle

Conus elasticus

Mucous glands

Fig. 16-3. Half of frontal section of larynx of monkey. (×10.)

The epithelium of the true vocal cords is of the nonkeratinized stratified squamous variety and does not contain mucous glands in the lamina propria. Above and below the true vocal cords the epithelium is ciliated pseudostratified columnar with goblet cells, and many mucous glands are present in the lamina propria. Patches of the stratified squamous type are sometimes found in this region.

Lower parts of the respiratory tract

Morphologists have differentiated the lower parts of the respiratory tract on the basis of gross dissection and by the injection of low melting point alloys into the passageways. Thus there are lobes and lobules of the lung (Fig. 16-4), with their attendant blood and lymphatic circulation, containing various air tubules. Ordinarily one does not utilize more than a small portion of a lobule for study. In addition, the former tendency to utilize the diameter of a tubule as a criterion for identification is no more valid here than it is for blood vessels. In routine histology the salient features to observe in the tubules and lungs are (1) the epithelial makeup, (2) the presence or absence of cartilage and its disposition (that is, location, shape, and extent), (3) the glands and their disposition, (4) the disposition of the muscles, and (5) the relation of the parts to each other at the microscopic level. The student should attempt to visualize how each component appears in cross section and longitudinal section.

TRACHEA

The trachea consists of (1) mucosa, (2) submucosa, and (3) a layer of cartilage and muscle that corresponds to the muscularis of the digestive tract (Fig. 16-5). External to the

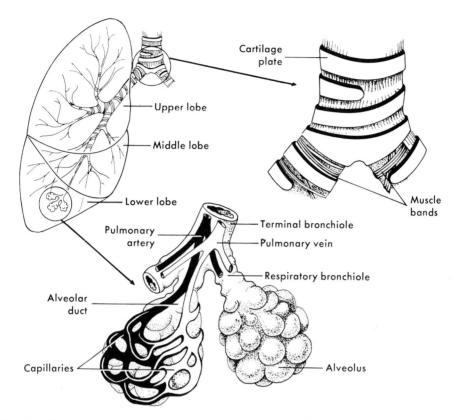

Fig. 16-4. Gross structure of respiratory passages showing detail of one respiratory unit. (Drawing by Emily Craig.)

Fig. 16-5. Transverse section of trachea of child.

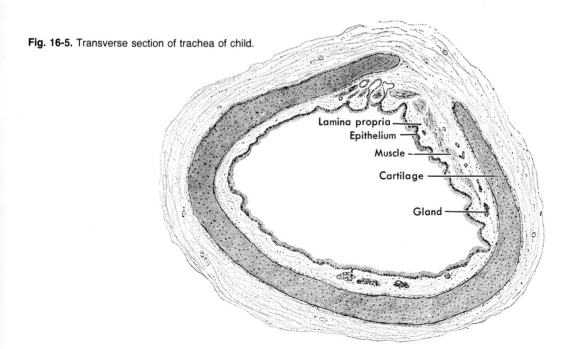

Adipose tissue   Submucosa   Epithelium

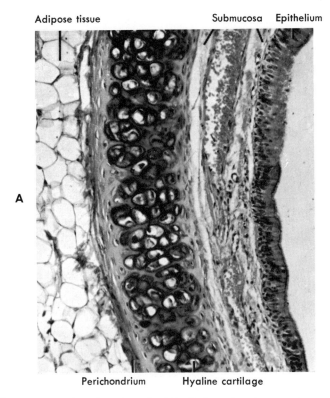

Perichondrium   Hyaline cartilage

Fig. 16-6. A, Transverse section of trachea of rabbit. **B,** Scanning electron micrograph of epithelial lining of rat trachea. (**A** ×40; **B** ×400.) (**B** courtesy Dr. H. Nakahara.)

perichondrium of the cartilage is a fibrosa or adventitious layer of connective tissue, which fuses with the tissue of the mediastinum and the similar layer enclosing the esophagus. This layer is usually destroyed during dissection of the trachea.

1. The *mucosa* consists of (a) a ciliated pseudostratified columnar epithelium with numerous goblet cells bounded by (b) a prominent basement membrane, which is part of (c) the lamina propria, consisting mainly of reticular or fine areolar tissue containing many elastic fibers (Fig. 16-6). At the outer edge of the lamina propria, coarse elastic fibers are oriented longitudinally to form (d) a relatively compact elastic membrane or lamina. The latter is said to be comparable to the muscularis mucosae of the digestive tract and the similar elastic layer in the upper part of the esophagus. In the epithelium small patches of the stratified squamous variety are

encountered, especially in older animals or those with chronic inflammations.

2. The *submucosa* is areolar tissue. It contains fat cells, blood vessels, and the secreting portions of mixed glands, with some units exhibiting prominent serous crescents. In longitudinal sections, dense clusters of these glands are seen in the triangular regions between the adjacent cartilage rings, to be described later.

3. In cross sections of the trachea the *cartilages* appear as a single C-shaped or U-shaped crescent with the open end or prongs directed posteriorly toward the esophagus. The prongs may branch so that more than one piece of cartilage may appear near the open side of the crescent. Bands of smooth muscle fibers transversely arranged appear between the prongs and at times may be observed inserting in the perichondrium, either inside or outside the crescent. External

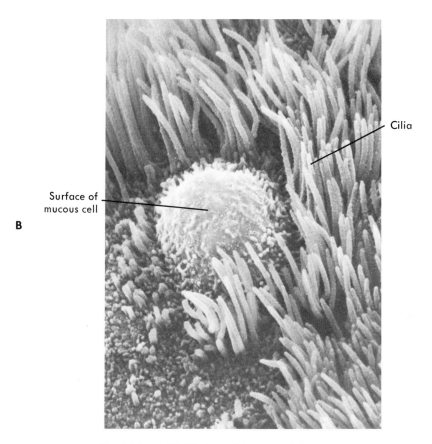

B

Surface of
mucous cell

Cilia

Fig. 16-6, cont'd. For legend see opposite page.

to this *muscle band* one may observe the cut ends of longitudinally and obliquely arranged muscle fibers and their associated elastic fibers. The tracheal glands frequently penetrate the muscle layers. In longitudinal sections the cartilages appear as two rows of ovoid bodies. Occasionally two adjacent cartilages may fuse or be connected by a small longitudinal bar of cartilage. In the region between cartilages there are longitudinal bands of tough dense connective tissue, which merge with the perichondria of the cartilages. In older animals some cartilages may appear to contain fibers or to be partly calcified.

BRONCHI

The extrapulmonary or primary bronchi are histologically identical with the trachea in practically all details except size. In the lungs the cartilages of the bronchi are arranged in a series of overlapping crescentic plates, which completely encircle these structures. Deeper in the lung these soon give way to irregular masses of cartilage with more or less rounded edges (Fig. 16-7) and may or may not overlap when viewed in cross section. The intrapulmonary bronchi differ from the trachea as follows: (1) the elastic membrane of the tracheal lamina propria is replaced by a layer of smooth muscle, which completely encircles both epithelium and the elastic, fiber-containing lamina propria; (2) mucous and seromucous glands are more numerous and more generally distributed in the bronchi than in the trachea and often extend through the muscle and between adjacent cartilage plates; (3) the single crescent-shaped cartilage is replaced by a concentric ring of overlapping crescents. These eventually give way to smaller irregular masses of cartilage, which

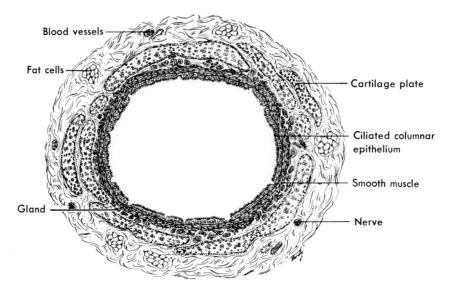

Blood vessels

Fat cells

Cartilage plate

Ciliated columnar epithelium

Smooth muscle

Gland

Nerve

Fig. 16-7. Transverse section of bronchus.

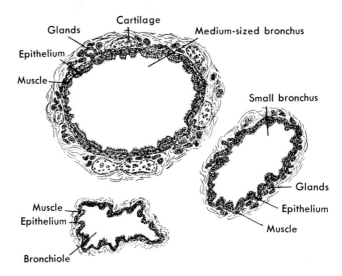

Glands

Cartilage

Medium-sized bronchus

Epithelium

Muscle

Small bronchus

Glands

Epithelium

Muscle

Muscle

Epithelium

Bronchiole

Fig. 16-8. Terminal intrapulmonary passageway of respiratory tract.

continue to diminish in size until the tubules are completely devoid of cartilage. In the smallest bronchi only glands may be seen, and the cartilage is completely absent (Figs. 16-8 and 16-9). As the tubules become smaller, the muscle bands that encircle the lumen become more prominent, with the concomitant reduction of the other structures. The muscles are arranged, however, as two opposing spirals, which tend to form looser helices as the tubule branches and narrows. In cross section the looser spirals in smaller

tubules appear as gaps between muscle bands at the same level. At death, contraction of the spiraling circular muscles throws the pseudostratified columnar epithelium into longitudinal folds, carrying along with it folds of elastic lamina propria. Classification of large, medium-sized, and small bronchi on the basis of definitely overlapping crescentic plates of cartilage, circles of nonoverlapping plates, or no cartilage at all introduces as many problems as it solves and is not a satisfactory criterion to use for identification.

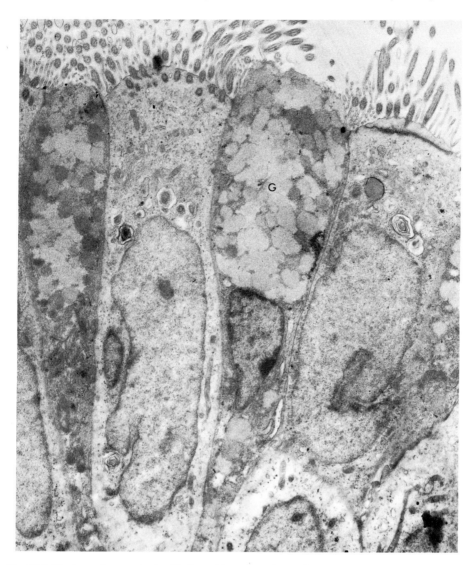

Fig. 16-9. Electron micrograph of epithelium of bronchus of cat. This epithelium is typically ciliated and exhibits numerous goblet cells, *G,* filled with mucous droplets. (×7,600.)

BRONCHIOLES

Bronchioles contain neither glands nor cartilages (Fig. 16-8). The lumen is lined by ciliated simple columnar epithelium, which lacks goblet cells. The lamina propria is elastic and thin and is surrounded by the same type of loosely spiraling, smooth muscle bands found in the bronchi. It is interesting to note that ciliated cells are found beyond the point where glands are no longer in evidence. It has been postulated that this is a protection against the accumulation of mucus in the respiratory portion of the lungs. Subdivision of bronchioles into different types according to size is not histologically feasible and accordingly is not elaborated on in this text.

RESPIRATORY BRONCHIOLES

In the first part of the respiratory bronchiole the epithelium is of the ciliated low columnar or cuboidal type. Distally the epithelium becomes nonciliated cuboidal. The lamina propria is a thin layer of diffuse reticular, collagenous, and elastic fibers. The spiraling muscle bands are prominent, but, between adjacent muscle bands in the region where the lamina propria is not in evidence, one can observe thin walls composed of simple cuboidal epithelium supported on a few helical elastic fibers. Some authors consider this to be respiratory epithelium, and from the appearance of these flattened plates the name respiratory bronchiole has arisen. It should be noted that in some sections the cells are so attenuated that the nuclei in these plates are not visible. In addition, pulmonary alveoli may arise directly from the

walls of the respiratory bronchiole so that they appear as pockets in the tubule wall. Near their termini, respiratory bronchioles flare out and give rise to two or more alveolar ducts (Fig. 16-10).

ALVEOLAR DUCTS

The alveolar ducts (Figs. 16-4 and 16-10) are similar to the respiratory bronchioles from which they branch. The walls of the ducts are provided with so many openings into the alveoli that the wall appears discontinuous. Small bits of the branching, spiraling muscle fibers are seen around the open-

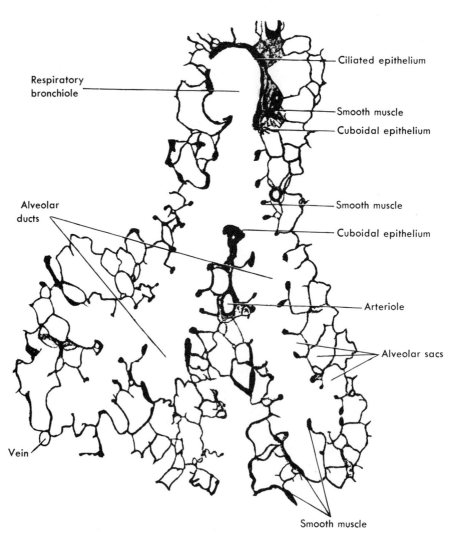

Respiratory bronchiole

Alveolar ducts

Vein

Ciliated epithelium

Smooth muscle

Cuboidal epithelium

Smooth muscle

Cuboidal epithelium

Arteriole

Alveolar sacs

Smooth muscle

Fig. 16-10. Section through respiratory bronchiole and two alveolar ducts of human lung. (After Baltisberger; from Maximow, A. A., and G. Bloom. 1952. Textbook of histology. W. B. Saunders Co., Philadelphia.)

ings into the alveoli or the chambers that lead into the alveoli.

Alveoli

In the alveoli of the lung are respiratory epithelium and elastic tissue. To understand the arrangement of the former, one must remember that all the tubules of the fetal lung are lined with cuboidal epithelium and are embedded in embryonic connective tissue. When respiration begins, at birth, some of the epithelium is stretched into the form of thin plates described previously in this discussion. However, at the angles between alveoli, areas remain where the cells are not flattened. The surrounding connective tissue is reduced to a network of elastic fibers and a few fibroblasts between the alveoli. One may see, therefore, in a section of lung, regions where the cells are reduced to a mere line and other regions where they are polygonal and evidently nucleated.

The original shape of each alveolus or air sac is round. The mutual pressure of adjacent sacs, however, alters the shape, and they appear as irregular polygonal spaces open on one side. They are grouped so that several of them open into a common central space or atrium, which in turn opens into an alveolar duct.

In humans the atria are rare, and in other animals they are an inconstant feature, and so this term may well be considered superfluous.

The true relation of the parts described previously is not often clear in a section of the lung. Occasionally one may have the good fortune to see an area in which the relations of respiratory bronchioles, alveolar ducts, atria, and alveoli appear, as in Fig. 16-10.

With the light microscope one may observe that there are capillaries and some connective tissue between the air spaces of adjacent alveoli (Fig. 16-11). The fine structure of the alveolar wall has now been resolved, and it has been shown to consist of three basic cell types (Fig. 16-12).

1. The most numerous cells of the alveolar wall are the *endothelial cells* of the capillar-

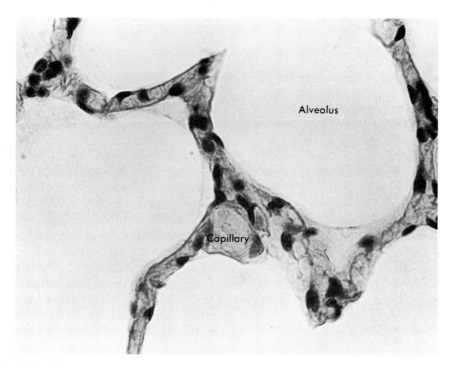

Fig. 16-11. Photomicrograph showing parts of several alveoli of lung. Most nuclei shown in alveolar septa are those of endothelium. (×640.)

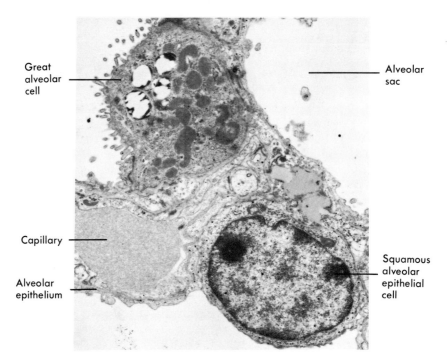

Great alveolar cell

Alveolar sac

Capillary

Alveolar epithelium

Squamous alveolar epithelial cell

Fig. 16-12. Electron micrograph of part of alveolar wall of mouse lung. (Original × 14,000.)

ies. The nuclei of these cells are usually smaller and more elongated than those of epithelial cells.

2. Thin attenuated epithelial cells *(squamous alveolar epithelial cells, type I cells)* fit together and form a continuous lining of the alveolar spaces. This lining is so thin that it is not observable at the light level. The cytoplasm is devoid of an endoplasmic reticulum but contains a variety of other organelles.

3. *Great alveolar cells (type II cells)* appear to be epithelium. They are cuboidal or rounded and are less numerous than the squamous alveolar cells (only five to eight per alveolus). They usually occur at the junction of the walls of several alveoli but may make up part of the air sac as well. They are much larger than the squamous epithelium cells, averaging 15 to 20 μm in diameter in comparison to 0.5 μm width for type I cells. At the light microscope level the cytoplasm appears vacuolated, and the nuclei are large and vesicular. These cells have microvilli on their free borders, and the cytoplasm contains osmiophilic inclusions called cyto-

somes, which consist of peculiar lamellar arrangements of membranes. Since the development of the inclusions coincides with the beginning of surfactant secretion in the fetal lung, the cells may either secrete surfactant or phagocytose it. Surfactant is a surface film that serves to lower the surface tension of the fluid covering the alveolar wall and thus helps hold these small air channels open. It has also been suggested that the great alveolar cells may give rise to alveolar macrophages, which are different functionally from the usual tissue macrophage in that they do not rely on glycolysis for energy but require oxygen instead.

Another group of large cells is found in the terminal bronchioles. They are called Clara cells, contain whorls of endoplasmic reticulum, and are packed with mitochondria. They appear to be active secretory cells, and it has been suggested that they are the source of surfactant.

The barrier or wall between the alveolar air and the blood is extremely thin (about 1 μm) and consists of the capillary endothelium, a connective tissue space, the base-

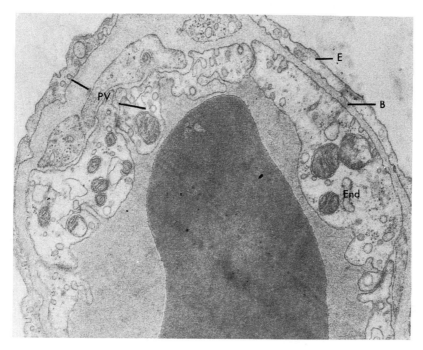

Fig. 16-13. Electron micrograph of alveolar membrane of mouse. Alveolar air is separated from blood by thin epithelium, *E;* basement membrane, *B;* and capillary endothelium, *End.* Pinocytotic vesicles, *PV,* are present in epithelium and endothelium. (×28,000.)

ment membrane of the capillary, and the alveolar epithelium (Fig. 16-13). The wall is readily permeable to gases and water, less so to salts, and least of all to proteins. The main barrier to absorption from the alveolar sac into the blood is the alveolar epithelium. This barrier must serve the dual function of preserving a highly permeable membrane for gaseous exchange and maintaining sufficient strength to hold the wall together. It must also include a defense system against foreign particles and invasive organisms that reach the alveolus in the inspired air (see the last heading of this chapter). The alveolar wall is renewed continuously and is completely replaced every 35 days or so.

In the thicker sections of the alveolus, the basal laminae of the capillary and the epithelial cells are separated by reticular and elastic fibers that tend to increase the resilience of the wall. Fibroblasts and other cells can be found in the thickest parts of the wall. The functional unit of the lung is the respiratory bronchiole with its branching al-veolar ducts and terminal alveoli (Fig. 16-4).

The entrance into each of these units at the mouth of a respiratory bronchiole is narrow and is a vulnerable area because of the possibility of becoming clogged with mucus during inflammatory reactions. It is also a transitional point in the lung defense system, having neither a mucous-ciliary escalator to remove debris nor a good local macrophage population capable of phagocytizing debris. It is accordingly a frequent site of invasion by infectious agents such as viruses.

BLOOD SUPPLY OF THE LUNGS

The lungs have a dual blood supply: (1) the pulmonary arteries and (2) the bronchial arteries.

1. The *pulmonary arteries* carry deoxygenated blood from the right ventricle to the lungs. The pulmonary artery gains access to the lung with the corresponding chief bronchus. It follows the branching of the bronchus, and, on reaching the alveolar duct, the artery divides into a capillary

plexus located in the alveolar walls. Veins arise from these capillaries, which pass first through the septa, then along the bronchioles to the root of the lung.

2. The *bronchial arteries* arise from the aorta. They accompany the bronchi and supply them, as well as the connective tissue of the lung, with oxygenated blood. These vessels terminate in capillaries, which anastomose with capillaries of the pulmonary plexus. Part of the blood carried by the bronchial arteries reaches the pulmonary veins through this anastomosis, the remainder by way of the bronchial veins.

Lymph supply of the lungs

Two groups of interconnected lymphatic vessels are present in the lung. One, a superficial or pleural group, occurs in and drains the pleura; the other deep group follows the bronchi, pulmonary artery, and vein. All drain centrally to the hilum, where they communicate with the efferent vessels of the superficial group.

NERVE SUPPLY OF THE LUNGS

The lungs are supplied by branches of the vagus nerve and also fibers of the thoracic ganglia. The fibers that supply the constrictor elements are derived chiefly from the vagus. Those that innervate the dilators of the bronchi are, in the main, sympathetic in character; they are said to arise from the inferior cervical and upper thoracic ganglia.

• • •

DEFENSE SYSTEMS IN THE RESPIRATORY TRACT

Small dust particles are dangerous only if they reach the alveoli. To prevent this, there are two basic adaptations of the air-conducting passageways: the mucociliary escalator and the tortuosity of the channels themselves. Particles 5 to 10 μm or larger are filtered out in the nasal cavities as air swirls past the turbinate bones, which project from the walls of the nasal cavity. They are swept into the oral pharynx by the ciliary movement of a mucous sheet. Many of the smaller particles are deposited on the mucosa of the larger tubes such as the trachea and large bronchi and are cleared from the tract by moving along with the mucus as it is swept up toward the pharynx by the cilia on the lining cells. These cilia move mucus up toward the pharynx (a mucociliary escalator) at the rate of 1 to 3 cm/min in the larger bronchi and more slowly in the bronchioles (0.1 cm/min). The surface coat that is moved along is about 5 μm thick and is made up of a watery film covered by a thick viscous layer of mucus. This mucus is produced by the goblet cells located in the mucosal lining of the wall and by mixed seromucous glands located beneath the epithelium (about one per square millimeter).

Small particles 0.1 to 2 μm in size probably reach the alveoli. Some of these are innocuous but some, particularly industrial dusts such as coal dust, silica, and asbestos, may result in considerable damage to lung tissue. Insoluble particles such as silica or carbon are retained permanently and accumulate in local macrophages (appropriately called dust cells), where they may elicit a slow inflammatory reaction leading to the accumulation of fibrous tissue in the walls of the respiratory passageways. There are around seven dust cells in each alveolus, lodged in small niches near the capillaries. Dust does not usually accumulate in the cells lining the alveolar wall. The macrophages in the lung may come from the bloodstream, but there is also a small area between the blood and the air sacs that seems to serve as a compartment for cell division and maturation of new macrophages from alveolar type II cells. There are no lymphatics in this space. The lymphatics penetrate only as far as the alveolar ducts, yet dust particles entering an alveolus may reach the lymphatic circulation quickly. It is not certain how this occurs. The efficiency of the alveolar macrophages in defending against local accumulation of dust particles and infectious agents is much diminished by hypoxia.

17

Urinary system

ACID-BASE + FLUID BALANCE REGULAT᷎ᵃ.

KIDNEY

The basic function of the kidneys is to clear or clean the blood plasma of the end products of metabolism as these substances pass through the elaborate capillary beds of the kidney. The kidney also adjusts the composition of body fluids by selectively retaining or excreting many plasma constituents.

The kidney filters between 10% and 30% of the plasma as blood passes through the highly coiled renal capillary beds (glomeruli), and the ultrafiltrate (plasma devoid of large proteins and particulate matter) enters the tubules of the nephrons, the functional units of the kidney. As the filtered fluid passes along the tubules, unwanted by-products of metabolism, such as urea and creatinine, remain in the tubule, whereas valuable substances such as water, electrolytes, glucose, and amino acids are selectively returned to the blood (the process of reabsorption). As the urine is formed, the tubule walls also secrete some substances into the lumen. The final urine is formed by a process of filtration and secretion, and adjustments are made in urine composition all along the tubule passage by a process of resorption. The kidney contains within it sensing devices (juxtaglomerular apparatus) for comparing the electrolyte composition of body fluids with the content of the urine, and final adjustments can be made to allow the retention or excretion of electrolytes such as sodium, potassium, and chloride or hydrogen ions. The kidney therefore is an important organ in the regulation of acid-base and fluid balance.

Gross structure of the unilobar kidney

The kidney of the rabbit is a bean-shaped gland covered by a fibrous tunic or renal capsule, which involutes into the kidney parenchyma along the medial aspect to form the kidney sinus. The external orifice of the sinus is called the hilum or hilus. The ureter expands into an extrarenal pelvis, which enters the kidney sinus and gives rise to an intrarenal pelvis (Fig. 17-1). The distal portion of the latter is expanded into a trumpet-shaped cup or calyx. The lateral walls of the calyx fuse with the tissue lining the sinus. In addition to the ureter, the renal sinus contains a prominent fat pad, nerves, lymphatics, and branches of the renal artery and vein. (The highly vascularized perirenal fat body in the abdominal cavity functions to cushion and support the kidney.)

A rabbit kidney sliced lengthwise is seen to be composed of a single, large, mushroom-shaped lobe (unilobar kidney) (Fig. 17-1). The cap of the structure appears granular and is known as the kidney cortex. The stemlike portion appears triangular, striated, and in three dimensions resembles a pyramid (from which it derives its name). The tip of the pyramid is called the papilla, and it is this part that projects into and is received by the calyx. In the unilobar, unipyramidal kidney the term medulla applies to the pyramid itself, whereas the region near the base of the pyramid in the cortex is called the juxtamedullary region. Examination of the juxtamedullary region reveals fine strands of medullary substance penetrating and subdividing

275

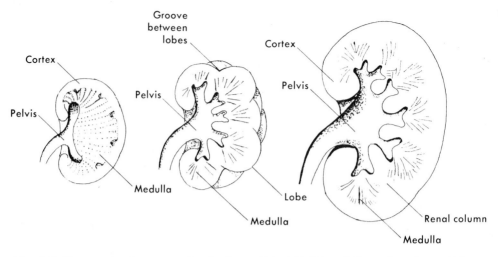

Fig. 17-1. Diagram showing topography of unipyramidal rabbit kidney (left), newborn human kidney (middle), and adult multipyramidal human kidney (right). (Drawing by Emily Craig.)

the cortical parenchyma. The former are called *medullary rays* (rays of Ferrein) and the latter are the *cortical labyrinths*. Also found in the juxtamedullary region are arched blood vessels running parallel to the base of the pyramid, which give rise to radial branches supplying and draining the cortical labyrinths (Plate 5).

Each lobe is subdivided into *lobules*. Most authors describe a lobule centered about a medullary ray and bounded by *interlobular arteries* running parallel to the ray in all the adjacent cortical labyrinths (Plate 5, medullary ray lobule). Valid reasons have been given for supporting the idea that the artery located in the cortical labyrinth should be considered the center of the lobule (Plate 5, vascular lobule), which is then bounded by the centers of adjacent medullary rays. In the vascular lobule the artery becomes a *lobular artery*, which is synonymous with the interlobular artery of the previous system.

Gross structure of the multilobar kidney

Examination of the external aspect of the kidney of a 6-month-old infant reveals remnants of many lobes (twelve to eighteen). With maturation, the external evidence of lobation in humans is obliterated. In the larger mammals, for example, the ox, elephant, or seal, the lobes are externally visible, and each one appears to act like a separate kidney. Humans have a multilobed, multipyramidal kidney (Fig. 17-1).

The kidneys are paired organs that lie behind the peritoneum in the posterior aspect of the abdomen on each side of the vertebral column. Located on the medial or concave side of each kidney is an indentation or hilus through which pass the renal artery and vein, lymphatics, a nerve plexus, and the renal pelvis.

In humans the intrarenal pelvis branches into three anterior and posterior tubes called the *major calyces*, which in turn branch to form a total of eight *minor calyces* (Plate 6). Each minor calyx receives a papilla from a single pyramid or a papilla formed by the fusion of two or more pyramids. As a result of fusion, there are fewer papillae (four to thirteen) than pyramids (eight to eighteen). In multipyramidal kidneys, trabeculae of the cortical parenchyma fill in the spaces between adjacent pyramids and are called the *renal columns*, or columns of Bertini or Bertin. The physiologist considers only the renal pyramids and medullary rays as medulla and the cortical labyrinths and renal columns as constituting the cortex of the kidney.

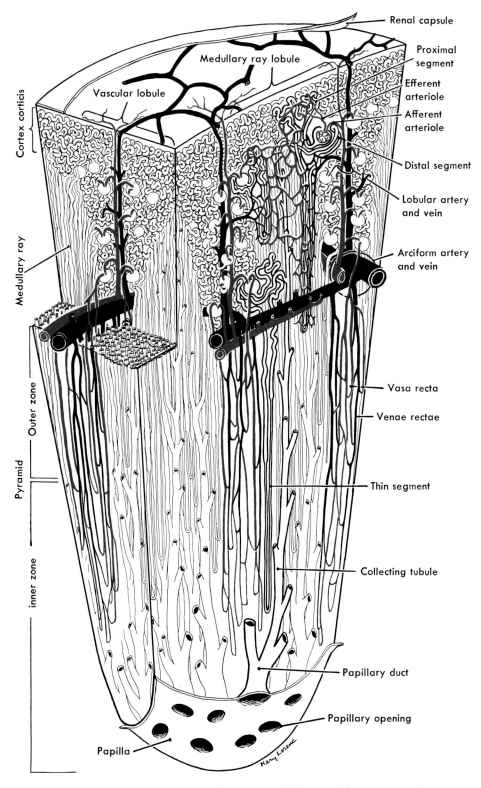

Plate 5. Details of renal pyramid and cortex. (From Smith, H. W. 1956. Principles of renal physiology. Oxford University Press, Inc., New York.)

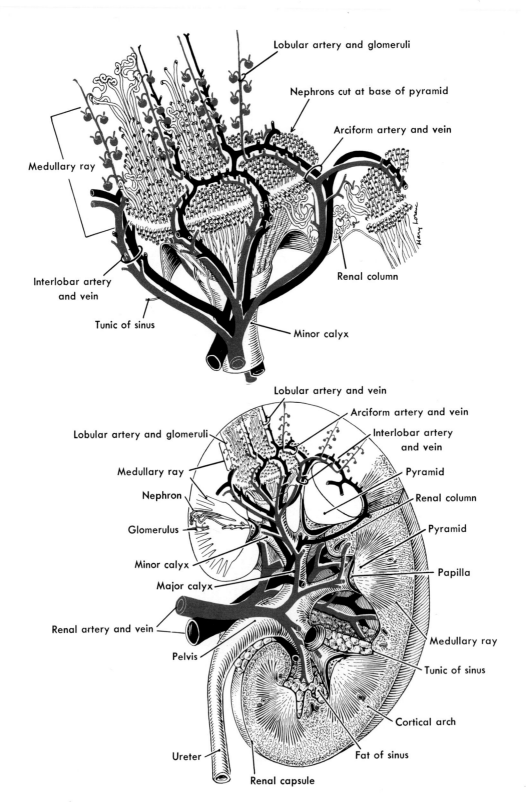

Plate 6. Circulatory plan of kidney. (From Smith, H. W. 1956. Principles of renal physiology. Oxford University Press, Inc., New York.)

Circulation

Each kidney receives approximately 10% of the blood pumped into the systemic circulation each minute by the heart and as a consequence the rate of blood flow through kidney tissue is among the highest in the body. Since the main function of the kidney is to control the composition of body fluids, the high blood flow is understandable, and a knowledge of the architecture of the kidney vasculature is crucial to an appreciation of how the kidney works.

Each kidney (Plate 6) is normally supplied by a single renal artery arising from the abdominal aorta. As the renal artery passes through the hilum it divides into an anterior and posterior branch, which supply the anterior and posterior segments of the kidney, respectively. The two main branches continue to divide into trunks that supply segments of the kidney. No collateral circulation has been demonstrated between these segmental or lobar arteries. The *lobar arteries* then divide

into a series of *interlobar arteries* that ascend to the corticomedullary junction between adjacent pyramids or between a pyramid and an adjoining renal column. Each lobe of the kidney receives six to fourteen interlobar arteries. These arteries curve abruptly in the juxtaglomerular region to form incomplete arterial arches called *arciform* (arcuate) *arteries*. Along their entire path over the base of the pyramid, the arcuate arteries give rise to radial or perpendicular interlobular arteries, which supply the cortical labyrinths. Within the renal cortex the interlobular arteries rise toward the subcapsular area giving off numerous short, straight afferent arterioles, which supply the tufts of blood vessels called glomeruli, in which plasma is filtered into the blind-ending kidney tubules (nephrons). As the lobular arteries approach the capsule, they become progressively smaller and finally break up into a plexus of arterioles and capillaries, which supply part of the capsule.

The blood flow leaving the glomeruli dif-

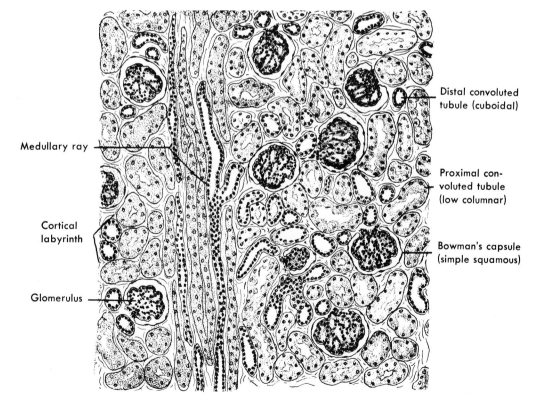

Fig. 17-2. Section of part of cortex of human kidney.

Distal convoluted tubule (cuboidal)

Medullary ray

Proximal convoluted tubule (low columnar)

Cortical labyrinth

Bowman's capsule (simple squamous)

Glomerulus

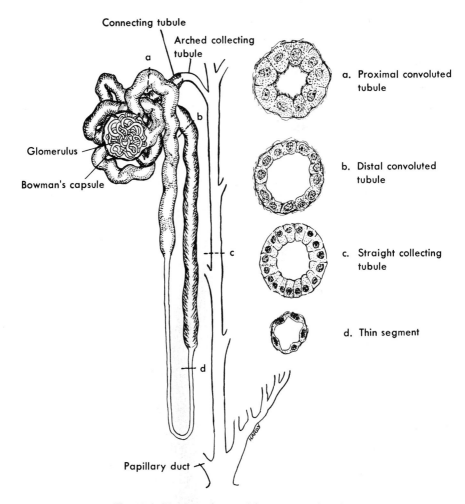

Connecting tubule
Arched collecting tubule
a
Glomerulus
Bowman's capsule
b
c
d
Papillary duct

a. Proximal convoluted tubule

b. Distal convoluted tubule

c. Straight collecting tubule

d. Thin segment

Fig. 17-3. Diagram of essential structures of nephron.

fers according to the location of the latter. Each of the *cortical glomeruli* (outer two thirds of the cortex) gives rise to an *efferent arteriole* having a diameter smaller than that of the afferent vessel (Fig. 17-5). The efferent arterioles soon divide shortly to form a *peritubular capillary network* within the cortical labyrinths and medullary rays found in the cortical region.

Only in the most superficial nephrons does this peritubular network invest primarily the tubule derived from the nephron supplied by that glomerular tuft. In midcortex, efferent arterioles may run either toward superficial or deep regions of the cortex, ultimately surrounding nephrons distant from the parent glomerulus. Near the corticomedullary junc-

tion are two main types of efferent arterioles. One type is referred to as a corticomedullary efferent. This vessel is a thin-walled arteriole that divides into a capillary network in the immediate area and within the outer rim of the medulla. The other type is the medullary efferent arteriole, a larger vessel at least as large as the afferent arterioles, which contains smooth muscle arranged in an intermittent circular pattern. These efferent arterioles penetrate the pyramid and divide there into a series of long, straight parallel blood vessels passing into the papilla. They are collectively referred to as the *vasa rectae*, and they form the main blood supply to the outer rim of the medulla. These vessels are arranged with parallel ascending and descend-

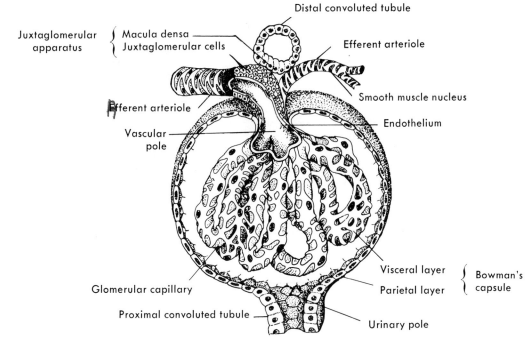

Juxtaglomerular apparatus { Macula densa
Juxtaglomerular cells

Distal convoluted tubule

Efferent arteriole

Smooth muscle nucleus

Efferent arteriole

Endothelium

Vascular pole

Visceral layer } Bowman's capsule
Parietal layer {

Glomerular capillary

Proximal convoluted tubule

Urinary pole

Fig. 17-4. Representative drawing of renal corpuscle. (Redrawn and modified from Bailey.)

ing vessels connected by a hairpin loop or sharp bend so that blood runs in opposite directions in the two limbs. This is where countercurrent exchange occurs, thus maintaining osmotic equilibrium. Careful observation is necessary to differentiate these from ordinary capillaries. An incomplete inner elastic membrane may occur in afferent arterioles but not in the efferent or glomerular vessels. The smooth muscle elements of the efferent arterioles may be lacking or replaced at intervals by groups of contractile pericytes or Rouget cells.

If the renal capsule is stripped away carefully, one may observe that a series of subcapsular blood vessels merge at certain points. Such vessels give the impression that the kidney surface is covered by several star-shaped blood vessels. These are the so-called *stellate veins*, and the central point of fusion marks the beginning of the *lobular vein* (interlobular vein). The lobular veins pass through the cortical labyrinths together with the lobular arteries. The freely anastomosing peritubular capillaries drain into short cortical veins (intralobular veins), which in turn join the lobular veins. In the juxtamedullary region the lobular veins join the *arciform veins* (arcuate veins). In contrast with the arciform arteries, the arciform veins form complete arches over the surface of the pyramidal base (Plates 5 and 6). The papilla is drained by a series of straight blood vessels, the venae rectae (vasa rectae). The walls of these veins contain smooth muscle spirally arranged and have a thinner endothelial lining than do the descending vessels. The vasa rectae and venae rectae are extensions of the peritubular capillary network that penetrate deeply into the medulla in association with the long loops of Henle of the juxtamedullary nephrons and return toward the cortex in a hairpin loop. They are concerned with exchanges of water and salt between the loop of Henle and the blood. The venae rectae drain directly into the arciform veins in the juxtamedullary region.

Glomerular capillaries   Afferent arteriole   Efferent arteriole

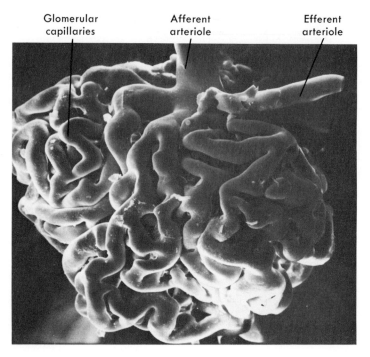

Fig. 17-5. Scanning electron micrograph of injected glomerulus from mouse kidney. (×960.) (Courtesy Dr. H. Nakahara.)

Fine structure of the kidney

The urinary functions of the kidney are carried out by three groups of structures: (1) the glomeruli, (2) the nephrons, and (3) the collecting tubules and papillary ducts. Urine is formed by the activity of the nephrons, described as the functional units of the kidney. There are about 1 million nephrons in each human kidney.

Glomeruli. The glomerulus is that portion of the nephron responsible for the production of an ultrafiltrate of plasma. The total filtration surface of all glomeruli combined is about 1 square meter. The glomerulus is composed of a capillary network lined by endothelial cells, a central region of mesangial cells (also called the centrolobular region, stalk region, or intercapillary region) and the layers of Bowmans' capsule with associated basement membrane. In tissue sections each glomerulus is observed as an oval or rounded body consisting of a mass of capillaries containing many red blood cells and bounded by a small space (Figs. 17-2 to 17-4). The space

is the cavity of Bowman's capsule and is formed by invagination of the capillary into an enlargement of the end of the nephron. Thus Bowman's capsule is a double-layered epithelial structure composed of squamous epithelium, with nuclei bulging into the capsular space. The inner layer of Bowman's capsule is known as the *visceral layer* and invests the exposed surfaces of the glomerular tuft. The *parietal layer* forms the outer boundary of the capsule. A prominent basement membrane is visualized by the PAS technique and is located around the parietal layer of the capsule and between the visceral layer and the glomerular capillaries.

The side of the glomerulus where the afferent and efferent arterioles enter and leave and approximate each other forms the vascular pole of the glomerulus. The end directed toward the tubular portion of the nephron is known as the urinary pole of the glomerulus (Fig. 17-4). As the afferent arteriole approaches the vascular pole, it gives rise to the juxtaglomerular apparatus (Fig. 17-4), a

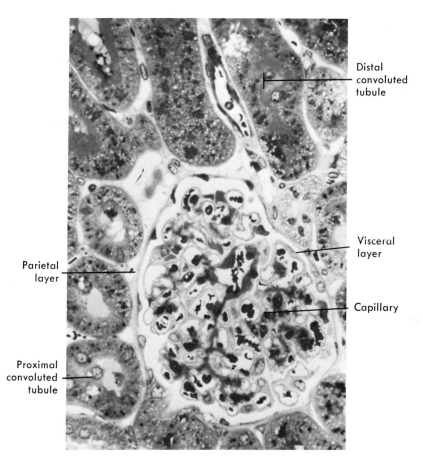

Distal convoluted tubule

Visceral layer

Parietal layer

Capillary

Proximal convoluted tubule

Fig. 17-6. Section of glomerulus and associated structures from mouse kidney. (×400.) (Courtesy Dr. H. Nakahara.)

site where the chemical composition of the forming urine in the tubule can be compared to the blood that is about to be filtered. As it enters Bowman's capsule, the afferent arteriole loses its inner elastic membrane and gives rise to from four to eight primary capillaries that branch and form several anastomosing secondary capillaries. They, in turn, merge to form primary capillaries draining into the efferent arterioles. As a result of this arrangement of capillaries, the glomerulus is described as *lobulated* (Fig. 17-4). In section, however, the mass of capillaries observed in glomeruli rarely appears lobulated (Fig. 17-6).

The glomerulus together with Bowman's capsule forms the *Malpighian* (renal) *corpuscle.* Although they vary considerably in size, the juxtamedullary glomeruli appear to be larger and in humans may average approximately 0.2 mm in diameter. Glomeruli are limited to the cortical labyrinths and renal columns and are not ordinarily found in the medullary rays or pyramidal tissue of the kidney (Plates 5 and 6). *Note:* Many lower chordates, for example, certain fishes, possess aglomerular kidneys.

Nephron. On an anatomical basis the nephron consists of four parts: Bowman's capsule, proximal convoluted tubule, loop of Henle, and distal convoluted tubule (Fig. 17-3). Bowman's capsule has been described previously as an invaginated dilation of the nephric tubule. The parietal layer leads into a small necklike constriction, which contains ciliated cells in submammalian forms but not in human beings. The tubule leading from the capsule almost immediately begins a twisted and tortuous path through the cortical labyrinth and is accordingly named the proximal convoluted tubule. In sections this is indicated by tubules cut in several planes (Figs. 17-2 and 17-6); most, however, appear in transverse or tangential section.

The proximal tubule enters a medullary ray at the site where it bends toward the papilla and forms a relatively straight tube, the *descending arm* of Henle's loop. This extends for a variable distance and then reverses its direction to form the so-called *ascending arm*

of Henle's loop, which is approximately parallel to the descending arm. In the region of the actual curvature the tubule becomes extremely thin, giving rise to the *thin segment* of Henle's loop. The thin segment is a variable structure, since it may be located on the ascending side, the descending side, or both. Thin segments of nephrons arising from cortical glomeruli are abbreviated or lacking entirely, whereas nephrons originating in the juxtamedullary region bear long thin segments penetrating deeply into the pyramids (Plate 6). In summary, the loops of Henle are located entirely within the medullary rays

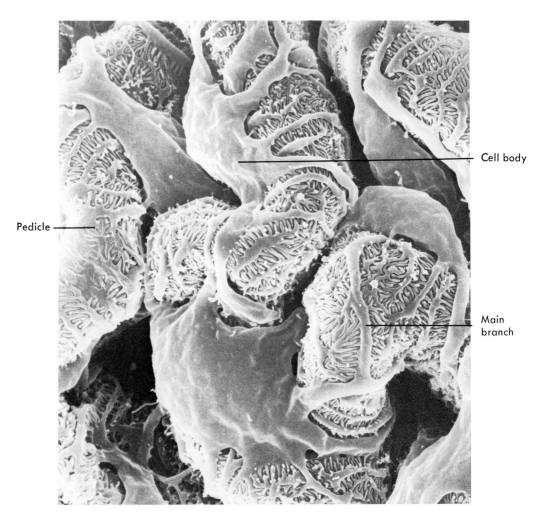

Cell body

Pedicle

Main branch

Fig. 17-7. Scanning electron micrograph showing podocytes from visceral epithelium of rat glomerulus. This three-dimensional micrograph shows the manner in which the pedicles from adjacent podocytes interdigitate with one another. (×4,700.) (Courtesy Dr. P. M. Andrews.)

and pyramids. They consist of a thick descending limb; a thin segment, which varies in location and length; and a thick ascending limb.

The ascending limb enters the cortical labyrinth slightly below the level of the glomerulus of origin, passes between the afferent and efferent vessels, and makes tangential contact with the vascular pole of the glomerulus. The region of tangential contact is specialized to form the *macula densa* (Fig. 17-4). The portion of the tubule extending beyond the vascular pole is known as the *distal convoluted tubule.* It is less convoluted than the proximal tubule. The distal tubule leads to an arched tubule, which enters the medullary ray to join the system of collecting tubules.

On a cytological-physiological basis, only four subdivisions of the nephron are designated: Bowman's capsule, a proximal segment, a thin segment, and a distal segment.

Bowman's capsule. The *parietal* layer of Bowman's capsule consists of squamous epithelium with prominent nuclei that protrude into the capillary space (Fig. 17-6). The inner

or *visceral* epithelium forms a thin sheet over the loops of the glomerular capillaries. This fact was not clearly demonstrated until observed by electron microscopy. Studies utilizing the electron microscope have shown that the cells comprising the visceral epithelium are branching cells called *podocytes* (Fig. 17-7). Each cell consists of a central mass containing a nucleus and several radiating processes or branches, which, in turn, give rise to smaller processes known as *foot processes* or *pedicles* (Fig. 17-8). The pedicles make contact with the basal lamina of the capillary. Pedicles from adjacent cells interdigitate and leave slits (filtration slits) that communicate with the larger spaces between major extensions. They all empty into the capsular (urinary) space.

The endothelium of the capillaries is composed of thin flattened cells with a mass of cytoplasm in the area of the nucleus. In the thinner portions they exhibit a specialization that consists of numerous round openings (fenestrations), which are regularly arranged and lie near one another (Fig. 17-8).

The glomerular tuft and Bowman's capsule

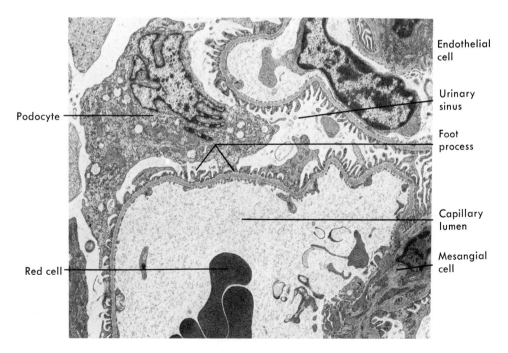

Fig. 17-8. Electron micrograph of portion of renal corpuscle of rat. (×6,000.) (Courtesy Dr. H. Nakahara.)

form the filter through which the fluid component of blood is forced under hydrostatic pressure to form an ultrafiltrate that then passes into the proximal convoluted tubule. Large molecules in the circulation do not pass this barrier. Numerous attempts have been made in recent years to identify the anatomical components of the capillary wall that form the filter which prevents passage of large molecules from the capillaries into the urinary space. Experiments designed to follow the movement of large identifiable molecules through the glomerulus led to the view that there are three barriers in series. The endothelial cells of the capillary wall were regarded as a coarse filter that serves primarily to keep large particles away from the basement membrane; the basement membrane was believed to be a relatively coarse filter; and the slits between the epithelial

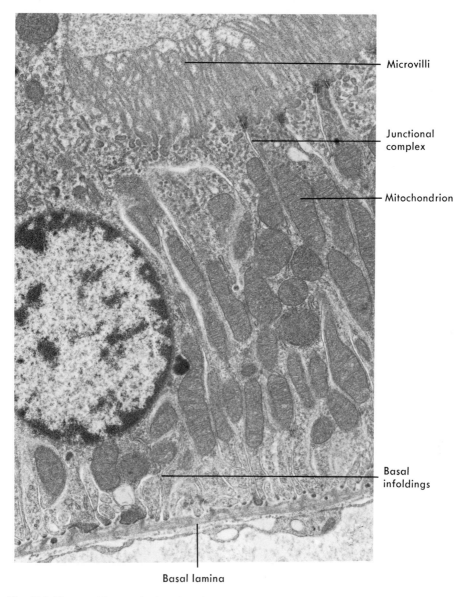

Microvilli

Junctional complex

Mitochondrion

Basal infoldings

Basal lamina

Fig. 17-9. Electron micrograph of portion of epithelial cell of proximal convoluted tubule of mouse kidney. (×8,000.) (Courtesy Dr. H. Nakahara.)

cells of Bowman's capsule, which coat the glomerular capillaries, were thought to be responsible for controlling the composition of the ultrafiltrate by almost completely blocking the passage of any molecule larger than 4.4 nm in radius. Recent evidence, however, suggests that the basement membrane itself is the fine filter, and the functions of the cell processes are as yet unknown.

Another component of the glomerulus consists of cells and intercellular matrices that occupy a position between the capillary loops, known as the *mesangium*. The mesangial (intercapillary) cells lie at the branching of the capillary loops (Fig. 17-8). They were described as having a dense cytoplasm and radiating cytoplasmic processes and tonofilaments. Since they have been shown to contain a myosin-like protein by immunofluorescent techniques, these cells are probably contractile. They maintain close contact with the macula densa of the distal tubule by means of cellular interdigitations. In addition to their supportive role, mesangial cells are phagocytic. They probably serve to clean the glomerular filter by removing protein and debris that accumulate on the basement membrane or between the cell processes.

Proximal segment. The proximal segment consists of a convoluted portion in the cortical labyrinth and a straight descending limb in the medullary ray and pyramid. The proximal segment is composed of a tubule with low columnar epithelium (Fig. 17-3) bearing a brush border at the free surface and basal striations in the subnuclear position. Inasmuch as adjacent cells interdigitate freely, the cell outlines are rarely seen in cross sections of the tubule. The coarsely granular eosinophilic cytoplasm bulges into the lumen, and the nuclei are basally located. The brush border is not ordinarily well preserved; accordingly, the free edge of the cell appears rounded and slightly ragged. The

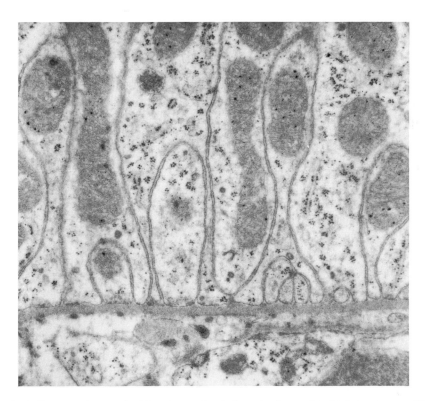

Fig. 17-10. Electron micrograph of basal part of cell of proximal convoluted tubule of mouse kidney. Note extensive infolding of cell membranes enclosing densely packed mitochondria and scattered ribosomes. (×25,000.)

basal striations become less distinct as the thin segment is approached.

At the electron microscope level the brush border is shown to consist of numerous thin microvilli (Fig. 17-9). Frequently, small vesicles appear between the bases of the microvilli, and it has been suggested that tubular reabsorption may be accomplished in part by pinocytotic activity. A Golgi complex located in the supranuclear position is a constant feature of these cells.

A prominent feature of the cells of the proximal tubule is the basal portion that is divided into compartments by prominent infoldings (Figs. 17-9 and 17-10). These compartments contain numerous elongated mitochondria and polyribosomes. They rest on a continuous basal lamina, which separates them from the walls of the surrounding (peritubular) capillaries. The cells of the proximal tubule are held together by junctional complexes.

Until recently, it was assumed that the tight junction of the proximal convoluted cells could restrain the passage of both solutes and water between the lumen and the intercellular space beneath the tubular epithelium, but it is now believed that this path is "leaky" and that there is a shunt pathway between the cells that may play a role in the reabsorption of solute and water in the proximal tubule. By the time the ultrafiltrate reaches the end of the proximal tubule, approximately 70% has been reabsorbed and returned to the bloodstream. The final adjustments in composition and volume of the urine will occur in the distal parts of the tubule. One of the main functions of the proximal convoluted tubule and to a lesser extent the tubule's straight part *(pars recta)* is recapture of filtered substances—albumin, other small proteins, and nonproteins such as carbohydrates. This is accomplished by a process called endocytosis in which the proteins become enmeshed in the surface coats of the tubule cells and are then taken up in fluid-filled vesicles by pinocytosis. The materials are then ingested into the cell, broken down by lysosomes, and the processed materials returned to the blood on the sublumi-

nal side by exocytosis. In addition, sodium is actively transported across the cell into the lateral cellular spaces where the high sodium buildup serves to produce a high osmotic gradient that also facilitates passive water flow. The fluid in the spaces is driven into the capillaries by a combination of osmotic (oncotic) pressure and hydrostatic pressure.

Thin segment. The thin segment (Fig. 17-3) is a tubular structure consisting of squamous cells. The cytoplasm appears agranular, and the nucleus is slightly compressed. In transverse section it may be confused with capillaries and arteriolae rectae, especially since red blood cells are sometimes forced into the thin segment during preparation of the tissue. It is distinguished from capillaries by the more extensive protrusion of nuclei into the lumen and the greater number of cells present in cross section of a tubule.

The transition from the terminal proximal tubule to the thin ascending limb of Henle occurs in the medulla. The loop descends into the medulla, then makes a sharp turn and rises toward the outer medulla. In the short loops that arise from cortical nephrons one wall thickens as the hairpin turn occurs. A smaller number of juxtamedullary nephrons have longer loops that penetrate deeply into the medulla. As the thin loops descend, they are accompanied by the arterial and venous vasa recta; as these loops turn and ascend, they are associated with the collecting duct and capillary plexuses. The thin ascending and descending segments of Henle's loop appear to play an important role in the concentration of urine. The parallel arrays of tubules and the vasa recta are thought to be actively involved in the passage of sodium and chloride first into the interstitial fluid and then into the circulation by a process known as countercurrent multiplication.

Thin segments are demonstrable in profusion in the deeper portions of the pyramids, since they extend almost to the papillae. Thin segments of the kind described are lacking in reptiles, most birds, amphibians, and fishes.

Distal segment. The thin segment turns in

a loop (the loop of Henle) and thickens before it joins the distal segment, which is composed initially of low cuboidal cells with indistinct boundaries. As the ascending limb approaches the cortex, the cells are taller but are still cuboidal and bear irregular projections into the lumen. On entering the cortical labyrinths, the tubule passes the vascular pole of the glomerulus of origin and makes tangential contact with the afferent arteriole. At the point of contact the cuboidal cells become more closely packed so that the cells appear taller (sometimes columnar), and many nuclei are visible and crowded together to form the *macula densa* (Fig. 17-4). Beyond this structure the tubule becomes convoluted, consisting of smaller cuboidal cells, the free surfaces of which are smooth. These cells are less eosinophilic (or more basophilic) than are those found in the proximal tubule. The cells do not bear a striated or brush border or basal striations (Fig. 17-11); neither do they exhibit definite cell boundaries in sectioned material. The basement membrane is prominent along all parts of the tubule except in the region of the macula densa. Since the convoluted portion is short, fewer sections through this segment are observed in the cortical labyrinths.

A number of functions have been assigned to the distal tubule, including reabsorption of bicarbonate and water, transport or secretion of ions: hydrogen, sodium, chloride, ammonia, calcium, and magnesium. Because of difficulties in sampling from different regions of the tubule, it is uncertain whether these processes take place in the convoluted distal tubule, the initial part of the collecting tubule, or both. It is clear, however, that the distal tubule and collecting tubule are the site for the final adjustment of urine composition and volume.

Collecting tubules and papillary ducts. At the termination of the distal convoluted tubule a short connecting tubule can sometimes be observed. It contains a mixture of the cuboidal cells characteristic of the distal segment and occasional isolated large granular (intercalary) cells. This is supposedly the region of embryonic fusion between the nephron and the collecting tubule.

The connecting tubule is continuous with the *arched collecting tubule* that passes into the medullary ray where it joins the *straight collecting tubule* (Fig. 17-3). The straight tubules, along with Henle's loops, lie in parallel bundles and occupy most of the medulla, with the exception of the papilla. The cells of the collecting tubules have distinct boundaries, spherical nuclei at approximately the same level in the cell, and relatively agranular cytoplasm (Fig. 17-12). Eventually the straight tubules (Plate 5) reach the papillary region and fuse to form relatively large ducts, the *papillary ducts* (ducts of Bellini). The latter are lined by tall columnar cells. In each papilla there are sixteen to twenty papillary ducts, which penetrate the apex of the papilla to form a sievelike region or *area cribrosa* (Plate 5). From this site the urine formed in the nephrons is drained into a minor calyx (Fig. 17-1).

Juxtaglomerular apparatus. The juxtaglomerular apparatus is made up of four basic elements: (1) the terminal portion of the afferent arteriole just prior to its entry into the hilum of the glomerular tuft; (2) the macula densa, a specialized segment of the distal tubule; (3) the mesangial region; and (4) the efferent arteriole of the glomerulus (Fig. 17-4). The juxtaglomerular apparatus thus represents a complex anatomical arrangement of vascular and renal tubule components. At the vascular pole of the glomerulus (Fig. 17-4) the media and adventitial reticulum of the afferent arteriole are replaced by cells that vary from cuboidal to columnar. These form a thickening or cuff around the arteriole (periarteriolar pad). Numerous cells may spill into the cleft between the afferent and efferent vessels to form an asymmetrical cap (Polkissen or polar cushion). The polar cushion and periarteriolar pad both may be in contact with the macula densa, and their region of contact is marked by the absence of a PAS-positive basement membrane. The Polkissen cells of certain rodents exhibit some large epithelioid cells containing brilliant fuchsinophil granules. In canines and humans the cells are small and agranular.

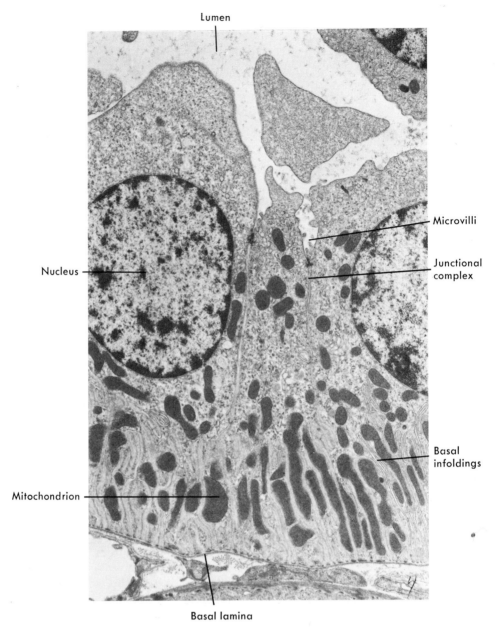

Lumen

Microvilli

Junctional complex

Nucleus

Basal infoldings

Mitochondrion

Basal lamina

Fig. 17-11. Electron micrograph of portions of two epithelial cells of distal convoluted tubule of mouse kidney. (×7,000.) (Courtesy Dr. H. Nakahara.)

The nature of the points of contact between the distal tubule and the vascular components has been a source of controversy. Two types of contact appear to exist. One is a simple apposition of basement membranes, which may be reversible, and another is a more complex interdigitation between the cells. The distal tubule is more closely connected to the efferent arteriole and mesangial region than with the afferent arteriole. Its anatomical arrangement allows for a comparison between the chemical composition of

Cuboidal cells   Basement membrane

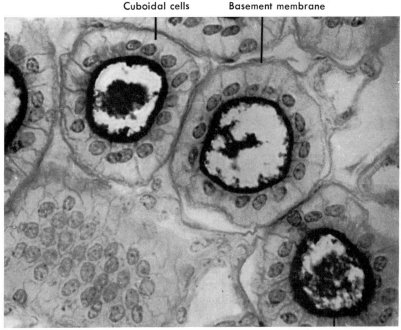

Alkaline phosphatase

Fig. 17-12. Section of kidney of skate. Collecting tubules treated to show localization of enzyme alkaline phosphatase. (×640.)

blood perfusing the tubule and the urine entering the distal tubule where a final adjustment of salinity and volume can be made. The juxtaglomerular apparatus plays a major role in the regulation of sodium excretion by the kidney and as a consequence is a major element in the control of overall body salt and water balance. The juxtaglomerular apparatus is not demonstrable in humans for the first 2 years of postnatal life. The presence of epithelioid cells similar to those found in certain endocrine organs suggests an endocrine function. Physiological experiments indicate that these cells produce renin. Renin is a proteolytic enzyme secreted by the juxtaglomerular apparatus that reacts with a precursor in the blood to form an active vasopressor substance, angiotensin II, which, in addition to its effect on blood pressure, influences the release of aldosterone from the adrenal cortex. Aldosterone in turn facilitates sodium retention by the kidney. Present techniques have not adequately demonstrated whether renin is made in the macula densa of the distal convoluted tubule, the juxtaglomerular (JG) cells of the afferent arteriole, or cells between them. Current evidence favors the juxtaglomerular cells as the source of renin, but the cellular membranes of the juxtaglomerular cells and the macula densa cells interdigitate, and some exchange of materials between them is likely.

Lymphatic circulation. The lymphatic plexuses are found in three main regions as follows. (1) A network of lymphatic capillaries permeates the cortex and renal columns; these capillaries form an anastomosing network around blood vessels, especially the larger arteries. The plexus drains into the lymphatic vessels leaving the hilum of the kidney; then it passes into the lateral aortic nodes (2) beneath the renal capsule in intimate association with the stellate veins and subcapsular plexus of blood capillaries. This group communicates with (3) the lymphatics draining the perirenal fat body. The perirenal lymphatic plexus drains into the lateral aortic nodes.

Lymphatics are lacking in the renal pyramids and glomeruli and do not enter the tubules. No specific function has been demonstrated for the kidney lymphatics, and our knowledge of their distribution is severely limited.

Nerve supply. The nerve supply to the kidney arises largely from the celiac plexus, although some fibers are also contributed by other plexuses. Both adrenergic and cholinergic fibers enter the renal parenchyma along the routes taken by the arterial supply. Only the juxtaglomerular portion of the nephrons and the efferent glomerular arterioles appear to be richly innervated, providing a route by which neural input can adjust salt and water balance. Nerve endings have not been observed in the glomerulus itself or on other parts of the nephrons. The blood flow through the kidney is maintained relatively constant despite changes in perfusion pressure, but this process does not require either innervation or humoral mechanisms from outside the kidney. The most likely explanation for autoregulation of kidney blood flow is the myogenic theory, according to which changes in pressure directly alter the tone of the smooth muscle in the kidney vascular bed.

Connective tissue. The renal capsule is formed of a dense fibrous connective tissue that is primarily collagenous, with some elastic fibers and a few scattered smooth muscle cells. A thin inflexion of this capsule lines the renal sinus and fuses with the adventitia of the blood vessels and epineurium of the larger nerves. It also disperses into fine strands in the fat body of the renal sinus. The renal capsule is easily stripped from normal kidneys because of a lack of trabeculae from the capsule.

The basement membrane envelops all parts of the nephron and collecting tubules except as previously noted. The ground substance of the basement membrane is PAS positive, and the reticular fibers are typically argyrophile and fine. In the pyramids the reticular fibers form an extensive network, binding ducts and blood vessels together.

Excretory passages. The excretory passages consist of the calyces, renal pelvis, ureter, bladder, and urethra. All these structures, with the exception of the urethra, have a similar basic structure. The wall consists of

Adipose tissue   Muscularis

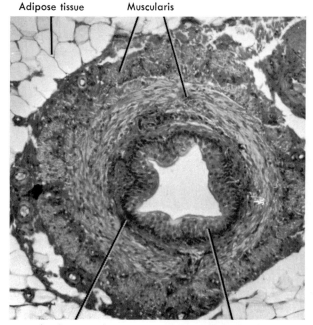

Fig. 17-13. Ureter of cat. (×160.)

Lamina propria   Transitional
                        epithelium

an inner mucosa lined with transitional epithelium, a middle muscular layer that becomes thicker as the ureter reaches the bladder, and an outer adventitia that blends into the surrounding connective tissue. There is no distinct submucosa (Fig. 17-13).

URETER

Urine collects in the pelvis of the kidney and passes into the ureter, a thin duct leading to the bladder.

Mucosa. The mucosa includes an epithelium of the transitional type resting on a lamina propria of reticular and fine areolar tissue. The basement membrane separating the epithelium from the lamina propria is not distinct, although one can be detected at higher magnification. The epithelium is two or three cell layers thick in the renal pelvis; it gradually increases to six or more layers in the undistended bladder. When the organ is stretched, the cells flatten and interdigitation between the cells is reduced. The epithelium lining the ureter and bladder is reduced to a layer approximately three cells thick in the distended state. The muscularis mucosa is lacking.

Muscularis. In the muscularis the usual arrangement of coats is reversed, there being an inner longitudinal and an outer circular layer. The lower portion of the ureter contains a third layer of muscle, longitudinally disposed, outside the circular layer. All three layers are somewhat loosely arranged, with a great deal of areolar tissue among the muscle fibers.

Adventitia. The adventitia is formed of loose connective tissue (Fig. 17-13).

URINARY BLADDER

The wall of the urinary bladder is composed of the same elements as those of the lower part of the ureter, that is, transitional epithelium, lamina propria, three layers of muscle, and adventitia (Fig. 17-14). In the bladder the epithelium (transitional) varies

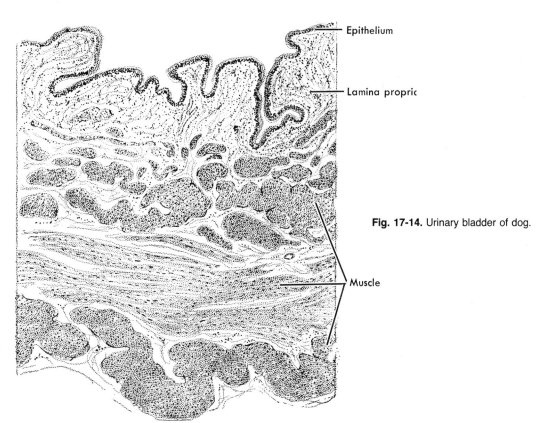

Epithelium

Lamina propric

Fig. 17-14. Urinary bladder of dog.

Muscle

in thickness according to the degree of distention of the organ. The muscular layers of the bladder are not as regular in their arrangements as those of the ureter, but they form a thicker layer (Fig. 17-15). Where present, the adventitia is composed of fibroelastic tissue.

The primary function of the mammalian bladder is to retain urine produced continuously by the kidneys until it can be voided. The urine arriving in the bladder is frequently hypertonic and differs considerably from blood in both its organic and inorganic content. The blood capillaries lie just beneath the epithelium within the lamina propia so that the blood is within a few microns of the urine. If the lining of the bladder were semipermeable, water would be driven across the epithelium, and the urine would be quickly diluted. The unique properties of transitional epithelium permit it to serve as a barrier. The basal walls may be cuboidal or columnar and are similar to the base of other epithelial sheets. The cells rest on a thin uninterrupted basal lamina and are attached to it by half-demosomes at frequent intervals.

The intermediate cells are deeply infolded in the contracted bladder and are connected to each other by desmosomes. The surface layer is unique in transitional epithelium and consists of a layer of flattened squamous cells that form a continuous pavementlike covering held together by desmosomes and junctional complexes. The free luminal surface of the cells forms a thickened semirigid membrane composed of plaques covering up to 90% of the cell surface. They are separated by thinner regions that act like hinges to allow the surface to fold when the bladder contracts during micturition (the voiding of urine). The relative impermeability of the luminal membrane of the adult bladder presumably depends on the chemical composition of these placques, but much work must be accomplished before the barrier function of transitional epithelium will be fully explained.

URETHRA

The urethra of the female serves as an outlet for urine from the bladder, whereas that of the male functions also as the terminal

Lamina propria   Transitional epithelium

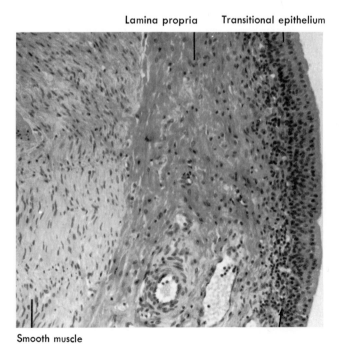

Smooth muscle

Fig. 17-15. Section of human urinary bladder showing mucosa and part of muscularis. (×40.)

portion of the ducts of the reproductive system. The organ is, therefore, somewhat different in the two sexes.

Female urethra

In the female the tube is composed of an epithelial lining, a connective tissue layer, and a muscular coat. The epithelium of the proximal part is like that of the bladder. This type is replaced further down the tube first by stratified or pseudostratified columnar epithelium and later, toward the distal end, by stratified squamous epithelium.

The connective tissue layer contains elastic fibers and a rich plexus of veins, which may be compared with the corpus cavernosum of the male urethra (to be discussed next), although it is much less extensive. The lumen of the organ is irregular, since the connective tissue and epithelium are thrown into longitudinal rugae. There are also small diverticula from the lumen (lacunae) into which open the mucus-secreting glands of Littré.

The muscularis consists of two sets of smooth muscle fibers intermingled with connective tissue. The fibers of the inner set are longitudinally placed; the outer have a circular direction. Note that this is different from the arrangement of muscle in the gut wall, where the inner muscle coat is circular and the outer is longitudinal. At the distal end of the urethra there is, in addition, a sphincter of striated muscle.

Male urethra

The male urethra shows modifications of the structure just described. It is divided into three portions: prostatic, membranous, and cavernous (Fig. 18-1).

Prostatic portion. The proximal end of the prostatic urethra is homologous to the female urethra and resembles it in structure as well as in function. As the tube passes through the prostate gland it receives the openings of the ducts from the testes and numerous small ducts from the prostate.

Membranous portion. The membranous portion of the urethra, which passes through the urogenital diaphragm, is also somewhat like the female urethra. The epithelium changes in or about this region from transitional to stratified or pseudostratified columnar, but the location of the change varies considerably in different individuals. Glands are more common than in the female urethra. The bulbourethral (mucous) glands of Cowper are situated in the muscle near the distal part of the membranous urethra, but their ducts enter the cavernous urethra.

Cavernous portion. The cavernous portion is the longest segment of the urethra, lying in the penis. The tissues surrounding it will be discussed more fully in Chapter 18. The epithelial lining of the urethra changes at the distal end to stratified squamous with well-developed connective tissue papillae. The lamina propria contains an extensive plexus of blood vessels, which forms the corpus cavernosum urethrae, and the glands of Littré are most numerous in this portion of the tube. The muscular coat is broken up into scattered groups of fibers.

Blood and nerve supply of the excretory passages

The blood supply of the ureter, bladder, and urethra comes from arteries that penetrate the muscular coats of the organs and form plexuses in the deeper layers of the lamina propria. From here, vessels continue inward, forming other plexuses just below the epithelium. The deeper layers of the connective tissue and probably the muscular layers have a rich lymphatic supply.

Plexuses of myelinated and nonmyelinated nerves occur in the walls of the ureter and the bladder. The nonmyelinated nerves supply the muscles; the myelinated, the mucosa. Numerous ganglia are present in the connective tissue.

18

Male reproductive system

The male reproductive system consists of (1) the testes, which produce sperm and male hormones, (2) the system of ducts that carry the sperm from the testes to the urethra and in which sperm continue their maturation, (3) several accessory glands associated with the duct system that secrete components of the seminal fluid, and (4) the penis (Fig. 18-1).

TESTIS

The testis is covered by a two-layered connective tissue capsule. The outer layer, the tunica albuginea, is composed of dense collagenous fibrous tissue; the inner or vasculosa layer is of looser areolar tissue richly supplied with blood vessels. From the capsule, trabeculae extend inward to a central mass of connective tissue, the mediastinum, which contains the proximal portions of the duct system. The parenchyma of the testis is thus divided into many pyramidal lobules, which contain the closely packed coils of the seminiferous tubules and a stroma of interstitial connective tissue (Figs. 18-2 and 18-3). In the connective tissue are blood vessels and groups of endocrine cells called the *interstitial cells* of the testes *(Leydig cells)*, which produce steroid hormones.

The convoluted seminiferous tubules are lined with germinal epithelium that may contain as many as five layers of cells (Fig. 18-3). This epithelium is composed of spermatogenic or sperm-forming cells and *Sertoli* or *supportive cells* (Fig. 18-3). These two cell groups are generally believed to be derived from two independent cell lines. At birth, the testes contain recognizable spermatogonia, but within a few months they disappear, reappearing again at the onset of puberty. When sexual maturity begins, the Leydig cells become more prominent (Figs. 18-3 and 18-4), and spermatogenic cells in diverse stages of development appear within the tubules (Figs. 18-2 and 18-3). The epithelium rests on a thin basement membrane which, in turn, is surrounded by a capsule consisting of fibroelastic connective tissue (Fig. 18-5). Most closely applied to the outside of the wall of the tubules are the spermatogonia or primordial germ cells separated from the wall by fine Sertoli cell processes. These germ cells are small, cuboidal, or rounded with vesicular nuclei. Proceeding toward the lumen one observes the primary spermatocytes (Fig. 18-5). They are larger cells and exhibit dense clumps of chromatin in the nuclei. Next in order are the secondary spermatocytes, which are rarely seen but are similar in appearance to the primary spermatocytes except somewhat smaller. Superimposed on these are the spermatids, which are much smaller cells with vesicular nuclei. Bordering on the lumen one may observe the fully formed spermatozoa, possessing dark, elongated nuclei and flagella (Fig. 18-6).

The process involved in the development of the spermatozoa consists of (1) a reduction of the chromosomal number from the diploid or somatic number (forty-six in humans) to

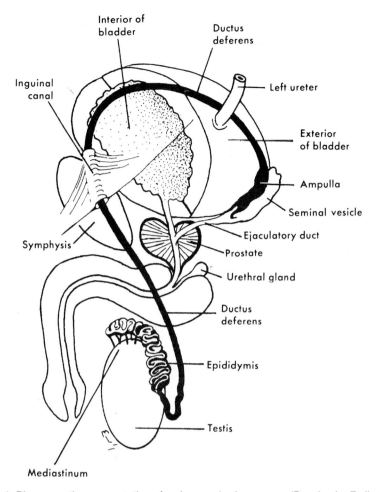

Fig. 18-1. Diagrammatic representation of male reproductive organs. (Drawing by Emily Craig.)

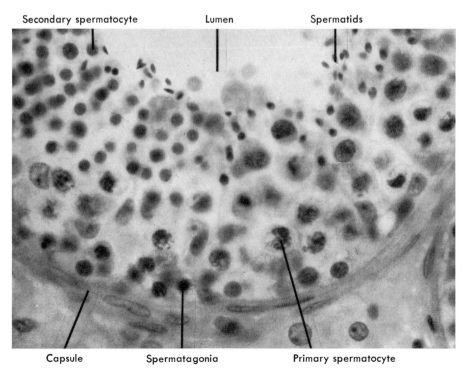

Fig. 18-2. Section of portion of human seminiferous tubule. (×640.)

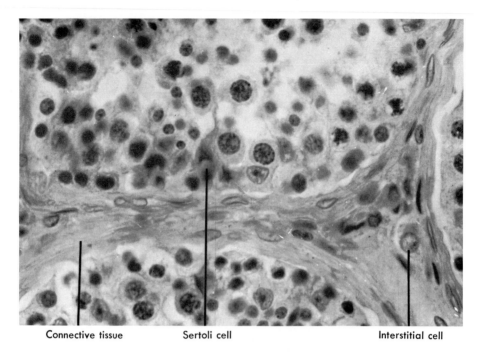

Connective tissue   Sertoli cell   Interstitial cell

Fig. 18-3. Section of human seminiferous tubules showing interstitial (Leydig) cells between adjacent tubules. (×640.)

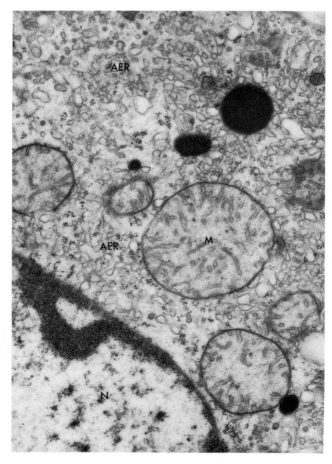

Fig. 18-4. Electron micrograph of part of interstitial cell of mouse. Note abundant, tubular, agranular endoplasmic reticulum, *AER. N,* Nucleus; *M,* mitochondrion. (×23,000.)

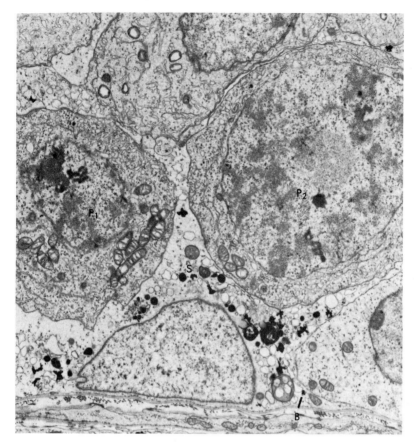

Fig. 18-5. Electron micrograph of part of seminiferous tubule of mouse. *B,* Basement membrane; $P_1, P_2,$ primary spermatocytes in prophase; *S,* Sertoli cell. (×7,000.)

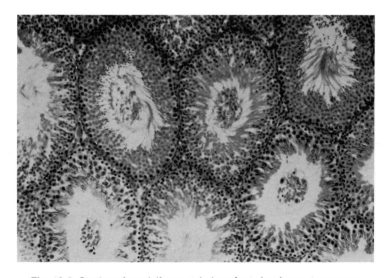

Fig. 18-6. Section of seminiferous tubules of rat showing mature sperm.

the haploid or germ cell number (twenty-three) and (2) the formation of elongate, tail-bearing motile cells from the primitive oval spermatogonia. In males, chromosomal redistribution (meiosis, spermatogenesis) occurs before the cell becomes differentiated (spermiogenesis). In females, the egg is formed while the cell is in the first stage of meiosis, and the egg remains arrested in meiosis until approximately the time of ovulation. In ordinary cell division (mitosis) the chromosomal material is replicated before the onset of nuclear division. Following this, each daughter cell then receives one full set of chromosomes. The number of chromosomes in each mitotic cell is constant and characteristic for each species of animal. In humans there are forty-four autosomes and two sex chromosomes (X and Y), mak-

ing a total of forty-six. This number is also found in the nucleus of spermatogonia and is replicated during division of the spermatogonia. Mature sperm have the haploid number of chromosomes. To achieve the duplication and distribution of chromosomes in meiosis, two divisions (maturational divisions) are required. In the first maturational division, which occurs in primary spermatocytes (Fig. 18-7), the forty-six chromosomes become arranged as twenty-three homologous pairs, each chromosome being joined by its replicate. One member of each pair, accompanied by its replicate, is distributed to each daughter cell. The resulting cells are the *secondary spermatocytes*, which almost immediately enter the second maturational division. In this stage, each daughter cell receives one copy of the twenty-three

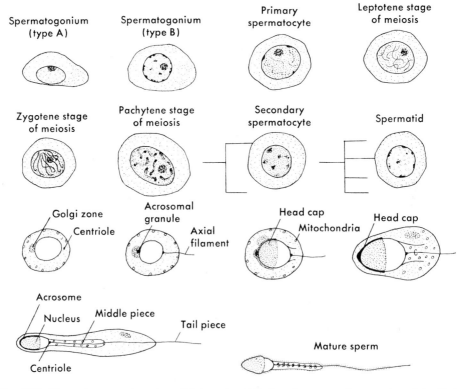

Fig. 18-7. Stages in sperm formation. It takes about 74 days for group of spermatogonial cells to progress through stages of sperm formation to mature sperm with head and tail. Large numbers of spermatogonia tend to enter maturational process together and to divide synchronously. New groups of spermatogonia enter cycle before older "generations" have completed their sequence, resulting in patchwork arrangement of cell communities with youngest generations next to wall of seminiferous tubule and more mature cell clusters near lumen. (Drawing by Emily Craig.)

chromosomes contained in the primary spermatocyte. The resulting daughter cells, called spermatids, contain the haploid number of chromosomes and have completed the first step in the formation of a mature sperm. Each spermatid will now mature to form a sperm cell.

The female germ cell also undergoes meiosis, but the timing of the events is different (Chapter 19). The result of meiosis is to produce spermatozoa and ova containing twenty-three chromosomes. When these two gametes unite, the resulting zygote is provided with the original number of chromosomes (forty-six) contained in all body cells other than germ cells. Since the chromosomes are the bearers of hereditary charac-

teristics, their distribution is of great interest to geneticists.

Spermiogenesis is the process whereby the maturation of the spermatids form spermatozoa. This occurs, after meiosis is complete, in a series of orderly changes that transform the small, round spermatid into the elongated, tail-bearing spermatozoan (Fig. 18-7). The stages in this process, which are shown diagrammatically in Fig. 18-7, consist in (1) the formation of an acrosome (a derivative from the Golgi apparatus), (2) a change in the shape and degree of condensation of the nucleus, (3) the formation of a flagellum that will later become motile, and (4) an extensive remodeling of the cytoplasm, including the formation of an elabo-

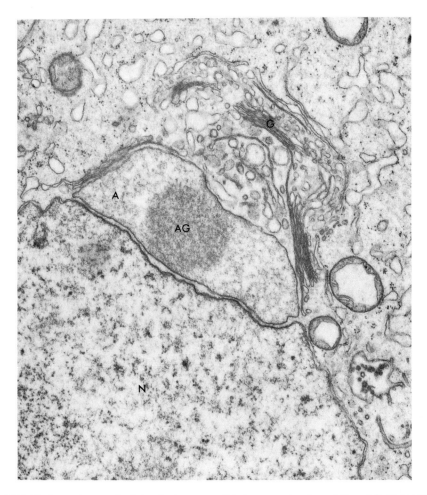

Fig. 18-8. Electron micrograph of developing spermatid of mouse showing relation of Golgi apparatus, *G*, to acrosome. *A*, Acrosomal vesicle; *AG*, acrosomal granule; *N*, nucleus. (×28,000.)

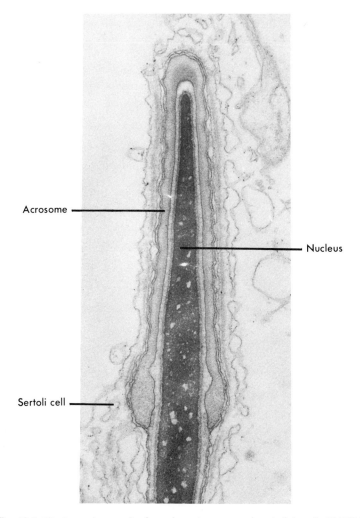

Acrosome

Nucleus

Sertoli cell

Fig. 18-9. Electron micrograph of nearly mature sperm head of dog. (×18,000.)

rate mitochondrial sheath surrounding the flagellum beneath the sperm head.

The spermatid exhibits a large centrally located nucleus, numerous mitochondria, and a pair of centrioles. The prominent supranuclear Golgi apparatus consists of numerous lamellae and vesicles. Granules that appear in these vesicles coalesce to form the *acrosome* within the acrosome vesicle (Fig. 18-8). The acrosome contains enzymes necessary for sperm penetration of the egg. The acrosome and its vesicle lie between the Golgi apparatus and nuclear membrane. The vesicle enlarges and eventually envelops approximately half of the surface of the nucleus; finally it collapses and forms a closely

applied membrane covering the acrosome, known as the acrosomal or *head cap* (Figs. 18-9 and 18-10). During the formation of the acrosome at one pole of the nucleus, one of the centrioles becomes modified into a slender flagellum at the opposite pole. Further differentiation consists in the application of a filamentous sheath around the axial filaments of the flagellum. Meanwhile, the other centriole migrates toward the surface of the cell and gives rise to the annulus encircling the longitudinal axial filaments (Fig. 18-12). The nucleus decreases in size, becomes flattened and elongated, and is then known as the sperm head. Development of the tail consists in a shift of the cytoplasm and a re-

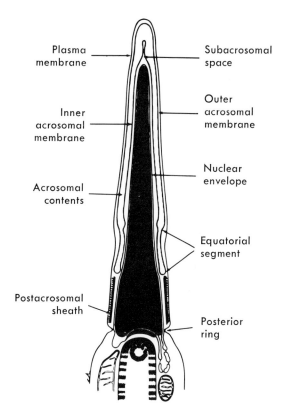

Plasma membrane

Subacrosomal space

Outer acrosomal membrane

Inner acrosomal membrane

Nuclear envelope

Acrosomal contents

Equatorial segment

Postacrosomal sheath

Posterior ring

Fig. 18-10. Diagrammatic representation of principle components seen in sagittal section of primate sperm head. Posterior ring marks junction of head and neck. (From Fawcett, D. 1975. The mammalian spermatazoon. Dev. Biol. **44:**394-436.)

arrangement of the mitochondria to the region between the basal centriole and the annulus. In this region, the mitochondria become aligned in helical fashion and make up the mitochondrial sheath of the middle piece of the developing sperm. As differentiation continues, the excess cytoplasm is shed as the residual body; thus, eventually the spermatozoon is covered by a very thin layer of cytoplasm (Fig. 18-9).

The cells taking part in spermatogenesis tend to occur in cell associations, with the deepest layer near the wall of the tubule that is one of the early stages of spermatogonia formation. Progressing toward the lumen one observes stages in diverse states of maturation. In the human there are six such cell associations (Fig. 18-11). The cells in a given

part of the tubule progress through each set of associations in an orderly sequence called a cell cycle. In humans the stages of this cycle are more difficult to observe than in other mammals. The length of time necessary for a complete cell cycle of sperm formation to be completed is estimated to be 16 days, based on the time observed for the incorporation of ^{3}H-thymidine by germ cells. This cell cycle refers to the series of changes or cell differentiations in a given area of the tubule between two successive appearances of the same developmental stage or cellular association. This wave of differentiation proceeds down the tubule. It takes approximately 64 days to produce a mature sperm cell after an initial type A spermatogonium enters a cell cycle. The maturation of sper-

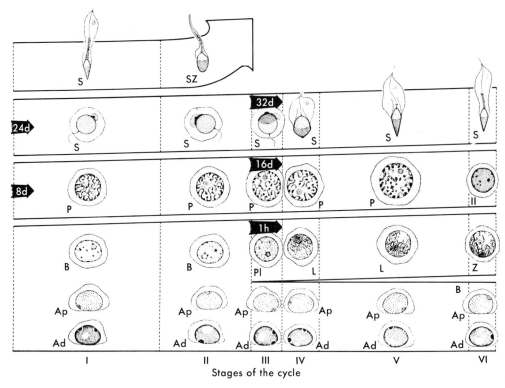

Fig. 18-11. Diagram showing cells found associated together in six stages of cycle of human semi-niferous epithelium. Stages are indicated by Roman numerals (*I* to *VI*). After stage VI, cycle starts again at I. *Ad,* Dark spermatogonium; *Ap,* pale type A spermatogonium; *B,* type B spermatogonium; *PL, L, Z, P,* preleptotene, leptotene, zygotene, and paclytene primary spermatocytes, respectively; *II,* secondary spermatocyte; *S,* spermatid; *SZ,* spermatozoan. Arrows refer to most advanced cell types labeled at various times after intratesticular injection of 3H-thymidine. (From Clermont. In Rosenberg, L., and Paulsen, A. [eds.] The human testis. Plenum Publishing Corporation, New York.)

matozoa occurs in a series of irregularly shaped zones in which all the cells are in the same stage. For this reason, a transverse section through the testis will show some profiles of seminiferous tubules in which all six stages are visible and others in which only three or four stages are observed.

The mammalian sperm is comprised of three main components: the head, neck, and tail (Figs. 18-10 and 18-12). The head consists mainly of a dense nucleus that is surmounted by a small crescentic acrosome. The acrosome contains a number of hydrolytic enzymes and is assumed to play a role in penetration of the egg by the spermatozoon. The cell membrane overlying the acrosome is shed during fertilization.

Behind the posterior margin of the acrosome is the region of the sperm head where attachment and fusion of the sperm with the egg membranes takes place. Underneath the cell membrane at this site is a dense layer running parallel to the membrane, which is called the *postacrosomal sheath* (Fig 18-10). The envelope surrounding the sperm nucleus is unusual in several respects. The entire surface under the acrosome is devoid of nuclear pores, and the two envelopes that make up the nuclear membrane are separated by less than 10 nm. Behind the posterior ring (Fig. 18-10) is a loop of nuclear envelope extending down into the neck region. Here the membranes are separated by the usual 40 to 60 nm and nuclear pores are seen. It is tempting to speculate that the absence of pores over most of the nucleus protects its contents, as mentioned earlier. The motor apparatus of the sperm

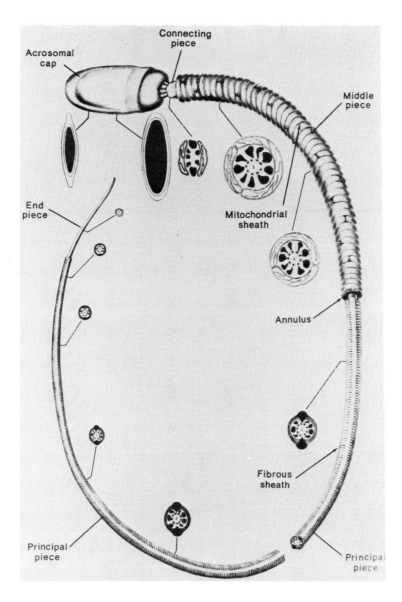

Fig. 18-12. Schematic representation of typical mammalian spermatazoon as it would appear with cell membrane removed to reveal underlying structural components. (From Fawcett, D. 1975. The mammalian spermatazoon. Dev. Biol. **44:**394-436.)

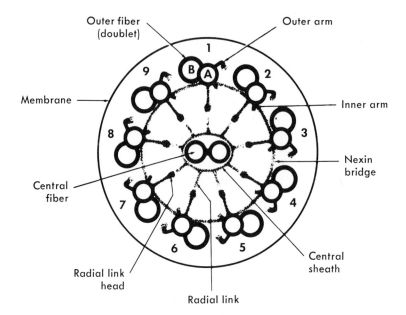

Fig. 18-13. Schematic representation of current interpretation of organization of contractual apparatus (axoneme) of cilia and flagella. (From Fawcett, D. 1975. The mammalian spermatazoon. Dev. Biol. **44**:394-436.)

tail (*axoneme* or *axial filament complex*) consisting of two central microtubules surrounded by a row of nine evenly spaced doublet microtubules (Fig. 18-13). This arrangement of a 9 + 2 pattern of tubules is found in cilia and flagella everywhere in the body. External to these fibrils are nine outer, coarse fibers of uneven size and shape (Fig. 18-14), which extend varying distances down the tail, enclosed by a helical mitochondrial sheath.

In front of the neckfold of the nuclear envelope is another region where the pores are again absent and the membranes narrow down to a distance of less than 10 nm. The region is called the *implantation fossa* and is the site of attachment of the sperm tail to the head (Fig. 18-10). The fossa is lined by nuclear membrane covered by a thick layer of dense material called the *basal plate*, which provides sites for the attachment of a number of fine filaments that reach it from the articular surface of the connecting piece (called the *capitulum*) (Fig. 18-12). Connected to the basal plate are nine

segmented columns which overlap the tapering anterior margins of the nine dense fibers of the flagellum with which they are closely associated. A proximal centriole occupies a niche in the connecting piece just below the capitulum. As the sperm develop, a distal centriole is also found at the base of the *axoneme* (the column of fibrils in the sperm tail) at a right angle to the proximal centriole but as the sperm tail develops the distal centriole disappears, sometimes leaving remnants of its nine triplet microtubules behind.

The neck region is slender and devoid of organelles except for the porous fold of nuclear membrane. In the presence of a fertilizable egg, the sperm undergoes the *acrosomal reaction*. The membrane overlying the apical and lateral segments of the acrosome fuses at several points with the cell membrane overlying it, and the enzymes of the acrosome are released. This process continues until the inner layer of the acrosome is open to the environment.

The mitochondrial sheath of the middle

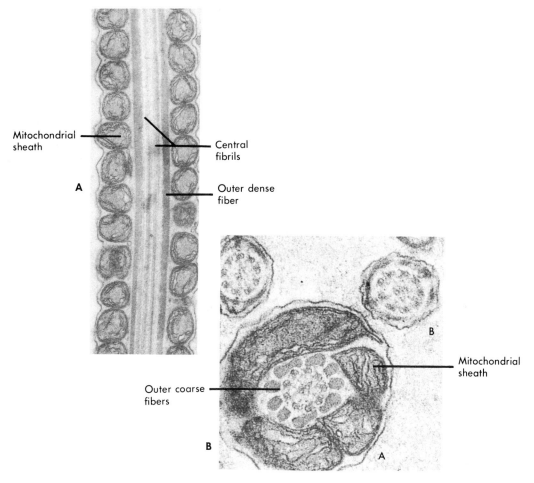

Mitochondrial sheath

Central fibrils

A

Outer dense fiber

Outer coarse fibers

Mitochondrial sheath

B

B

A

Fig. 18-14. A, Electron micrograph of part of middle piece of sperm tail of mouse. **B,** Electron micrograph of transverse section of tail of mouse sperm. *A,* Middle piece; *B,* principal piece. Middle piece shows internal core of one central pair and nine peripheral pairs of fibers surrounded by nine outer coarse fibers enclosed by mitochondrial sheath. (**A,** ×38,000; **B,** ×60,000.)

piece is believed to provide the energy for sperm locomotion. The mitochondria are arranged end to end to form a tight spiral around the longitudinal fibers of the tail. The end of the middle piece is marked by an *annulus* (Fig. 18-12). At the annulus a fibrous sheath begins that consists of a series of ribs oriented lengthwise along the tail to form two columns. These columns pass along its length, with circumferential ribs forming a framework between the columns (Fig. 18-12). Presumably these ribs and columns affect the kinds of motion that the sperm tail can perform.

Regulation of sperm production

Little is known about the regulation of sperm production. The process, however, can be considered in two stages for the purpose of understanding its control. These stages are (1) the maintenance of a continual source of cells to enter spermatogenesis and (2) the progressive passage of cells through the steps of sperm formation. The first process involves the continued renewal of the stem cell population (spermatogonia) by repeated mitotic proliferation. The type A sperm cells, which can be distinguished by the presence of dustlike oval nuclear chromatin, divide to produce some cells that begin sperm production. The remainder persist in the basal layers of the germinal epithelium and continue to provide a stem cell population. There is no definite information concerning the mechanism of control of the rate of stem cell proliferation. The number of stem cells that enter sperm formation and the number that survive to form mature sperm constitute the second process in sperm production. This process is regulated by FSH (follicle-stimulating hormone) from the anterior pituitary gland and by local androgen (male sex hormone) concentration.

Sertoli cells

In addition to the cells that represent stages of spermatogenesis, the seminiferous tubule has in its wall supporting cells, the sustentacular or Sertoli cells. These are irregular elongated cells, the bases of which lie against the basement membrane and the apices of which border on the lumen (Figs. 18-3 and 18-5). The nucleus, located either basally or somewhat removed from the base of the cell, is ovoid in shape, appears pale, and contains finely dispersed chromatin and usually one or more prominent nucleoli that stain unevenly with a central acidophilic core and a basophilic rim. The nuclear membrane may exhibit a longitudinal spiral groove. Above the nucleus, in addition to mitochondria and other cytoplasmic inclusions, an unusual spindle-shaped crystalloid structure is often present in the human Sertoli cell only. The processes of Sertoli cells form a barrier between the layer of spermatogonia and the upper layers of spermatogonia and spermatids. As spermatogonia enter the sperm-providing sequence, they must pass through this barrier to enter the compartment near the lumen (the adluminal compartment). The spermatids become embedded in the Sertoli cell cytoplasm and are anchored there during development. It is assumed that the later stages of spermiogenesis are under metabolic regulation by the Sertoli cells.

The Sertoli cells can bind the pituitary hormone, FSH (follicle-stimulating hormone), and are therefore probably under direct pituitary control. In addition to maintaining their intimate connection to the spermatids, Sertoli cells appear to produce a special protein that binds the male hormone, testosterone. This binding protein may be transferred to the lumen to provide the basis for a local response to androgen. Both FSH and testosterone can influence the number of cells that become mature sperm cells, perhaps by influencing the metabolic status of Sertoli cells.

In the mature testis there are fewer Sertoli cells than germinal cells, and the former tend to be evenly spaced around the seminiferous tubule. The Sertoli cells (Fig. 18-3) are fairly resistant to many noxious agents such as x-irradiation and to the effects of aging. Two types of Sertoli cells may be seen, one that stains darkly and another that stains lightly. The functional significance of these staining differences is unknown.

Leydig cells

The spermatogenic tubules lie coiled in a stroma of loose connective tissue. In the latter and separated from the tubules are groups of cells either aggregated in clusters or arranged in thin layers along blood vessels. These are the Leydig cells. They are the source of testicular androgens (the male hormones) and trace amounts of female hormones such as estrone and estradiol. The cells are fairly large and ovoid or polygonal in shape. The nuclei are large and eccentrically placed. The cytoplasm near the nucleus is dark and granular, whereas peripherally it is vacuolated and stains lightly. Pigment granules (lipochromes) and crystalloids (of Reinke) may be present (Figs. 18-3 and 18-4).

The most striking feature of the cytoplasm of the Leydig cells, like that of most steroid-secreting cells, is the presence of an extensive smooth endoplasmic reticulum composed of interconnecting tubules that extend throughout much of the cytoplasm (Fig. 18-4). The mitochondria are rod shaped and of variable diameter; the cristae appear to consist of fenestrated lamellae. The Leydig cells of the human secrete a moderate amount of steroid in comparison with some other mammals.

The size and secretion of the Leydig cells is under the control of the pituitary hormone LH (luteinizing hormone), which is also called ICSH (interstitial cell–stimulating hormone) in males. The action of male hormones has been ascertained by direct observation and by many experimental procedures involving castration at various stages of sexual maturity. Briefly, it has been shown that male hormone is necessary for the appearance of the so-called secondary sex characters in the developing mammal. If castration is performed after sexual maturity has occurred, the effect on already established secondary sex characteristics is less pronounced than in the developing individual. In the latter situation, involution of the epithelium of the genital ducts and accessory glands is the most constant feature observed.

Passage of sperm from testes

From the convoluted seminiferous tubules the spermatozoa pass into the proximal part of the duct system of the testis, which lies in the mediastinum of the organ (Fig. 18-1). They traverse the straightened necks of the seminiferous tubules (called tubuli recti or straight tubules) into the rete testis, consisting of a network of fine spaces occupying part of the mediastinum. The walls of the straight tubules and rete testis are lined with a low cuboidal epithelium. The surrounding connective tissue is tightly woven and extremely vascular. Scattered strands of smooth muscle can be found next to the tubules but do not form a definite coat. The rete drain into eleven to twenty efferent ductules that penetrate the tunica to form the head of the epididymis. Each tubule is arranged as a tightly woven cone held together by loose connective tissue. The separate efferent ductules are lined with alternating groups of high columnar cells having motile cilia and shorter columnar cells without cilia. The nonciliated cells can be classified into functional groups on the basis of their ultrastructural appearance as either secretory or absorptive. It has been suggested that these cells, which

are derived from the primitive kidney (mesonephros), may absorb fluids secreted by the seminiferous tubules and also may aid in sperm transport by setting up a continuous current of fluid flow. The tubules are surrounded by smooth muscle responsible for the production of peristaltic waves that pass along the tubules at the rate of about one every 15 seconds. It has been estimated that the time necessary for the sperm to traverse the male duct system and reach the ductus deferens is approximately 1 to 3 weeks. The sperm traversing the efferent ductules empty into a single duct, the ductus epididymis. During their passage, sperm are relatively immobile and must be transported by a combination of muscular contraction and fluid motion. The swirling action of the cilia in the tract provides continual mixing of the sperm with the fluid secreted by the testes and the duct system.

EPIDIDYMIS

The epididymis lies near the testis and is surrounded by a fold of the tunica vaginalis, which is enclosed within a connective tissue capsule (Figs. 18-15 to 18-17). It consists of one long extensively coiled tubule, the ductus epididymis, which if stretched out would measure over 20 feet in length. The part of the epididymis into which the efferent ductules empty is called the *head* (*caput* or beginning) and the part that blends with the ductus deferens is called the *tail* (end). A slide prepared from this region of the tract will show a great number of tubule profiles cut tangentially, transversely, or longitudinally (Fig. 18-15). The epithelium is pseudostratified columnar and contains small rounded basal cells, as well as tall columnar cells that together form a smooth luminal surface. The surface cells contain secretory granules and are involved in both secretion and absorption. Their free surfaces exhibit projections that resemble cilia but lack axial filaments. The sperm spend from 1 to 3 weeks in the epididymis, and during this time changes occur in appearance, motility, size, membrane permeability, temperature sensitivity, and metabolic function.

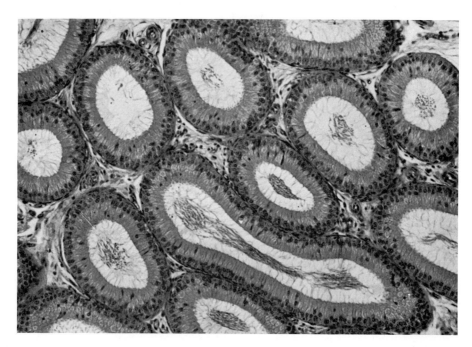

Fig. 18-15. Section of epididymis of dog showing several sections through the ductus. Stereocilia are prominent and lumen contains spermatozoa. (×160.)

Sperm in lumen   Smooth muscle fibers

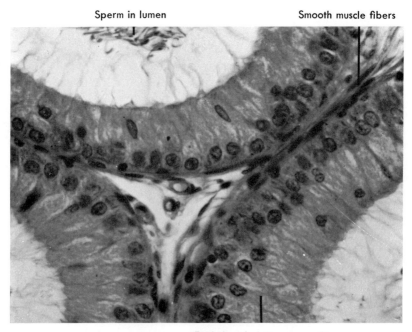

Epithelium bearing stereocilia

Fig. 18-16. Section of epididymis of dog. (×640.)

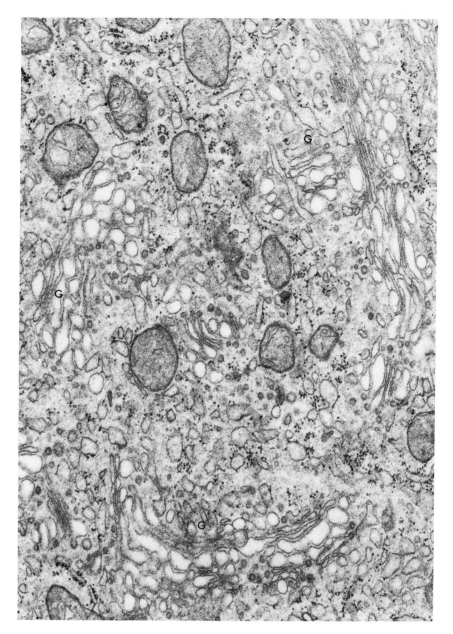

Fig. 18-17. Electron micrograph of part of epithelial cell of mouse epididymis showing prominent Golgi complex, G. (×38,000.)

In some as yet unspecified way, the environment of the epididymis contributes to the maturation of sperm. It has been established that the sperm of several species, including the rabbit, *must* pass through the epididymis to develop the capacity to fertilize an egg. The importance of epididymal residence for the maturation of human sperm is unclear. The role of the epididymis in con-

tributing to sperm maturation is androgen-dependent and the principle columnar epithelial cells that line the epididymis require androgen to maintain both their form and secretory and absorptive functions. Sperm do not develop full functional capacity until they have spent a period of time in the female tract where they undergo a process called *capacitation*. Capacitation confers on the sperm the ability to undergo a coordinated acrosome reaction that is necessary for fertilization, but the mechanism of this conditioning by the female tract is poorly understood. The composition of the secretions of the epididymis changes from the beginning to the end of it, and the epithelium gradually gets taller in the region of the ductus deferens. A corresponding change occurs in the thickness of the muscle coat, which is maximum as the epididymis leads into the ductus deferens (Fig. 18-1). The blood supply of the head and tail of the epididymis is more abundant than in more proximal parts of the male reproductive tract and supports active fluid secretion by the cells lining the lumen.

DUCTUS (VAS) DEFERENS

The vas deferens is a continuation of the ductus epididymis. It is lined by a somewhat lower epithelium. The epithelial cells lack cilia and rest on a well-developed lamina propria. The muscularis has three layers: a thick intermediate circular layer and two thin longitudinal layers, one on the inner and the outer surfaces, respectively (Fig. 18-18). On reaching the prostate gland, the ductus deferens dilates to form the ampulla, a thin-walled structure with a complexly folded mucosa. As it passes into the substance of the prostate, the ampulla narrows again to form the ejaculatory duct that opens into the prostatic part of the urethra.

ACCESSORY GLANDS

Many cells in the epithelial lining of the male reproductive tract are secretory. In addition, all male mammals have several specialized glands associated with specific regions of the reproductive tract. These glands elaborate the major portion of the seminal fluid. Usually the secretory epithelium of these glands is characterized by infoldings of the mucosa and loosely arranged subjacent connective tissue. These structural features facilitate expansion of the gland and an increase in the surface epithelium. There is also a mass of smooth muscle within the connective tissue that helps to empty the glands quickly during entrance of the seminal

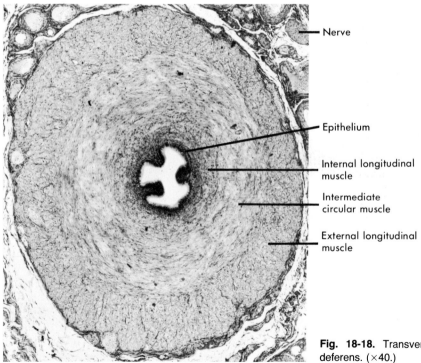

Nerve

Epithelium

Internal longitudinal muscle

Intermediate circular muscle

External longitudinal muscle

Fig. 18-18. Transverse section of human d deferens. (×40.)

fluid into the urethra (emission). The secretory activity of these glands depends on testicular hormones, and the appearance and function of the cells varies greatly with hormonal status.

The two major accessory glands in man are the seminal vesicles, which are derived from the mesonephric or Wolffian duct, as are the ductus deferens and the prostate. In addition, a pair of small compound tubuloalveolar glands called the bulbourethral or Cowper's glands empties into the proximal urethra. These glands, similar to mucous glands, elaborate a fluid believed to function as a lubricant during intercourse. Opening into the urethra along its entire length are also small mucous glands (glands of Littré).

Seminal vesicle

The paired seminal vesicles are elongated saccular organs lying near the ampulla of the ductus deferens leading from each testis and opening into the ductus at the point where it narrows to form the ejaculatory duct. When uncoiled they extend 15 cm. The most striking histological characteristic of the seminal vesicle is the folding of its mucosa (Fig. 18-19). In sections this produces a great number of projections and pockets; since the latter are often tangentially cut, there appear to be follicles in the mucosa much like those occurring in the gallbladder.

The epithelial cells of the seminal vesicle are columnar. They have a prominent, centrally located nucleus and at times exhibit several vacuoles and granules. At the electron microscope level additional cytologic details observed consist of microvilli lining the lumen, numerous scattered mitochondria, rough endoplasmic reticulum, and a large prominent supranuclear Golgi complex. Scattered secretory granules and vacuoles are transitory structures (Fig. 18-20). The seminal vesicle contributes to seminal fluid a thick, yellowish secretion. It is slightly alkaline and a rich energy source (fructose) for sperm metabolism. It contains coagulating enzymes that cause seminal fluid to congeal in the female tract after it is deposited. The seminal vesicles also produce pros-

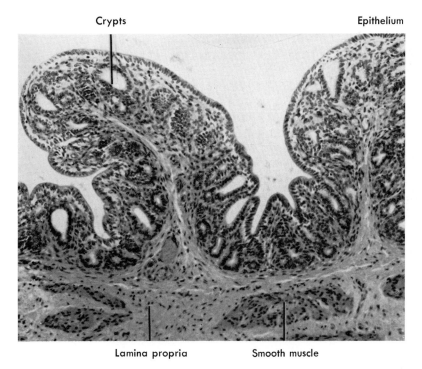

Fig. 18-19. Mucosa of seminal vesicle of cat. (×160.)

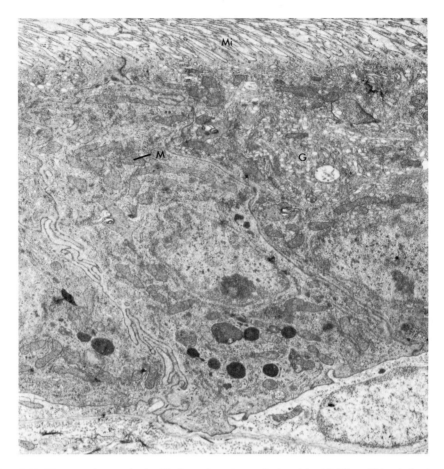

Fig. 18-20. Electron micrograph of epithelium of mouse seminal vesicle. *Mi,* Microvilli bordering lumen; *M,* mitochondrion; *G,* Golgi complex. (×10,000.)

taglandins, substances that affect muscular contraction and may influence sperm transport in the female tract.

Prostate

The prostate (Fig. 18-21) is a bean-shaped structure consisting of clusters of glandular tissue surrounding the urethra at the site where it emerges from the bladder. The firm grandular tissue is surrounded by a thin connective tissue capsule containing some smooth muscle. The gland as a whole is composed of secretory channels (50%), smooth muscle (25%), and fibrous tissue (25%). The bulk of the glandular tissue consists of thirty to fifty large glands that open into the urethra at the seminal colliculus along with the ejaculatory ducts. In addition, there are some small mucosal and submucosal glands that contribute to the prostatic secretion. The gland can be divided rather imperfectly into lobes produced by the passage of the ejaculatory ducts through the glandular mass. The lobes are further subdivided into lobules, each drained by a duct that empties into the urethra. The lobes are of interest; some of them tend to be the site of prostatic tumors (posterior and dorsal lobes) and others may give rise to benign hypertrophy (anterior and ventral lobes). The glands are of the tubuloalveolar type and show considerable infolding of their epithelium to accommodate the distention required during storage of prostatic fluid. The secretory portions of the gland are lined with columnar epithelium superimposed on a few flattened cells. With-

Alveolus

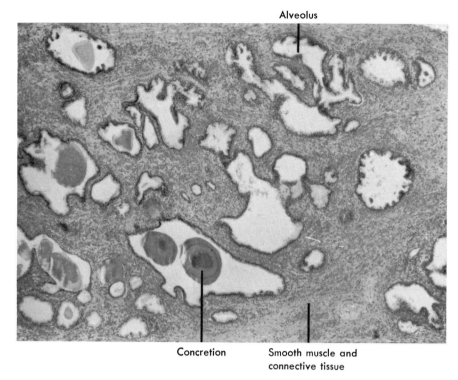

Concretion

Smooth muscle and
connective tissue

Fig. 18-21. Section of human prostate gland. (×40.)

in the contorted, large irregular lumina of these glands one can sometimes observe lamellar bodies that stain red with eosin. These are called *prostatic concretions*. The epithelium of a lumen containing a prostatic concretion is often flattened. These concretions are often calcified, especially in older men. A characteristic feature of the prostate is the presence of scattered fibers of smooth muscle in the connective tissue surrounding the glands. The muscle does not form organized layers around the glandular portions but is distributed in groups or strands of fibers running in various directions.

The prostate produces most of the fluid that is contributed to the seminal fluid during sexual arousal and ejaculation. Prostatic secretions are watery, slightly acidic (pH 6.5), and rich in enzymes (acid phosphatase, fibrinolysin). At the time of ejaculation, sympathetic discharge to the prostate, the

seminal vesicles, and the ductus epididymis projects fluid into the urethra.

Bulbourethral glands

The bulbourethral glands are small glands similar to mucous glands, and open by way of long ducts into the membranous urethra. These glands discharge their secretion first during sexual arousal, and their fluid may act as a lubricant or an early neutralizer of the acidic lumen of the urethra.

Seminal fluid

The fluid in which the sperm are suspended originates from several accessory glands as well as from the isolated secretory cells lining the male reproductive tract, including the epididymis, ductus deferens, seminal vesicle, prostate, and bulbourethral glands. It is different in composition from blood plasma and other body fluids. It has, for example, a high concentration of fructose

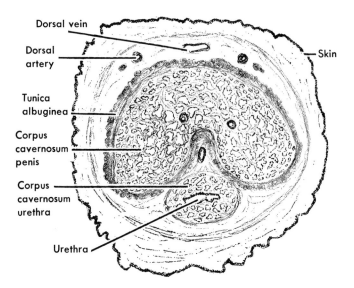

Fig. 18-22. Transverse section of penis of newborn infant.

and certain amino acids, as well as several unique substances such as spermidine, an amine with a characteristic odor. At emission, prostatic secretion enters the urethra first, followed by the ampullar sperm and then the secretions of the seminal vesicle.

PENIS

A section of the penis shows, under low microscopic power, three large masses of erectile tissue, each of which contains a great number of anastomosing blood vessels (Fig. 18-22). The two dorsal masses of erectile tissue, connected by a bridge of the same kind of tissue, are the *corpora cavernosa penis*. The smaller ventral mass surrounding the urethra is the *corpus cavernosum urethrae*, called also the *corpus spongiosum*.

The cavernous bodies are surrounded by a sheath of dense connective tissue, the tunica albuginea. Outside this is a stroma of loose connective tissue containing blood vessels, nerves, and Pacinian corpuscles. There is no well-defined corium of the skin covering the penis, and it has a thin epidermis.

Blood is brought to the penis by the arteria penis, which branches to form the dorsal artery and the paired deep arteries. The dorsal artery sends branches to the tunica albuginea and to the large trabeculae of the cavernous bodies. Such branches break up into capillaries from which blood passes into the lacunae of the erectile tissue and then to a plexus of veins in the albuginea. The deep arteries run lengthwise, giving off branches that open into the cavernous spaces. During times of sexual excitement the flow of blood into the cavernous spaces is greatly increased, especially that coming from the deep arteries due to parasympathetic dilatation of the helicine arteries that supply the erectile tissue. The veins that drain the blood spaces leave at an oblique angle. The central spaces are filled first, and their distention compresses the peripheral spaces and obstructs the flow of blood through the angular openings into the veins, thus producing rigidity of the penis. In the flaccid condition of the organ, the incoming flow of blood is less and the passage into the veins remains open.

The penis has an abundant supply of spinal, sympathetic, and parasympathetic nerve fibers and many sensory end organs.

19

Female reproductive system

The female reproductive system consists of the ovaries, the fallopian tubes (oviducts), the uterus, and the vagina. Because of its functional relation to the reproductive tract, the mammary gland is discussed with the group of genital organs.

OVARY

The ovary, like the testis, is concerned with the formation of gametes and with the development and maintenance of the secondary sexual characteristics. In this latter function the ovary serves as an endocrine gland.

The paired ovaries are slightly flattened, ovoid structures lying within the pelvis near the fringed open ends of the oviducts. They are attached to a strand of connective tissue, the *broad ligament*, by a fold of mesentery called the mesovarium, which in turn inserts into the ovary at its stalk or hilus. The hilus is the margin of the ovary that serves as an entrance point for nerves, blood vessels, and lymphatics. A section through the whole ovary shows that it is divided into a wide outer cortex and a smaller inner medulla (Fig. 19-1). The central deep zone or medulla consists of a loose connective tissue stroma rich in elastic fibers in which are embedded many large, coiled blood vessels, a rich lymphatic bed, and a nerve supply. Occasionally vestiges of fetal tissue, the rete ovarii, may be observed. Closely associated with the nonmyelinated nerves and vascular spaces along the length of the hilum and occasionally trailing onto the adjacent mesovarium are the hilus cells. These cells re-

semble the Leydig cells of the testis in the appearance of the nucleus and cytoplasm and also in the presence of lipids, lipochromes, and crystalloids. They are believed to secrete androgens, and overgrowth of the hilus cells can cause masculinization in women.

The cortex is a broad peripheral zone consisting of a compact cellular stroma punctuated by fluid-filled follicles containing maturing ova. The connective tissue cells of this zone are long and spindle shaped, with elongate nuclei resembling those of smooth muscle. The stromal cells are embedded in a matrix of delicate collagenous fibers. The matrix also contains clusters of interstitial cells, especially prominent during pregnancy and lactation. These cells may produce progesterone and androgens. The ovary is covered by a simple columnar epithelium called the germinal epithelium because formerly it was held that the oogonia or germinal cells were derived from this epithelium. Immediately underneath the germinal epithelium is a denser stroma, the tunica albuginea, which contains a few scattered cells amid tightly packed collagenous fibers (Fig. 19-2).

Origin of ova and follicles

The germ cells of the female are derived from cells that migrate into the developing ovary from the endoderm of the primitive yolk sac. The oogonia thus formed continue to divide during early fetal life and in some species such as the pig continue to divide for as long as several weeks postnatally. In humans the process of oogenesis (the forma-

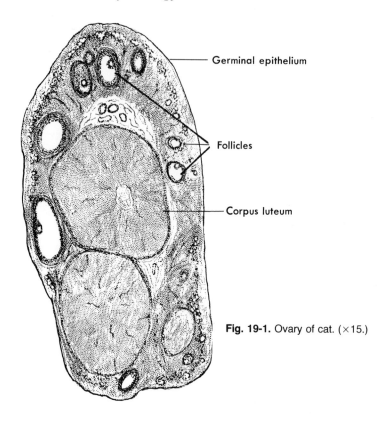

Germinal epithelium

Follicles

Corpus luteum

Fig. 19-1. Ovary of cat. (×15.)

Fig. 19-2. Cortex of ovary.

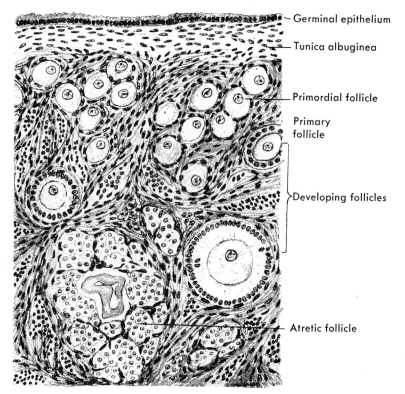

Germinal epithelium

Tunica albuginea

Primordial follicle

Primary follicle

Developing follicles

Atretic follicle

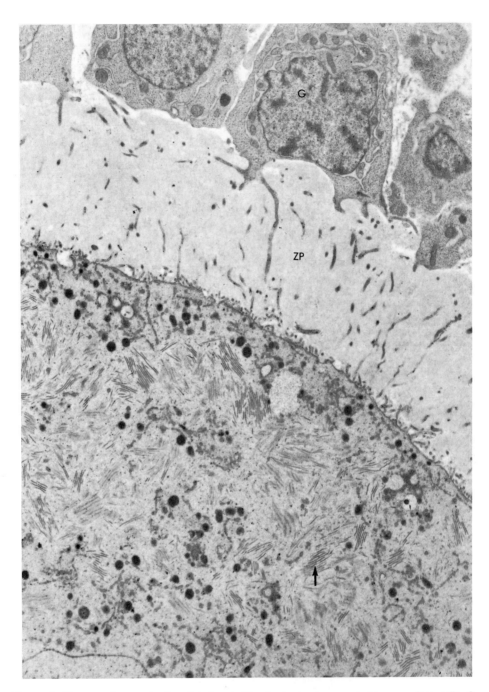

Fig. 19-3. Electron micrograph of ovulated, unfertilized rat ovum surrounded by granulosa cells, *G,* whose processes extend through zona pellucida, *ZP.* Note abundance of protein plaques (linear structures) in ovum (arrow). (×6,100.) (Courtesy Dr. A. C. Enders.)

tion of new germ cells by mitosis, in a manner comparable to the continuing process of spermatogenesis in males) is thought to be completed by approximately the fourth prenatal month. At this time the ovary may contain as many as 5 million oocytes. Each oocyte is surrounded by a single layer of smaller cells called the follicular or granulosa cells; each egg and its associated granulosa cells is called a primordial follicle (Fig. 19-2).

Growth of the follicles

Before an oocyte is released from the ovary (the process called *ovulation*) it will undergo marked changes in organization and size. The oocyte will grow from about 30 μm in diameter to about 120 to 150 μm. It will complete the first stage of meiosis and will enter the oviduct in the second stage of meiosis. Of the oocytes remaining in the ovary at birth, approximately 400 will eventually be

released, leaving the remainder to degenerate *(atresia)*.

The primordial follicle contains a small oocyte measuring about 20 μm in diameter (Fig. 19-2), with a large eccentric nucleus and relatively few organelles located near one pole of the nucleus. Surrounding the egg is a single layer of flat cells *(follicle cells)* attached to the cell membrane by desmosomes. Occasional outpocketings of ova cytoplasm indent the follicle cells (Fig. 19-3). Outside the follicle wall a thin basement membrane is present. As the oocyte begins to grow, the single layer of flat follicular cells becomes cuboidal or columnar, forming the *granulosa layer*. Continued development results in the formation of a nucleolus and a Golgi apparatus within the egg. The mitochondria form clusters called rosettes. The cell surface becomes coated with protein polysaccharides apparently secreted by the

Primordial follicles

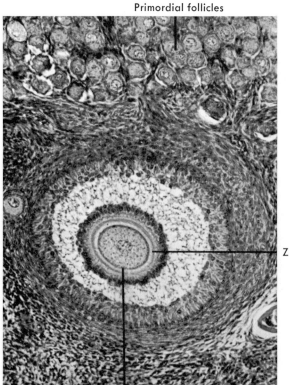

Zona pellucida

Developing ovum

Fig. 19-4. Section of cortex of rat ovary showing ovum within follicle. ($\times$640.)

follicular cells. This coat, the *zona pellucida*, remains as a covering for the oocyte even after fertilization (Fig. 19-4). It is finally shed shortly before blastocyst formation.

As the follicle cells divide, the oocyte becomes surrounded by a multilayered wall of cells and is now called a *secondary follicle*. The stroma around the follicle subsequently undergoes a change, in which the inner zone nearest the basement membrane separating the follicle wall from the surrounding connective tissue develops into a highly vascular region *(theca interna)* (Fig. 19-5). The outer, more densely organized connective tissue remains as the *theca externa*. Throughout the development of the follicle, the granulosa remains avascular. Once the follicle has reached the multilayered stage, its further growth is under hormonal regulation by the pituitary. Follicle-stimulating hormone (FSH) is required for further thickening of the follicle wall by mitosis and cellular enlargement. FSH also stimulates the granulosa cells to secrete the components required for formation of the zona pellucida. Luteinizing hormone (LH) is responsible for inducing the formation of the surrounding theca, the growth of a vascular supply to the follicle, and the development of steroid secretion by the follicle wall. Steroid secretion near the time of ovulation depends on cooperation between the theca interna under LH in-

fluence and the granulosa under FSH control. As ovulation approaches, the cells of the granulosa become steroid-secreting. LH is also required for the follicle to enter the next stage, in which it is prepared for rupture and release of the egg from the ovary *(ovulation)*.

In the secondary follicle, the cells of the granulosa are cuboidal and rather loosely attached to one another. The follicle gradually assumes an oval shape, and the egg shifts to an eccentric position on the far side of the follicle, opposite the region of eventual rupture of the wall that occurs at ovulation. Fluid gradually accumulates between the follicle cells and finally coalesces to form a vesicle of fluid called the *antrum*. In the human a follicle destined for ovulation takes about 12 to 14 days to reach maturity from the time that it begins its final maturation at the start of a new cycle. At maximum size the mature (Graafian or vesicular) follicle is a large fluid-filled vesicle about 10 to 20 mm in diameter that may span the entire thickness of the ovarian cortex and produce a bulge visible on the ovarian surface. As ovulation approaches, the cluster of cells surrounding the ovum (Fig. 19-4), called the *cumulus oophorus*, gradually is undercut as the cells swell and the matrix between them depolymerizes. Finally, the egg with a surrounding halo of cells (the *corona radiata*) floats free in the

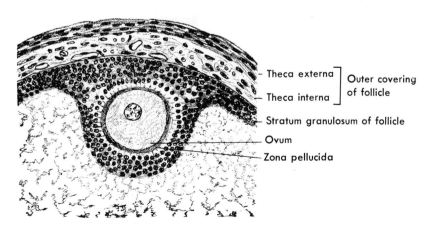

Fig. 19-5. Part of Graafian follicle showing ovum and surrounding structures.

antrum. About 36 hours before ovulation, the ovum completes its first maturational division and enters the second division of meiosis. It is currently believed that factors produced by the follicle wall, including the sex steroid estradiol and certain proteins, prevent completion of meiosis until this late stage in development. During the last few hours before ovulation, the wall of the follicle facing the surface of the ovary undergoes a reduction in thickness, and the cells separate from each other under the influence of luteinizing hormone (LH) secreted by the anterior pituitary gland. It is currently believed that LH stimulates the synthesis of local steroids such as progesterone that are involved in the breakdown of the follicle wall shortly before ovulation. At ovulation the ovum with its surrounding corona radiata passes slowly through the weakened and ruptured follicle wall onto the ovarian surface and is swept into the oviduct as the fringed ends of the oviduct sweep over the ovary.

The number of ova discharged at one time and the intervals between ovulations vary in different animals. In the human one ovum is usually discharged from the ovary every 4 weeks. In about 1% of cycles, multiple ovulations occur. In every cycle, three to thirty primary follicles will begin to mature. Those that do not undergo ovulation will become atretic.

The local ovarian mechanisms responsible for rupture of the follicle wall and the extrusion of the ovum are not known. Various explanations that have been proposed to account for this process are increased intrafollicular pressure (evidence fails to support this idea), enzymatic breakdown of the connective tissue matrix, local vascular changes, and smooth muscle contractility within the ovary.

Corpus luteum

After ovulation the majority of the follicular cells are retained in the ovary, and the wall of the ruptured follicle undergoes changes leading to the formation of the corpus luteum. Shortly after ovulation a blood clot forms from the ruptured vessels in the theca interna. The cells of the granulosa enlarge and begin to invade and resorb the clot. Ultimately, the follicular cells fill the center of the remodeled follicle with large, pale cells (Figs. 19-6 and 19-7). These cells secrete estrogen and progesterone.

The nuclei become vesicular, and the abundant cytoplasm, which at first appears granular, gradually accumulates lipid and yellow pigment granules. The granules are characteristic of these cells, known as the *granulosa lutein cells.*

At the electron microscope level the granulosa lutein cells exhibit a large prominent nucleus, numerous mitochondria, large numbers of scattered ribosomes, a prominent Golgi apparatus, and a supranuclear centrosome. Smooth-surfaced endoplasmic reticulum is also a prominent cytoplasmic organelle (Fig. 19-7).

The cells derived from the theca interna occur in groups located at the periphery of the lutein layer and are known as *theca lutein cells.* Although they also contain lipid granules and are similar in shape to the granulosa cells, they may be distinguished from the latter by their location in the periphery, their smaller size, and their denser appearing nuclei.

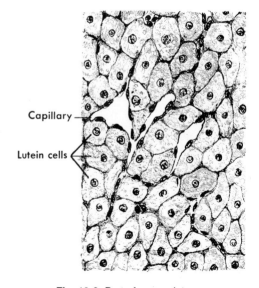

Capillary

Lutein cells

Fig. 19-6. Part of corpus luteum.

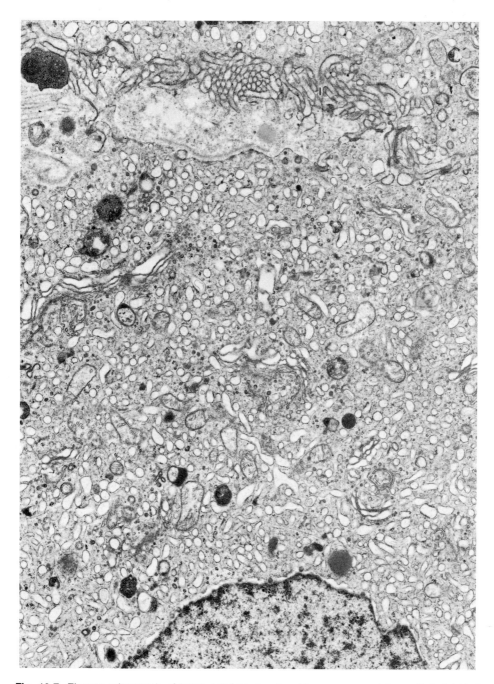

Fig. 19-7. Electron micrograph of lutein cell from functional human corpus luteum. Note infolded border of upper cell, *I,* and abundance of agranular endoplasmic reticulum. (×15,600.) (Courtesy Dr. A. C. Enders.)

The structure in a fresh specimen has a yellow color and is called the corpus luteum. The length of life of the corpus luteum and the size to which it grows depend upon the fate of the ovum that was discharged from the follicle. If the ovum is fertilized and becomes implanted in the uterine wall, the corpus luteum continues to grow and is called a corpus luteum (of pregnancy). If the ovum is not fertilized, the corpus luteum begins to degenerate about 14 days after ovulation. Such corpora lutea are soon replaced by scar tissue (corpus albicans).

Atretic follicles. In the preceding paragraphs the normal development of an ovum and its follicle was discussed. It often happens, however, that follicles which have developed to the Graafian stage degenerate rather than reach ovulation. The first step in atresia is the death of the ovum itself, which is followed by the degeneration of the follicular cells; the result is a mass of detritus left at the center of the follicle. The cells of the theca interna undergo a hypertrophy similar at first to that occurring in corpus luteum formation. It is, however, carried further so that the striking characteristic of an atretic follicle is the ring of enlarged theca cells surrounding it. At this stage these cells have some resemblance to the cells of the corpus luteum but are smaller, less eosinophilic, and not conspicuously vacuolated.

The theca cells gradually fill the space left by the degenerating ovum and follicular cells, thus forming a solid mass (Fig. 19-2). In this condition they may remain in the stroma of the ovary for some time.

Hormone secretion during the cycle

Each month a wave of follicle growth and development leads to the preparation of one or more follicles for ovulation. After ovulation the evacuated follicle is converted into a corpus luteum which functions in the ovary for two weeks, in a nonpregnant cycle, or for longer if pregnancy occurs. This regular succession of structures in the ovary is called the ovarian cycle. The cycle can be divided into two different phases on the basis of the structures functional in the ovary and the kinds of hormones being secreted. The first half of the cycle, which is dated from the time of menstruation, is occupied with follicle development and is referred to as the *follicular phase.* The period of time after ovulation during which a corpus luteum is functional is called the *luteal phase.*

During the follicular phase, estrogen secretion gradually increases as a number of follicles ripen. Estrogen initiates growth and repair of the uterine lining after menstruation, and as estrogen production increases, the reproductive tract is prepared for sperm and egg transport to facilitate the chances of fertilization. At midcycle, estrogen levels reach a peak and trigger a surge of FSH and LH from the pituitary. This surge results in ovulation.

After ovulation the ruptured follicle is transformed into a corpus luteum (luteal phase), which secretes estrogen and progesterone. Progesterone, acting on a tissue previously stimulated by estrogen, will induce further growth of the uterine lining and the initiation of secretion by the glands of the uterus. These conditions prepare the uterus for the reception of a fertilized ovum. If pregnancy does not occur, the corpus luteum degenerates, and the subsequent hormone withdrawal causes the lining of the uterus to be sloughed off, leading to a menstrual period.

FEMALE REPRODUCTIVE TRACT

The growth and function of the muscle and epithelium of the female tract are under hormonal influence and are conditioned by the progressive shifts in estrogen and progesterone secretion by the ovaries during the ovarian cycle. The oviducts (Fallopian tubes), uterus, cervix, and vagina are in extremely different functional states in the follicular and luteal phases of the ovarian cycle. During the early follicular phase, the tissues are remodeled and repaired in the aftermath of the preceding menstrual cycle. As estrogen levels rise, the tract as a whole becomes conditioned to facilitate sperm and egg transport. After ovulation, the tract is converted to a condition suitable for the establishment and maintenance of pregnancy. These changes entail shifts in muscle contractility, mucosal growth and repair, glandular secretion, and blood flow through the vascular bed of the tract.

Fallopian tube (oviduct)

When the ova are extruded from the ovary, they pass into the open end of the oviduct as it sweeps over the ovarian surface. The oviducts consist of a mucosa lined with a mixture of ciliated and nonciliated secretory cells, an underlying highly vascular lamina propria, and a subjacent muscularis having an inner circular and an outer longitudinal layer of smooth muscle (Fig. 19-8). There is no muscularis mucosa or submucosa. The tube is covered on the outside by a sleeve of peritoneum, a *serosa*, consisting of a thin sheet of squamous epithelium and a stroma of collagenous fibers (Fig. 19-9).

Functionally and structurally the tube can be divided into four segments that differ in (1) the complexity of folding of the lining mucosa, (2) the proportion of ciliated to nonciliated cells in the mucosa, and (3) the thickness of the muscle coat. These four segments are named the infundibulum, ampulla, isthmus, and intramural zones. The *infundibulum* (funnel) with its fringed ends (fimbriae) is the opening or mouth (ostium) of the oviduct near the ovary. Near the time of ovulation the fimbriae, which contain a tissue resembling erectile tissue, become turgid and motile. These thin-walled fringes hug the ovary and serve as an "egg catcher." The wall of the infundibulum is extremely thin and consists of a sheet of connective tissue interlaced with smooth muscle covered by a ciliated mucosa. The *ampulla* occupies the distal part of the tube, and it is here that fertilization takes place. The mucosa is covered in the main by ciliated cells. Also present is a thin muscle coat and a loose lamina propria that undergoes swelling at the time of ovulation.

A longer segment of the oviduct called the *isthmus* occurs between the ampulla and the uterus. This part of the tube is smaller and firmer and exhibits a larger lumen with a less complicated mucosa. Grossly, it is rather difficult to distinguish the isthmus from the broad ligament. Ciliated cells become less frequent and are confined to the crypts in

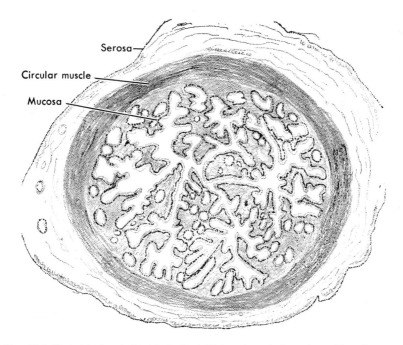

Serosa

Circular muscle

Mucosa

Fig. 19-8. Fimbriated end of oviduct of cat. Note extremely irregular outline of mucosa.

Columnar epithelium

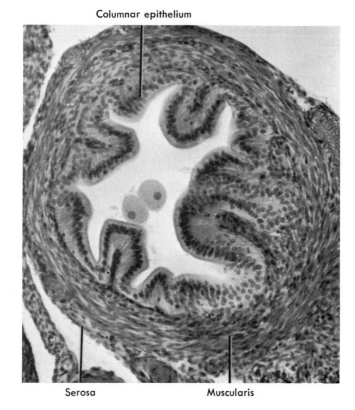

Serosa　　　　　　　　　Muscularis

Fig. 19-9. Section of Fallopian tube of mouse showing two fertilized eggs in lumen. (×200.) (Courtesy Dr. H. Browning.)

Gland

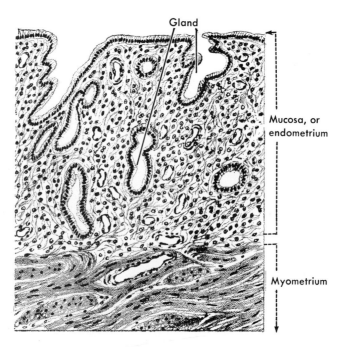

Mucosa, or endometrium

Myometrium

Fig. 19-10. Mucosa and part of muscularis of human uterus.

the mucosa as the tube approaches the uterus. The muscular coat is thick and prominent. The movement of the mucosal cilia and the peristaltic waves set up in the smooth muscle moves the egg slowly toward the uterus. It is not known how the oviduct can simultaneously transport an egg toward the uterus and sperm toward the ampulla. The muscular activity and ciliary beat are influenced by estrogens and by prostaglandins.

The junction of the oviduct with the wall of the uterus is called the *pars interstitialis* or *intramural zone*. This channel is short in humans, less than 1 mm at the most. An egg cannot pass through this narrow slit until it has been stripped of its halo of granulosa cells (corona radiata), a process that usually takes place as it travels down the oviduct. If fertilization occurs, the developing embryo is still within the confines of the zona pellucida at the time of its passage into the uterus, perhaps ensuring that it will not expand in size and block its own passage. Changes in the size of the slit of the intramural zone during the reproductive cycle may control entry of sperm into the oviducts. Changes in the contractility of the muscle of the oviducts may hold the unfertilized egg in place in the ampulla during the period when it is viable and then provide the basis for the slow, controlled passage of the ovum toward the uterus. One of the functions of the oviduct is to prevent entry of a fertilized egg into the uterine cavity prior to the development of the capacity of the mucosa to permit implantation.

UTERUS

The human uterus is a pear-shaped muscular organ having two parts, a body and a neck or cervix. At its upper, broader end it receives the oviducts; its lower end opens into the vagina.

Its wall consists of three layers: (1) the endometrium, which corresponds to the mucosa and submucosa; (2) the myometrium or muscularis; and (3) the perimetrium, a typical serous membrane. The myometrium is a thick layer of interwoven bundles of smooth muscle, forming three fourths of the uterine wall. At the lower end or cervix of the uterus the fibers are arranged in three fairly distinct layers; the middle layer is circular, and the outer and inner layers are longitudinal (Fig. 19-10).

The endometrium is lined by columnar epithelium that contains scattered groups of ciliated cells. It contains numerous tubular glands that open at the surface (Figs. 19-10 to 19-12). The mucosa undergoes cyclic variations, which are related to hormonal changes occurring during the ovulatory or menstrual cycle. Although the changes that occur in the endometrium are not abrupt, structural differences take place that have resulted in the classification of four morphologically distinct stages: (1) the proliferative, also known

Epithelium

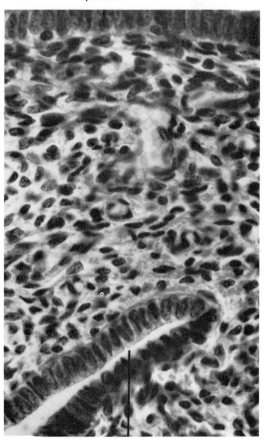

Gland

Fig. 19-11. Section of endometrial wall of human uterus. (×640.)

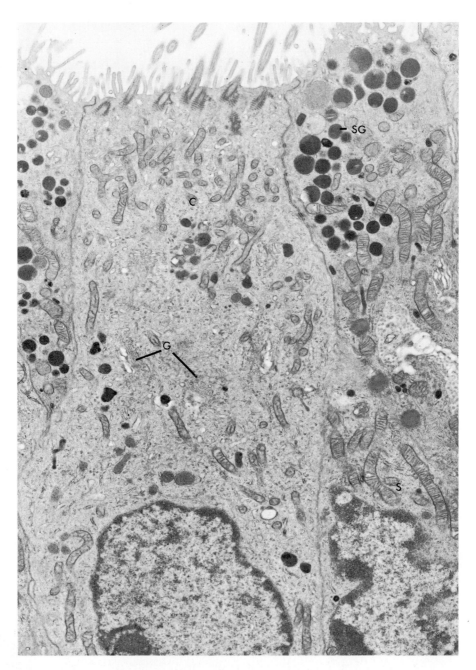

Fig. 19-12. Electron micrograph of endometrial cells from uterus simplex of armadillo, showing parts of two secretory cells, *S,* and a ciliated cell, *C. SG,* Secretory granules; *G,* Golgi apparatus. (×11,400.) (Courtesy Dr. A. C. Enders.)

as the estrogenic stage, (2) the progravid or secretory stage, (3) the premenstrual stage, and (4) the menstrual stage.

Proliferative stage. The proliferative phase of the cycle begins at the termination of the menstrual phase and continues until the thirteenth or fourteenth day of the cycle. It is characterized by the rapid regeneration of the endometrial wall and a replacement of epithelial cells to cover the surface of the mucosa (Fig. 19-13). Also, the gland cells increase in number, and the glands themselves increase in length. Vascularity of the tissue becomes more pronounced, and the endometrial cells are tightly packed. During this period, follicles are growing in the ovary and estrogen secretion increases. It is the action of estrogen that leads to growth and repair of the uterine lining.

Secretory (progravid) stage. The secretory stage is characterized by a marked increase in the hypertrophy of the endometrium, which is the result of proliferation of the glandular tissue, and a marked increase in edema and vascularity of the mucosa (Fig. 19-14). This stage begins on the thirteenth or fourteenth day of the cycle and continues until the twenty-sixth or twenty-seventh day. During this period there is a functioning corpus luteum in the ovary and the high progesterone levels, acting on a previous background of estrogen, lead to secretory changes in the uterine lining.

Premenstrual stage. In the premenstrual

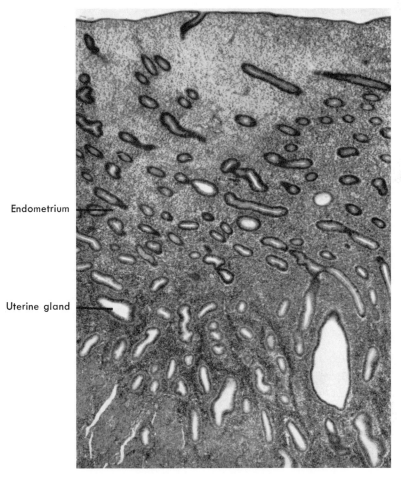

Endometrium

Uterine gland

Fig. 19-13. Section of human uterus in proliferative stage. (×40.)

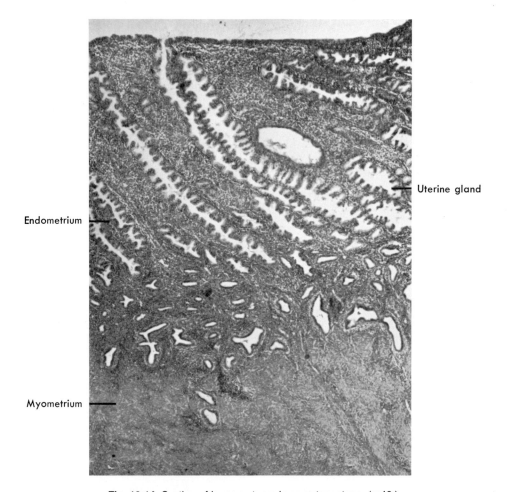

Endometrium

Uterine gland

Myometrium

Fig. 19-14. Section of human uterus in secretory stage. (×40.)

part of the cycle, changes occur in the vascular components, which result in a loss of the superficial portion of the mucosa. During this time fragmentation of the glands and the extrusion of blood and tissue debris into the lumen of the uterus occur. The premenstrual stage is confined to 1 or 2 days and is said to terminate at the first external signs of bleeding. At this time, the corpus luteum is reaching the end of its life span, and hormonal secretion declines. As steroid levels fall, hormonal support of the endometrium falls; as a result of hormone withdrawal, the outer layers of the endometrium down to the upper part of the stroma slough off.

Menstrual stage. The menstrual stage usually occupies 3 to 5 days of the cycle and is characterized by a considerable amount of endometrial destruction, which consists essentially in the sloughing off of the upper compact layer of the endometrium and small areas of the spongiosa. Rarely, desquamation extends nearly down to the muscularis. It involves the destruction of the epithelium and connective tissue and the rupture of blood vessels. Menstrual fluid consists of some blood and endometrial tissue debris, and on the average about 50 ml of blood are lost with each cycle.

Menstruation is caused by a change in steroid environment, which alters the blood flow through the spiral arteries that supply the functional zone of the endometrium. As the corpus luteum regresses and estrogen and progesterone levels fall, periodic contractions of the spiral arteries interrupt the

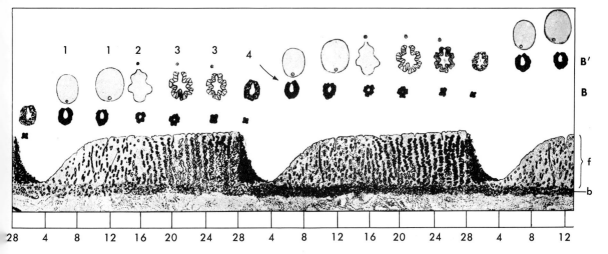

Fig. 19-15. Diagram illustrating relation of menstruation to ovulation. *A,* Cyclic changes in uterine mucosa; *B, B',* ovarian cycles; *b,* basal layer of mucosa; *f,* functional layer of mucosa; *1,* maturing follicle; *2,* rupture of follicle and discharge of ovum (ovulation); *3,* corpus luteum in full function; *4* and remaining figures, degenerating corpus luteum. Numbers at base indicate days of menstrual cycle. (After Schroeder.)

flow of blood. This leads to a shrinkage of the endometrium, a collapse of the vascular bed, and a shedding of the decidual layer of the endometrium. If ovulation does not occur, the continued secretion of estrogen during cycles of follicle development supports a continued endometrial hyperplasia, and the lining tends to erode in a patchy fashion, with small chunks breaking off at irregular intervals to produce excessive and prolonged or unpredictable menstrual flow (dysfunctional uterine bleeding).

Pregnancy. During pregnancy the structure of the endometrium undergoes marked hypertrophy to provide for the nutrition of the embryo. For a full description of the placenta the student should consult a textbook of embryology. Only as much as will explain the place of pregnancy in the female sexual cycle will be considered here. The changes that take place in the secretory stage are preparations for the implantation of a fertilized ovum. The endometrium is full of large irregular pockets, and in one of these the fertilized ovum becomes embedded. The surrounding tissues enclose it in a sac, from the walls of which the placenta develops. At first, while the embryo is small, the sac surrounding it is smaller than the cavity of the uterus. Later, the embryo and its membranes increase in size to completely occlude the uterine cavity. The part of the endometrium that first covered the ovum fuses with the wall of the opposite side, and the only space in the uterus is that immediately surrounding the fetus.

At the end of pregnancy (parturition) the muscles of the uterus contract and the fetus is expelled. Shortly after this another series of contractions dispel the placenta or so-called afterbirth. This includes the placenta and the upper layers of the endometrium. After parturition the uterus is in a condition similar to that which follows each menstruation, and it enters a period of repair similar to that of the postmenstrual period. From this stage it continues to the proliferative stage and to a renewal of the menstrual cycle. In Fig. 19-15 are shown the probable relations between the uterine cycle and the changes that occur in the ovary (ovulation and the formation of corpora lutea). The cycle represented is one in which there is no fertilization of the ovum. Ovulation occurs about the middle of the interval between menstrual periods (12 to 14 days before the beginning of the next menstrual flow). The unfertilized ovum travels slowly down the fallopian tube, reaching the uterus in from 5 to 8 days. In the meantime, the ruptured follicle is being transformed into a corpus luteum, and the endometrium is undergoing progravid hyperplasia. The ovum reaches the uterus when the latter is ready to receive a fertilized egg. But in the cycle under consideration the ovum is dead, and the endometrium enters the menstrual period, during which a part of its mucosa is sloughed off. The ovum also is expelled with the menstrual flow, and the corpus luteum begins to degenerate. If the ovum has been fertilized, it reaches the uterus, as before, when the latter is in the progravid condition. The endometrium provides a suitable place for the embedding of the ovum, which remains in the uterus for the 9 months of the gestation period. If pregnancy occurs, the corpus luteum does not undergo involution but grows larger and persists throughout pregnancy.

The regulating mechanism of the reproductive cycle resides in the ovary and its control system (the brain and pituitary), not in the uterus. The time of ovulation varies from one cycle to the next. It is now believed that ovulation is triggered by increased estrogen secretion, which, in turn, stimulates the pituitary to release FSH and LH. Ovulation takes place 24 to 36 hours later. Generally, the length of time between successive menstrual flows (the usual way the female cycle is timed) depends on the amount of time that it takes for a follicle crop to ripen. For the most part, the lifespan of a corpus luteum is definite, although occasionally short luteal phases do occur, perhaps because of inadequate preparation of the follicle before ovulation. More than 90% of adult female cycles during the most regular period of the reproduction life span (ages 25 to 35) falls between 23 and 35 days. Cycles at puberty and during the menopause are less regular, primarily because ovulation does not occur after every wave of follicle development.

Cervix

The most inferior and the narrowest portion of the uterus, differing in structure from the rest of the organ, is the cervix. It is a dense tube of connective tissue containing some smooth muscle. The cervix serves two main functions: (1) to secret mucus, which plays an important role in fertility (since it is the first secretion met by a sperm entering the female tract), and (2) to change from a narrow constricted channel to a dilated, soft tube at the time of parturition. This softening and dilation require considerable change in the matrix. The smooth muscle present may help to contract the cervix again after childbirth until the matrix has had time to reorganize.

The cervical canal is flattened anteroposteriorly with longitudinal ridges on the walls (the *plicae palmatae*, Fig. 19-16). The ridges are composed of long narrow folds of mucosa that make up cryptlike shelves in the wall. Over 100 such crypts are present and they produce 20 to 60 mg. of mucus per day, increasing to over 700 mg/day at the time of ovulation. The crypts are lined with secretory cells interrupted by an occasional ciliated cell whose beat helps to convey the mucus into the vagina. Occasionally the mouths of the crypts become occluded, leading to the development of cysts, often of considerable size. Beneath the mucosa is a cellular lamina propria that is less dense than the stroma of the uterine endometrium. It contains elongate fibroblast-like nuclei and a large amount of matrix.

The canal itself is lined with simple columnar epithelium, but near the external opening of the canal (Fig. 19-16) the epithelium changes abruptly to a stratified squamous epithelium that covers the vaginal wall as well. In humans the cervix undergoes changes in morphology during the menstrual cycle. Cyclic changes can be noted in the length and diameter of the cervical canal and isthmus and the appearance of the mouth (*os*). No striking histologic changes have been reported.

The chemical composition and the physical properties of cervical mucus change greatly during the menstrual cycle. Under estrogen influence at the midpoint of the ovarian cycle, mucus production is copious and a

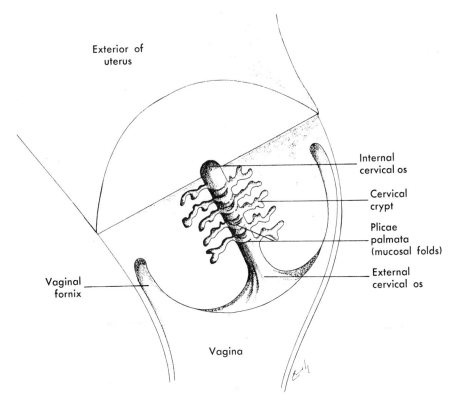

Exterior of
uterus

Internal
cervical os

Cervical
crypt

Plicae
palmata
(mucosal folds)

External
cervical os

Vaginal
fornix

Vagina

Fig. 19-16. Schematic drawing of human cervix showing mucosal folds. (Drawing by Emily Craig.)

thin, highly elastic fluid is produced. The proteins in this mucus are aligned in chains separating channels of fluid that facilitate sperm movement. Cervical mucus at mid-cycle provides a good medium for sperm transport, and the initial entry of sperm into the cervix is greatly facilitated by the composition of the mucus. At other times in the cycle, cervical mucus is thick, scant, and a poor medium for sperm movement.

Sperm traverse the cervix by means of their own forward swimming motions but appear to be carried beyond that point as a result of fluid movement and muscular contraction of the female tract. It has been suggested that the cervix plays a crucial role in weeding out defective sperm. In addition, sperm often swim into the cervical crypts and are then slowly released into the lumen. This serves to provide a steady movement of sperm up the female tract, a process that may provide that enough sperm reach the ampulla of the oviduct to ensure fertilization.

Vagina

The wall of the vagina includes a mucosa, submucosa, and muscularis. As in the oviduct and uterus, the mucosa and submucosa are blended. The epithelium is stratified squamous (Figs. 19-17 and 19-18); the muscularis is of interlacing fibers of smooth muscle that form somewhat indefinite circular (inner) and longitudinal coats.

The epithelium of the human vagina undergoes changes during the menstrual cycle, although they are less marked than those of the uterine mucosa. During the premenstrual period a zone of keratinized cells is formed in the middle layers of the epithelium. At the menstrual period the cells above this zone are sloughed off, and the keratinized cells are thus brought to the surface. In some mammals the changes are more marked so that vaginal smears furnish an indication of the stage of the estrus cycle of the animal from which they are made.

Stratified squamous
epithelium

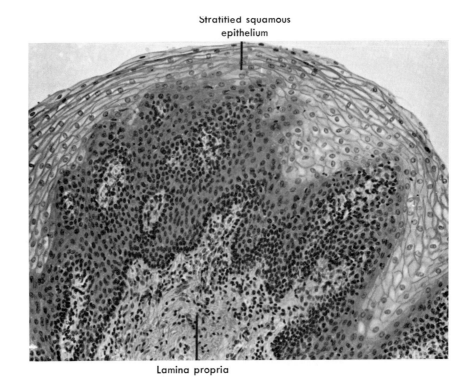

Lamina propria

Fig. 19-17. Section of mucosa of human vagina. (×160.)

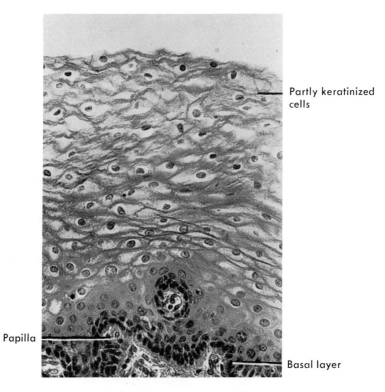

Partly keratinized
cells

Papilla

Basal layer

Fig. 19-18. Stratified squamous epithelium of vagina.

MAMMARY GLAND

The mammary gland is a compound alveolar gland that develops from the lower layers of the epidermis. It consists of from fifteen to twenty lobes separated by broad bands of dense connective tissue. The lobes are divided into lobules by connective tissue septa, from which strands extend into secreting units. The intralobular connective tissue is fine areolar. The alveoli of each lobule open into small intralobular ducts that unite to form interlobular ducts, and these, in turn, lead to the main excretory (lactiferous) ducts (Fig. 19-19). The inactive and active phases of the gland are marked by difference in appearance.

Resting gland. A section of the mammary gland during a period of inactivity hardly resembles a gland at all on first inspection. The secreting tissue is represented by scattered ducts, around the terminal portions of which one may see a few collapsed or small follicles and a few solid cords of epithelial cells (Fig. 19-20). Such groups of intralobular epithelial tissue lie in a thin investment of loose connective tissue, and this is surrounded by a dense mass of collagenous fibers. The connective tissue occupies by far the greater portion of the section. Examined under high power, the ducts are seen to be lined with two or three layers of cuboidal cells, whereas such follicles as may be found are composed of simple cuboidal epithelium.

Active gland. During pregnancy the epithelial portions of the mammary gland undergo a pronounced hypertrophy so that by the fifth month of gestation the organ presents a histological picture much different from that of the resting gland. Alveoli have developed from the cords of tissue that were to be seen before. The small areas of intralobular connective tissue have expanded, and the lobules appear as relatively large areas filled with alveoli and ducts. The amount of interlobular connective tissue is correspondingly reduced.

During the latter part of the gestation period the development of alveoli and ducts continues so that at childbirth they occupy the greater part of the organ. They are lined with an epithelium that varies from tall columnar in actively secreting units to low cuboidal in those that have been drained of milk (Fig. 19-21). The cells in active alveoli are filled with fat droplets, which distend them at the free surface and give an irregular

Excretory duct   Adipose tissue

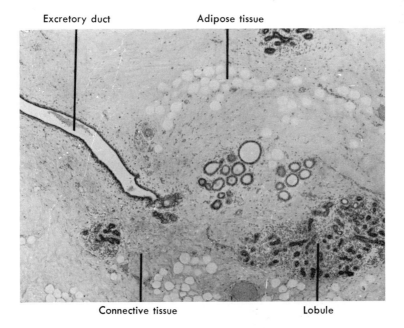

Connective tissue   Lobule

Fig. 19-19. Section of inactive mammary gland showing lobules made up chiefly of ducts. (×40.)

Duct

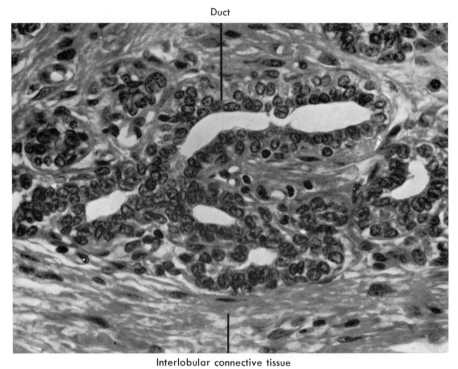

Interlobular connective tissue

Fig. 19-20. Lobule of resting (inactive) mammary gland of cat. (×160.)

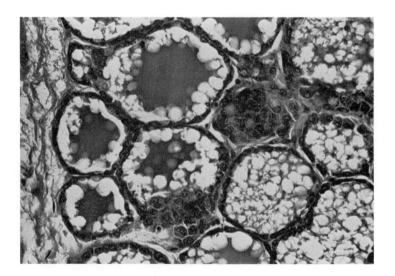

Fig. 19-21. Lactating mammary gland showing follicles and secretion.

outline to the lumen. The ducts leading from the alveoli are lined with low columnar cells and are wrapped around by contractile myoepithelial cells. The lining is replaced by pseudostratified epithelium in the excretory ducts. Near the nipple the epithelium changes to stratified squamous, which is continuous with the skin.

Hormonal control of secretion. The mammary glands are under the control or influence of several hormones. Although the glands undergo some development in the preadolescent state, this process is accentuated during adolescence and is under the influence of two ovarian hormones, estrogen and progesterone, the secretions of which are, in turn, regulated by hormones derived from the anterior pituitary gland.

The first stage in development of the glandular component of the breast during pregnancy requires estrogen for the ductal growth, progesterone to induce ductal branching and the formation of the treelike series of lobular division, and insulin and growth hormone to stimulate the cellular proliferation of the cells in the duct wall. During midpregnancy, cortisol from the adrenal cortex, followed by prolactin from the pituitary and insulin from the islands of Langerhans, induces the differentiation of the secretory alveoli so that clusters of alveoli form at the end of each duct and begin to produce a milklike secretion called colostrum. Although small quantities of colostrum can be expressed from the breasts during pregnancy, full-scale milk production is suppressed by the high levels of progesterone present. Once steroid levels drop at birth, milk production begins whether or not the breast is stimulated by a suckling infant, but milk synthesis will then gradually cease unless periodic surges of prolactin are released from the pituitary in response to suckling. As long as the breasts are regularly emptied of milk, prolactin secretion continues and milk production is adjusted to infant demand. The actual removal of milk is facilitated by a reflex release of oxytocin during suckling, which stimulates the myoepithelial cells. These cells contract and squeeze the alveoli and duct system, forcing milk into the ducts under pressure. Like many reflexes, oxytocin release can be conditioned and some women can respond to the sight or sound of their infants before the breast is stimulated.

The mammary gland remains in the active condition for a variable period after childbirth and then returns to the resting stage. After the menopause it undergoes involution in which the alveoli and parts of the ducts degenerate and their places are taken by connective tissue.

The mammary gland in the male. The early development of the mammary glands in males and females is similar, consisting of the formation of a bandlike thickening of epidermis, the *mammary line* or ridge, which is evident in the 7-week embryo. Along this ridge is a proliferation of epithelium, which sinks into the underlying mesenchyme and spreads radially to form a *mammary bud*. Androgens cause the mammary buds in males to separate from the surface to which they were previously attached by means of lactiferous ducts (galactophores). In females these duct connections remain intact. In males, the secretory tissue becomes isolated in separate cords. The development of this tissue reaches a maximum in males during adolescence and by age 30 the glands begin to regress. The first tissue to regress in males is the glandular (parenchymal) tissue, followed later by the stroma. At about 40 years of age some regrowth of parenchyma and connective tissue may occur. Under conditions of abnormal hormonal stimulation, duct tissue can increase in males (*gynecomastia*) and in rare cases some milk may actually be secreted (*galactorrhea*).

Blood vessels, lymphatics, and nerves. Blood is brought to the mammary gland by the intercostal, internal mammary, and thoracic branches of the axillary artery. The terminal branches of these vessels lie among the alveoli. Lymph vessels, which are numerous, drain chiefly toward the axilla. Nerves from the cerebrospinal and sympathetic systems supply the epithelial tissue and the blood vessels.

20

Endocrine organs

ENDOCRINE GLANDS

Secretory cells may be divided roughly into two categories: those that release their secretory products into a duct connected to a body or organ cavity (such as the salivary glands) and those that release their products directly into body fluids, by way of the capillaries or the lymphatics. Glands whose secretions are transported by ducts are called exocrine glands (Chapter 11); those without ducts are known as endocrine glands.

Both the endocrine glands (ductless glands, glands of internal secretion) and the exocrine glands arise from epithelial linings. The endocrine glands eventually lose contact with the surface and become isolated islands of epithelium embedded in a connective tissue matrix. The parenchymal cells of these glands secrete *hormones,* chemical regulators of specific tissue metabolism occurring elsewhere in the body.

Endocrine cells may occur singly or in groups making up separate glands. Single endocrine cells may be distinguished from unicellular exocrine glands by the fact that their secretory pole (the portion of the cell containing mature secretory products) is directed toward the capillary bed beneath an epithelium rather than toward the lumen of the organ lined by that epithelium (compare mucous cells and argentaffin cells in the gut wall) (Figs. 14-7 and 14-11). Typical endocrine glands consist of a collection of secretory cells arranged in sheets, cords, or small irregular nests of cells infiltrated by a

complex capillary or sinusoidal blood vessel network located in a thin connective tissue framework. The secretions of the cells of endocrine glands are released into the perivascular spaces and then enter the capillary bed. The term *endocrine gland* is usually reserved for glands that secrete hormones into the bloodstream, although in a functional sense an organ such as the liver that also secretes substances (glucose, blood proteins, and the like) that enter the blood indirectly might be considered in this category.

The cells of endocrine glands exhibit to some degree ultrastructural specializations correlated with the chemical composition of the hormones they secrete. Steroid hormone–secreting cells (Leydig cells of the testis, follicle wall and corpus luteum of the ovary, adrenal cortical cells) have large round nuclei, a prominent Golgi apparatus, extensive smooth endoplasmic reticulum with a sparse rough endoplasmic reticulum, numerous mitochondria often containing unusually shaped cristae, and many lipid and lipofuscin droplets in the cytoplasm. At the light microscope level the presence of abundant lipid material removed by routine tissue preparation produces a vacuolated appearance of the cytoplasm. Cells that produce polypeptide or protein hormones (such as the cells of the anterior pituitary, thyroid, and so on) resemble the classic acinar cell of the exocrine pancreas except for the fact that the secretory products do not accumulate at the apex of the cell. Numerous mitochondria are present, usually of a classical rod shape with transverse cristae. At the light microscope level the cytoplasm of these cells is usually basophilic and granular.

A general problem in endocrinology has been to isolate and identify hormonal substances and then to trace these hormones to their cells of origin. Until recently, only two methods of experimentation were in general usage. Both assessed the biologic effects of (1) removal of a suspected endocrine structure and (2) injection of substances derived from tissue extracts of that structure.

The first of these methods is not always practical. The second method may be questioned on the ground that extracts from organs do not necessarily represent the secretion elaborated by them. The use of the two methods may be illustrated by the work on the thyroid, which has yielded fairly clear-cut results. If this gland is removed from a laboratory animal, a marked retardation of the metabolic rate follows, but this becomes normal again when thyroid extract is administered. The extract also raises the metabolic rate of normal (unoperated) animals. Clinical and postmortem evidence also supports the belief that the thyroid contains a substance which influences, directly or indirectly, the rate of metabolism of the body. This effect is not produced by extracts of other glands. Moreover, the thyroid is a ductless organ composed of secreting epithelial cells so that its morphology supports the conclusion derived from experimental and clinical work that it secretes a hormone.

In recent years new techniques have been utilized. These methods are based on (1) correlation of histological and ultrastructural changes with functional states in which hormone secretion is shown to be elevated or depressed, (2) histochemical localization of enzymes responsible for the synthesis of a hormone (restricted to those hormones whose pathways of synthesis have been worked out fairly well, such as the catecholamines and steroids), and (3) identification of hormone storage sites by means of immunofluorescent techniques in which an antibody to a proteinaceous hormone is tagged with a fluorescent compound and then made to react with a tissue containing the hormone antigen (immunocytochemistry).

Endocrine cells can be found in various types of organization, ranging from separate organs that contain several types of hormone-secreting cells to scattered endocrine cells located within an organ, such as the gut, whose primary function includes hormonal secretion.

The separate endocrine glands are the thyroid, parathyroids, adrenal, and pituitary (hypophysis). Pockets of endocrine tissue are found scattered within the pancreas (the islands of Langerhans, described in Chapter 15), the testes, and the ovaries. Two other organs, the pineal and the thymus, *may be* endocrine glands, at least in part, and can be included in this group.

The grouping of organs just described indicates a part, at least, of the confusion existing in this field. The complications of the physiological side of the science are great, since all members of the endocrine group are closely interrelated, and disturbance of one may be expected to affect some or all of the others. Fortunately the histology is less complicated than the physiology. We shall now discuss the thyroid, parathyroid, hypophysis, adrenal, and pineal glands. The islands of Langerhans and the gonads, also in good standing as endocrines, have already been described (see discussions on pancreas, testis, and ovary).

THYROID GLAND

The thyroid gland consists of two lobes and a connecting isthmus. It lies in the neck in contact with the upper part of the trachea and the lower part of the pharynx. The thyroid is enclosed in a connective tissue sheath derived from the cervical fascia. Inside this loose capsule is a second glandular capsule of fibroelastic connective tissue firmly attached to the gland. Trabeculae from the inner capsule penetrate into the gland to provide internal support. These partitions divide the gland into lobules and provide a pathway for the vascular and nerve supply of the gland. The connective tissue within the gland is largely reticular and is extremely rich in nerve and vascular plexuses, although these are not clearly evident at the optical level.

The functional unit of the thyroid is the follicle, which consists of a simple epithelium enclosing a cavity (the follicular cavity) that contains a colloid secretion (Fig. 20-1). Follicles average about 200 μm in diameter but may vary considerably in size. Twenty to forty follicles bound together by a sheet of connective tissue supplied by a single lobular artery make up a thyroid lobule. It is thought that a lobule may give rise to thyroid nodules, local enlargements of a follicle

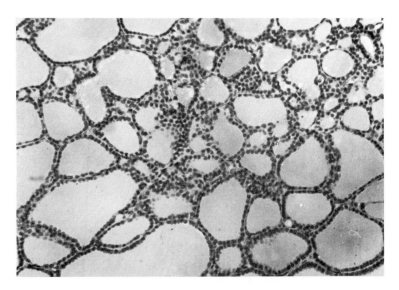

Fig. 20-1. Section of human thyroid gland showing variation in size of follicles. ($\times$40.)

Colloid

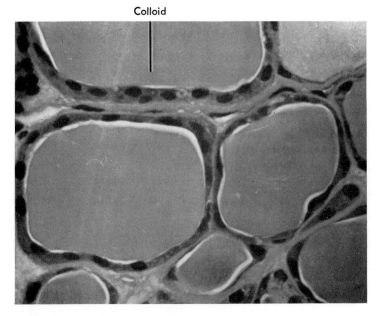

Fig. 20-2. Follicles of human thyroid showing epithelium of different heights and colloid secretion in follicles. ($\times$640.)

cluster observed in certain thyroid diseases.

The colloid, which appears structureless when stained with hematoxylin and eosin, is produced by the cells making up the follicle wall and is usually rich in iodine. It also contains thyroid hormones—thyroxine and triiodothyronine. In this respect the thyroid is different from other endocrine glands in that it stores an appreciable amount of hormone in an extracellular depot (the colloid).

The shape of the follicles, the appearance of the cells, and the amount and consistency of the colloid vary with different functional states of the thyroid. In the inactive state the follicles are round or oval and have regular outlines. At the other extreme, in the hyperactive state, the follicles are more folded and irregular in shape. The thyroid may contain as many as 3 million follicles in various stages of activity. In the newborn, most of the follicles are active and are made up of tall columnar cells, exhibiting a slightly basophilic colloid and vacuolated surfaces between the follicle cells and the colloid. This vacuolation was shown to be an artifact of fixation. In the adult most of the follicles are in the storage or inactive phase. In this state the follicle cells are cuboidal or flattened, the colloid is pink and viscous. The central zones of the gland tend to contain more active follicles, whereas the peripheral follicles are larger and inactive. In some mammals the cells of the follicles are uniform in size, but in humans the cells are variable in height (Fig. 20-2).

Fine structure of the thyroid follicular cells

The thyroid epithelium consists of two cell types: follicular cells and parafollicular cells (light cells, C cells). The follicular cells are the predominant cell type. They are polarized structurally, with their apices directed toward the lumen of the follicle, and their bases rest on a basement membrane that encloses the follicle wall. The prominent nucleus is usually located in the basal part of the cell. Rarely is a cell observed in mitosis; however, when stimulated by TSH, the cells are capable of division. Marked proliferation may occur following partial removal of the thyroid, in dietary iodine deficiency, or after treatment with antithyroid drugs.

The apical border of the cell exhibits microvilli whose height (Figs. 20-3 and 20-4) and number increase with cellular activity. The cell membranes of adjoining cells interdigitate. The cytoplasm contains ribonucleoprotein. The endoplasmic reticulum, which consists of numerous dilated cisternae studded with ribosomes, is usually extensive, especially in active cells. With the electron microscope the most characteristic features of the cell are the numerous dilated cisternae (Fig. 20-3). Mitochondria are scattered throughout the cytoplasm but are most numerous in the apical region. The Golgi apparatus is usually located in the supranuclear region and presents no special features. A centrosome is also present in the apical part of the cell. Several inclusions, which vary in number and size during different states of cell activity, are also present. They may be observed as colloid droplets, clear vacuoles, basal colloid vacuoles, and fine granules (Fig. 20-2).

Hormone secretion by the follicular cells

The function of the follicle cells is controlled by thyroid-stimulating hormone (TSH), a glycoprotein secreted by the anterior pituitary gland. TSH stimulation causes first an increase in the release of thyroid hormones by the gland, then growth of glandular tissue and enhanced hormone synthesis.

The process of thyroid hormone synthesis and release is complicated. Thyroid follicle cells take up iodine from the blood and combine the iodide ions with the amino acid tyrosine on the surface of a protein carrier, thyroglobulin. Two tyrosine molecules are coupled together to form the basic structure of the thyroid hormones, and the actual hormones secreted contain three (triiodothyronine) or four iodine molecules (thyroxine) attached to the thyroxine residues. The final step of hormone synthesis occurs on the microvilli that extend from the cell

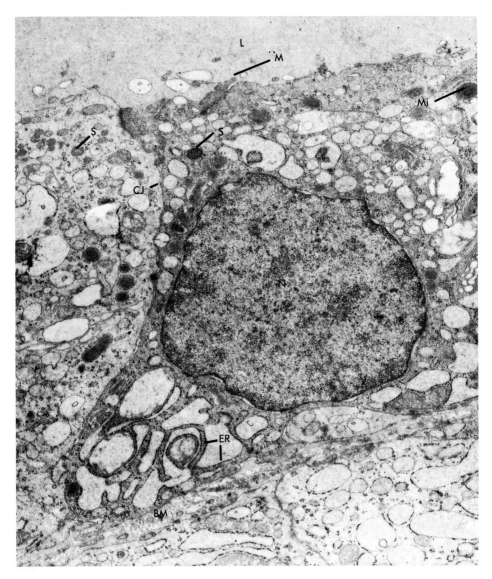

Fig. 20-3. Electron micrography showing parts of two follicle cells of thyroid of cat. *BM,* Basement membrane; *CJ,* cell junction; *ER,* cisterna of endoplasmic reticulum; *L,* lumen of follicle; *M,* microvillus; *Mi,* mitochondrion; *N,* nucleus; *S,* secretory granules. (×18,000.)

surface bordering the colloid. The completed hormone, still on thyroglobulin, is stored in the colloid. In this respect the thyroid gland is unique in that it stores several months' supply of thyroid hormone in a pool outside the cells.

When the thyroid is stimulated by TSH, the apical surface of the cells expand and develop fine pseudopods, which engulf portions of the colloid (Fig. 20-4). These membrane-bound colloid droplets migrate into the deeper areas of the cell where they fuse with lysosomes. The active thyroid hormones (thyroxine and triiodothyronine) are cleaved from their thyroglobulin carriers and released into the bloodstream; the residual membrane and colloidal material are retained within the cell and are probably broken down for reuse of their components. This process of breakdown of the secretory

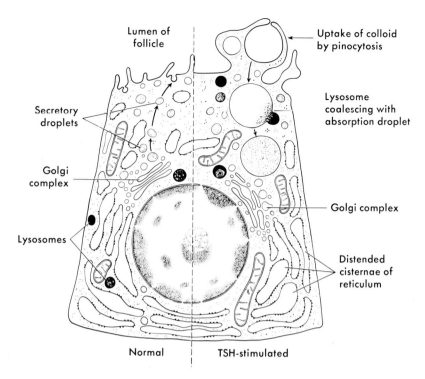

Lumen of
follicle

Uptake of colloid
by pinocytosis

Lysosome
coalescing with
absorption droplet

Secretory
droplets

Golgi complex

Golgi
complex

Lysosomes

Distended
cisternae of
reticulum

Normal | TSH-stimulated

Fig. 20-4. Diagrammatic representation of ultrastructural changes produced in TSH-stimulated thyroid follicle cells. (From Fawcett, D. W. 1969. Rec. Progr. Horm. Res. **25:**315.)

components and carriers of hormones and reuse of the components by the cell is referred to as *crinophagy*, a process that is thought to take place in other protein-secreting cells (such as the anterior pituitary) as a means of regulating the amount of stored hormone.

The thyroid is extremely labile in size and structure. Decrease in thyroid activity is associated with high temperatures, fasting, and aging; increase in activity occurs in cold temperatures, during pregnancy, and in periods of emotional stress.

Increase in the activity of the thyroid is associated with a decrease in follicle size and a reduction in the amount of colloid present. The cells become taller and the nuclei, which normally are centrally located in inactive follicles, migrate to the base of the cell. The amount of rough endoplasmic reticulum and free ribosomes increases, the Golgi apparatus hypertrophies, the height of the surface microvilli increases, and the number of intracytoplasmic colloid droplets increases (Fig.

20-4). Decreased activity is associated with an enlargement of the follicle, a flattening of the follicle epithelium, and storage of excess colloid. Prolonged stimulation by TSH may cause enlargement of the thyroid gland (goiter). A deficiency of iodine in the diet or the consumption of large amounts of goitrogenic foods, which inhibit utilization of iodine (cabbage, for example, contains thiocyanate, which inhibits iodine uptake by the gland), prevents formation of thyroid hormone. As a result, TSH secretion rises and a simple goiter results, consisting of a diffuse, nonnodular enlargement of the thyroid with signs of overactivity in the follicles. Such stimulation may also occur temporarily at puberty or during pregnancy.

Parafollicular cells

Most of the cells making up the epithelial wall of the thyroid follicles are derived from the floor of the pharyngeal gut and are concerned with the elaboration and secretion of thyroid hormones (thyroxine and triiodothyronine). A small percentage of cells (2% to 5%) are of different embryologic origin, arising from the fifth pharyngeal pouch of the embryo. These cells, called parafollicular cells, are derived from the ultimobranchial body, which is later incorporated into the thyroid gland. The parafollicular cells (C cells, light cells) are separated from the lumen of the follicle by slender cell processes derived from the neighboring epithelial cells. They are larger than epithelial cells and have a watery eosinophilic cytoplasm, a prominent Golgi apparatus, and many secretory granules. They were shown to be the source of the hormone *calcitonin*, a polypeptide that causes blood calcium levels to fall, apparently by stimulating the deposition of calcium in bone. It apparently serves to regulate the concentration of calcium in body fluids in combination with parathyroid hormone of the parathyroid glands and vitamin D, both of which elevate blood calcium. Parafollicular cells were conclusively demonstrated in the human thyroid; they are most abundant in the middle third of the gland. They are thought to give rise to medullary carcinomas that produce excess calcitonin.

PARATHYROID GLANDS

The parathyroid glands are paired and in man are usually four in number. They are surrounded by a framework of reticular tissue, which divides the gland into poorly

Capsule

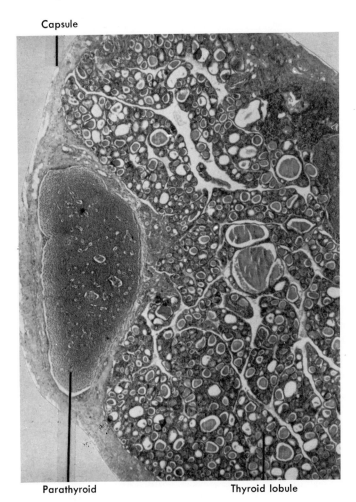

Parathyroid   Thyroid lobule

Fig. 20-5. Section of thyroid and parathyroid of cat. (×40.)

defined lobules (Fig. 20-5). The lobules are subdivided into sheets or cords by fine extensions of the trabeculae (Fig. 20-6). The connective tissue of the gland contains blood vessels, nerves, lymphatics, and adipose tissue. The cells of the gland are enclosed by a network of reticular fibers in which is found a dense network of capillaries.

The parenchyma of the parathyroid is made up of two kinds of cells in the adult human: (1) chief cells and (2) oxyphil cells, the former being most numerous.

1. The *chief cells* are polyhedral in shape and exhibit a round, centrally located nucleus and well-defined cell membranes. Chief cells are of two kinds—light and dark. The light cell is most numerous, is slightly larger, and exhibits a clear cytoplasm; both kinds contain glycogen and secretory granules. Evidence appears to indicate that the light cells may be an inactive form of the dark cells.

2. *Oxyphil cells* are larger and less numerous than chief cells. They exhibit small, dense nuclei and acidophilic cytoplasm. They can be found by scanning the gland for places where the nuclei appear widely separated, especially near the periphery of the gland. They have been observed only in humans, monkeys, and cattle; in man they do not appear until the fourth or fifth year of life.

Oxyphil cells interdigitate in a manner that differs from that observed in chief cells. They contain many mitochondria with densely packed cristae. The membrane systems of

Capillary

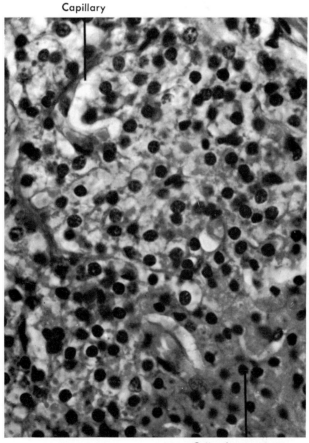

Cells of parenchyma

Fig. 20-6. Human parathyroid. (×640.)

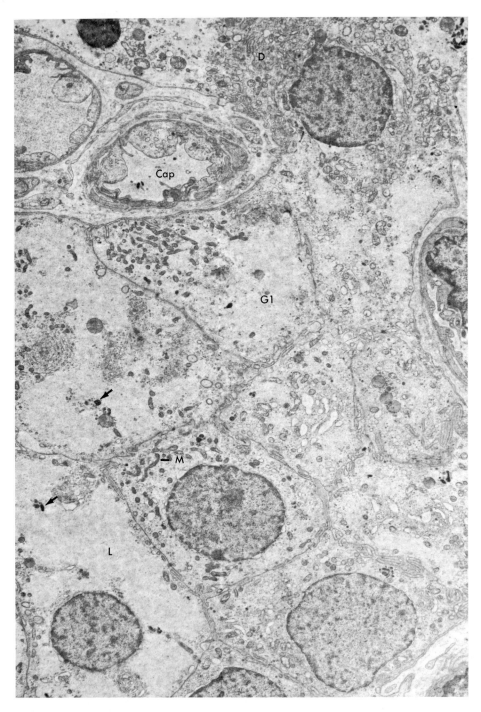

Fig. 20-7. Electron micrograph of human parathyroid showing chief cells. Most of these cells are "dark" variety, *D*. Light cells, *L*, show large lakes of glycogen, *Gl*, and relatively few organelles. *Cap*, Capillary; *M*, mitochondrion. Arrows indicate secretory granules. (×4,200.) (Courtesy Dr. B. Munger.)

the cells are reduced, and the Golgi complex occurs near the cell boundary.

Fatty infiltration of the gland is common in older individuals and at low magnification the gland might be mistaken for bone marrow because of the increase in the amount of adipose tissue, which may come to occupy 50% to 80% of the gland volume.

Fine structure of parathyroids

Active chief cells, the dark cells seen at the optical level, contain secretory granules, glycogen, a prominent perinuclear Golgi apparatus, numerous rod-shaped mitochondria, and occasional cilia (Fig. 20-7). The endoplasmic reticulum is a prominent feature of the dark cells.

In the light cells, secretory granules are few in number and glycogen is abundant. These cells generally do not exhibit a Golgi apparatus or endoplasmic reticulum.

Lipid granules are present in both dark and light cells (Fig. 20-7).

The cell membranes of all parenchymal cells are smooth, although in some instances examples of interdigitation are observed. Specializations of the membranes, desmosomes, occur in some areas.

Functions of the parathyroids

The parathyroid glands secrete a large amount of hormone per day (about 1 mg.) and, unlike the thyroid, store very little hormone. Parathyroid hormone (PTH) causes an elevation of blood calcium whenever the plasma level decreases. The plasma level of calcium in the normal mammal is remarkably stable, usually in the vicinity of 10 mg/100 ml. Removal of the parathyroids results in a decrease in blood calcium, followed by tetany and death in many mammals. The manner in which PTH produces an elevation in calcium is complicated and poorly understood. The best known effect of PTH is on bone. PTH inhibits collagen synthesis in active osteoblasts, enhances resorption of bone by osteoclasts, and probably hastens the maturation of precursor cells into osteoblasts and osteoclasts. The result is to stimulate bone resorption and release bone salts into the blood. The second major target is the kidney. PTH increases tubular reabsorption of calcium and magnesium, enhances potassium and phosphate excretion, and reduces the loss of hydrogen ions. The phosphate loss (phosphaturia) is a striking effect of parathyroid hormone. Parathyroid hormone has been purified and is known to be a peptide of low molecular weight (8,500) containing eighty to eight-five amino acids, the number depending on the species. Commercial preparations of PTH have not been used extensively for clinical treatment, since vitamin D and its related compounds are usually effective in treating hypoparathyroidism. The actual interaction of PTH, vitamin D and its derivatives, and calcitonin in controlling body calcium balance is an area of active research at the present time. The concept is developing that vitamin D (by way of its active metabolites) may be extremely important for the day-to-day control of calcium homeostasis.

HYPOPHYSIS

The hypophysis or pituitary gland consists of two lobes, each of which is again subdivided (Fig. 20-8). These lobes, unlike those of a secretory gland such as the parotid, are composed of tissues that differ from each other in function and (partially) in origin (Diagram 3). The gland is actually two organs intimately associated. One part of it, the glandular or *adenohypophysis*, develops from the roof of the oral cavity of the embryo; the other part, the *neurohypophysis*, develops as an outgrowth of the floor of the brain. The hypophysis is located in a fossa of the sphenoid bone, the *sella turcica*, and is invested by an extension of the dura mater. The buccal portion loses its connection with the oral cavity and becomes a solid mass of cells. In some animals the neural portion retains a cavity in its center.

The adenohypophysis (*pars anterior*) is divided by a lumen into two unequal parts. The *pars distalis* lies anterior to the lumen, and the *pars tuberalis*, an extension of the pars distalis, envelops the neural stalk. The third component, the *pars intermedia*, con-

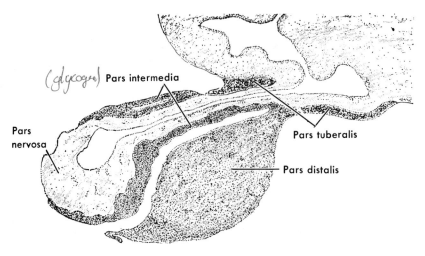

Fig. 20-8. Hypophysis of cat, midsagittal section, under low magnification to show topography.

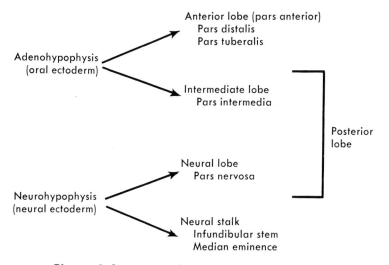

Diagram 3. Components of the pituitary gland (hypophysis).

sists of a thin cellular portion located posterior to the lumen. The term anterior lobe refers to the pars distalis and the pars tuberalis; the posterior lobe refers to the pars intermedia and the *pars nervosa* (the infundibular stalk and median eminence); and the intermediate lobe refers to the pars intermedia alone.

The pars distalis of the anterior pituitary gland is composed of glandular cells that are arranged in irregular clumps and cords that

are in intimate relation to vascular sinusoids. The anterior lobe is enveloped in a dense connective tissue capsule. Internally, fine reticular fibers arising from the capsule surround the cords of the parenchymal cells and serve to support them and the vascular elements.

The glandular cells are classified as *chromophilic* or *chromophobic* on the basis of their affinity or lack of it for routine dyes. The chromophil cells may be divided into

Connective tissue capsule   Basophil

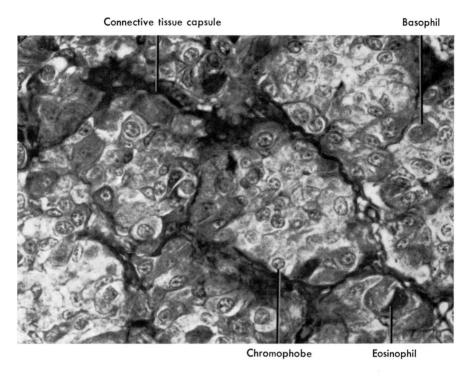

Chromophobe   Eosinophil

Fig. 20-9. Section of anterior pituitary of monkey showing several follicles. (Mallory-azan; ×640.)

two main categories, acidophils and basophils, on the basis of staining reactions following the use of hematoxylin and eosin (Fig. 20-9). Since the anterior pituitary gland secretes at least six different hormones, the classification of these cells as chromophobe, acidophil, and basophil is obviously rather nonspecific. The development of more discriminating dyes and the use of ultrastructural analysis have now permitted the identification of a cell type for each hormone known to be secreted by the anterior pituitary. In some cases it appears that the same cell may secrete two related hormones.

Chromophil cells

The acidophils are round or ovoid and measure from 15 to 19 μm in diameter. They possess a prominent Golgi apparatus, numerous rod-shaped mitochondria, and refractile granules that can be seen with the light microscope. The acidophils are of two types: somatotrophs and mammotrophs. The *somatotrophs* secrete growth hormone, and the *mammotrophs* secrete prolactin. Together

these two cell types account for approximately 35% of the cells of a normal anterior pituitary gland *(pars anterior).* The somatotrophs have dense spherical granules measuring as much as 350 nm in diameter and are arranged in clusters in the posterolateral region of the gland. They stain specifically with orange G. The mammotrophs can easily be distinguished from somatotrophs by the presence of large irregularly shaped secretory granules 600 to 900 nm in diameter (Fig. 20-10). In some species the two classes of acidophils cannot be distinguished by staining methods. In humans the mammotrophs stain with erythrosin or azocarmine. In the normal gland, mammotrophs tend to be sparse and poorly granulated. Mammotrophs are abundant in the gland of pregnant or lactating females. In males and in nonpregnant females most of the acidophils in the human anterior pituitary are somatotrophs, and the gland contains a large amount of growth hormone (milligram quantities in comparison to microgram amounts of other hormones). The majority of cells undergoing

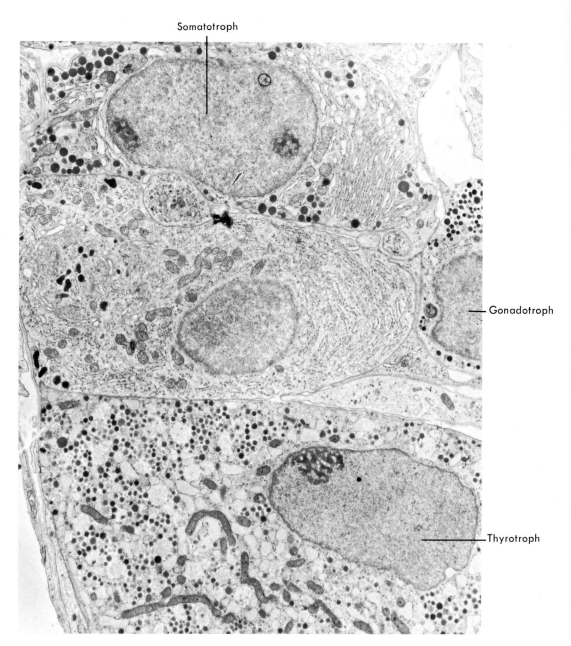

Fig. 20-10. Electron micrograph of rat pars distalis showing variation in appearance of different cell types. At the electron microscope level the size of the granules is the most important diagnostic criterion for the identification of different cell types. (× 7,000.) (Courtesy Dr. M. Farquhar.)

mitosis in the pituitary are somatotrophs.

The basophils represent 10% to 15% of the cell population of the anterior pituitary. They secrete the following glycoproteins: follicle-stimulating hormone (FSH), luteinizing hormone (LH), and thyrotrophin (TSH). The different types of basophils are more difficult to distinguish histologically than are the acidophil populations. In the human pituitary stained with aldehyde thionine PAS and orange G, the FSH-secreting cells take on a brick red color, the TSH-secreting cells (*thyrotrophs*) stain with aldehyde-thionine only, and the LH-secreting cells exhibit a pale pink color by reacting with both orange

G and aldehyde thionine. The LH-secreting cells contain fine granules and occasional lipid inclusions. There is still some doubt whether FSH and LH are secreted by separate cells. Some authors have identified two gonadotrophs ultrastructurally. FSH-secreting cells are said to be located along the periphery of the gland and have small (200 nm) granules. LH-secreting cells are relatively large, angular in shape, and more uniformly distributed. Both *gonadotrophs* (FSH- and LH-secreting cells) have granules of about the same size (Fig. 20-11). The cell that produces TSH contains smaller granules (150 nm) and is located peripherally. The thyro-

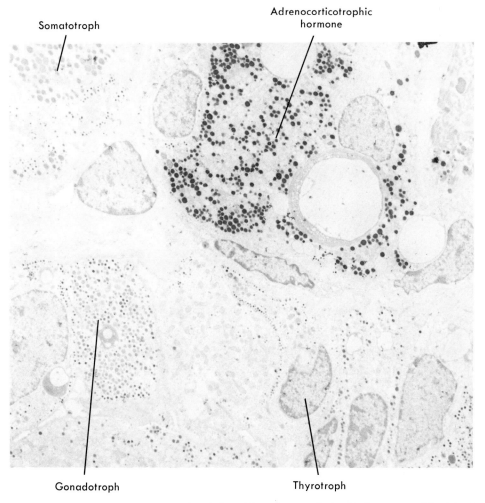

Fig. 20-11. Cell types of human anterior pituitary. The adrenocorticotrophic hormone cell is stained immunocytochemically for adrenocorticotrophic hormone. (×5,700.) (Courtesy Dr. G. Moriarty.)

troph cells are large, irregular, and polygonal in shape.

In general, basophils occur along the midline and anterior margins of the pituitary, whereas the acidophils are more centrally and posteriorly located.

Chromophobe cells

In general, chromophobes have less cytoplasm than chromophils and are often located in small clumps between sinusoids. In such clusters the nuclei appear close together because of the diminished amount of cytoplasm present. It has been suggested that the chromophobes represent a class of differentiating cells which give rise to the various chromophil cell types, but the evidence fails to support this. On the other hand, it now seems well established that one type of chromophobe, a large cell with 200 nm granules arranged around its periphery together with irregular long processes insinuating between other cells to reach a sinusoidal bed, may be the source of adrenocorticotrophic hormone (ACTH) (Fig. 20-11). These cells are weakly PAS positive (stain for 1,2 glycol groups in carbohydrate-containing substances, with periodic acid–Schiff base reaction) and strongly positive to aldehyde fuchsin. They can be found both in the anterior pituitary and the pars intermedia.

Hormones produced by the pars distalis

The pars distalis is known to produce six hormones, which consist of proteins or polypeptides.

Somatotrophic hormone (STH). One of the earliest hormones to be recognized was the growth or somatotrophic hormone (STH), which stimulates body growth, particularly that of the epiphyses of long bones. Hypophysectomy in growing animals results in a cessation of growth, which can be overcome by the administration of the hormone. Underproduction of the hormone results in dwarfism, overproduction in gigantism. If overproduction occurs when the epiphyseal plate has calcified, a thickening of the bones of the face, skull, hands, and feet occurs. This condition is known as *acromegaly*.

Thyrotrophic hormone (TSH). The thyroid-stimulating hormone maintains the integrity of the thyroid epithelium and is responsible for stimulating thyroid secretion. Hypophysectomy results in the atrophy of the thyroid, which, in turn, may be restored by administration of the hormone.

Adrenocorticotrophic hormone (ACTH). The adrenocorticotrophic hormone controls the secretion of the adrenal cortex. The growth of the adrenal cortex seems to be under different control, perhaps involving neural input. Hypophysectomy results in atrophy of the cortex, which can be alleviated by administration of ACTH.

Follicle-stimulating hormone (FSH). The follicle-stimulating hormone stimulates growth of the follicles in the ovary and spermatogenesis in the seminiferous tubules of the testis. Atrophy of the gonads following hypophysectomy can be partially alleviated and the gonads restored to their normal state by the administration of FSH, but complete restoration also requires some luteinizing hormone.

Luteinizing hormone (LH); interstitial cell–stimulating hormone (ICSH). After stimulation by FSH, the luteinizing hormone contributes to the maturation of the ovarian follicle and also to ovulation. In the male, ICSH stimulates the interstitial cells of Leydig in the testes to produce testosterone, which is responsible for the maintenance of the secondary sexual characteristics.

Prolactin (lactogenic hormone) (PRL). Prolactin initiates secretion of milk after hypertrophy of the mammary gland in response to stimulation of ovarian hormones during pregnancy. It also has been shown in the rat that prolactin initiates and maintains the secretion of progesterone; hence the synonym, luteotropic hormone (LTH).

Pars tuberalis

The pars tuberalis consists of a thin band of cells enveloping the infundibular stalk. The main cells are cuboidal or polyhedral; the cytoplasm is faintly basophilic and contains small granules. The cells arranged in cords or clusters are in intimate association

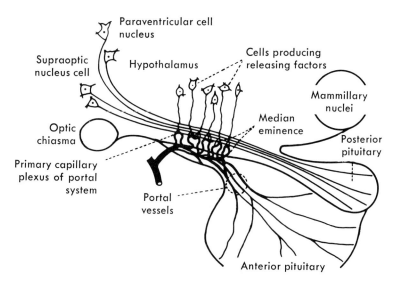

Fig. 20-12. Hypothalamic pituitary interactions showing relationship between neurosecretory neurons and pituitary. (Courtesy Dr. M. D. Mann and Mr. D. Martin.)

with a rich supply of blood vessels. Occasional small, colloid-laden vesicles occur among the cells. There are, in addition, undifferentiated cells and also small acidophils and basophils. The function of the pars tuberalis is not known.

Relationship between the anterior pituitary and the brain

The secretion of hormones by the anterior pituitary depends on stimulation or inhibition of the pituitary cells by polypeptides or transmitters synthesized in the hypothalamus and released into the vascular bed of the median eminence, the region of the hypothalamus overlying the pituitary stalk (Fig. 20-12). This vascular bed consists of a capillary network supplied by the internal carotid artery and the circle of Willis, which forms a ring around the infundibulum. Draining this bed are a series of long portal vessels that run through the stalk and on its surface make contact with the sinusoidal capillary bed of the anterior pituitary. Some short portal vessels also supply the posterior pituitary. The portal vessels provide a channel for chemical control of the pituitary by the central nervous system. It has been

difficult as yet to localize the cell bodies of the neurons that produce releasing and inhibiting hormones which regulate pituitary growth and function, but *heavy* accumulation of releasing hormones can be found in the terminals of cells in the median eminence (Fig. 20-13).

Pars intermedia

In humans the pars intermedia is rudimentary. It occupies a position adjacent to the residual lumen and is composed of cells and scattered follicles containing colloid. The cells are basophilic and blend with those of the pars distalis. The cells lining the colloid vesicles are frequently ciliated, and some secrete mucus. The colloid does not accumulate iodine.

The only known function of this part of the gland is the secretion of *melanocyte stimulating hormone* (MSH), but ACTH may also be produced here, possibly in the same cell.

Neurohypophysis

The neurohypophysis is composed of the infundibular process—the infundibulum and the median eminence of the tuber cinereum and the neural lobe (see diagram on p. 346).

Third ventricle

A

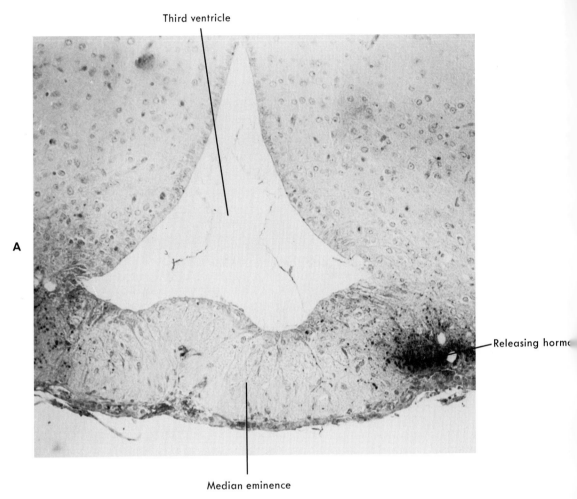

Releasing horm‹

Median eminence

Fig. 20-13. Section of median eminence of hypothalamus of rat treated to show localization of gonadotrophin-releasing terminals by means of immunochemical techniques. (Courtesy Dr. G. Campbell.)

The infundibulum and medium eminence of the tuber cinereum have in common the same type of cell, nerve, and blood supply and elaborate similar active substances. The cells of the neural lobe are small, have numerous processes, and are known as *pituicytes*. Unlike neuroglia, which they resemble, their cytoplasm contains fat and pigment granules. The nuclei of the pituicytes are round, and the cytoplasmic processes often extend to capillary walls or the septa of the gland.

The neurosecretory neurons in the supraoptic and paraventricular nuclei of the hypothalamus elaborate secretory products, which are transmitted by nerve fibers that

run through the infundibular process to the neural lobe where the hormone is stored in nerve fiber terminations known as *Herring bodies.*

A neurosecretory neuron is a nerve cell that combines the properties of a neuron with the properties of an endocrine cell. Neurosecretory neurons resemble neurons in that they have dendrites, a cell body, and axonal terminals containing neurotransmitters; they resemble endocrine cells in their ability to manufacture, package, and secrete hormones.

Two active fractions have been isolated from the neurohypophysis. They have been identified as polypeptides. One of these,

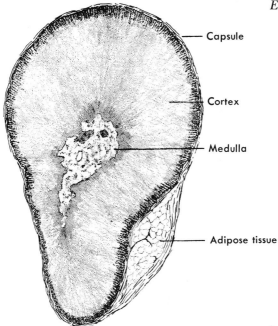

Capsule

Cortex

Medulla

Adipose tissue

Fig. 20-14. Section through adrenal gland of rabbit showing relation of its parts.

oxytocin, stimulates uterine contraction during late pregnancy and also activates the myoepithelial cells of the mammary gland, resulting in the flow of milk. The second fraction, *vasopressin*, is an antidiuretic (ADH) hormone. When administered in excessive amounts it also has the ability to raise blood pressure. Both hormones are produced in the cell bodies of neurosecretory neurons in the supraoptic and paraventricular nuclei (Fig. 20-12) and are transported down the axons of these neurons in secretory packets in association with carrier proteins called neurophysins. Because of the accessibility of these cells and their axons, the hypothalamo-hypophysial tract has been a model system for the study of neurosecretion.

ADRENAL GLANDS

The adrenal (suprarenal) gland is like the hypophysis in that it is in reality two glands having different functions and arising from different sources. One is the cortex, which is derived from mesodermal tissue. The other is the medulla of the organ, which comes from the same group of cells as those that form the sympathetic ganglia (Fig. 20-14).

The entire gland is surrounded by a capsule of connective tissue (Fig. 20-14). From the capsule, delicate connective tissue fibers pass into the cortex at the hilus. They continue into the stroma of the gland as reticular fibers supporting the arterioles and capillaries of the cortex and the sinusoidal vessels of the medulla. The capsule also gives rise to cells that replace those of the cortex.

Cortex

The cortex is composed of cords of cells, between which lie capillaries in a fine network of reticular tissue. Three zones are distinguishable, though they are not sharply delimited one from another. They are (1) the zona glomerulosa, (2) the zona fasciculata, and zona reticularis.

1. In the *zona glomerulosa* the cells are pale and columnar (Fig. 20-15); they are arranged in oval groups separated from each other by fine vascular connective tissue. The nuclei stain intensely, and the cytoplasm is faintly basophilic. The cells produce mineralocorticords.

2. The *zona fasciculata* is the widest zone

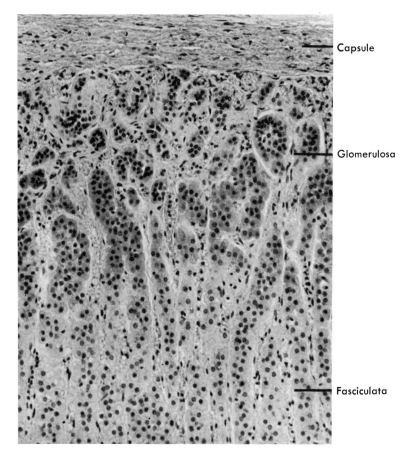

Capsule

Glomerulosa

Fasciculata

Fig. 20-15. Section of human adrenal cortex. (×160.)

Reticularis

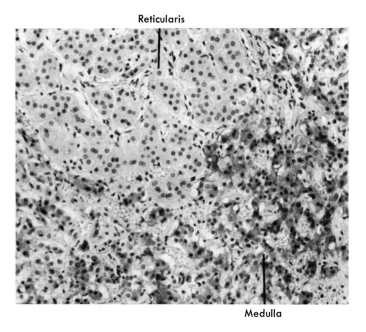

Medulla

Fig. 20-16. Section of human adrenal showing portion of reticularis and medulla. (×160.)

of the cortex and is composed of polygonal cells, in the cytoplasm of which fat (lipoid) droplets are present; cells in the zone are arranged in cords that radiate from the center of the gland (Fig. 20-17); the cords are usually two cells in width, being cuboidal and often binucleate. In the outer portion of the fasciculata the cells contain droplets of cholesterol and fatty acids. In the usual preparations these areas appear as vacuoles, giving the cell a spongy appearance. They are sometimes called spongiocytes. The cells reduce glucocorticoids.

3. In the *zona reticularis*, the innermost zone of the cortex, the cords of cells, rather than running in a radial direction, break up into a network. The capillaries are to be found in the spaces of this network. The cells of the reticular zone are somewhat smaller and darker than those of the fascicular zone (Figs. 20-16 and 20-17). Many cells have pyknotic nuclei and contain pigment granules. The cells secrete sex steroids.

Fine structure of cortical cells. Electron microscopy shows that the adrenocortical cells, like other steroid hormone–producing tissues, contain an abundance of smooth endoplasmic reticulum lying between the densely packed mitochondria (Fig. 20-18). Also present are scattered ribosomes, various dense granules, lipid droplets, and multivesicular bodies. The Golgi apparatus is not usually prominent and is often widely distributed throughout the cytoplasm.

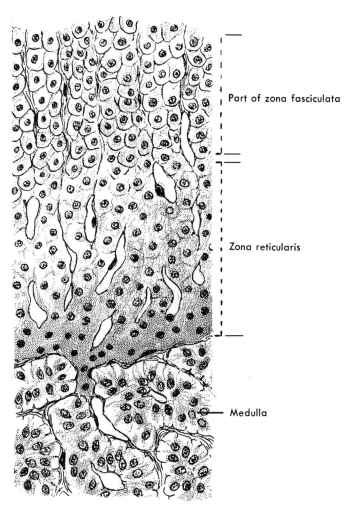

Part of zona fasciculata

Zona reticularis

Medulla

Fig. 20-17. Inner portion of cortex and part of medulla of adrenal gland of rabbit.

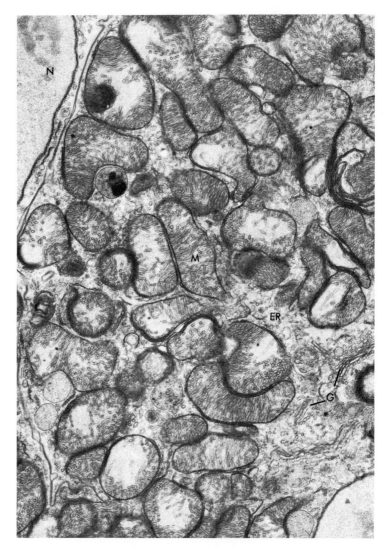

Fig. 20-18. Electron micrograph of fasciculata cell from cortex of adrenal gland of hamster. These cells have prominent nucleus, *N,* and cytoplasm is packed with large mitochondria, *M.* Between mitochondria are numerous profiles of smooth endoplasmic reticulum, *ER.* Also shown are laminar portions of Golgi apparatus, *G,* and granules of various kinds. (×17,880.) (Courtesy Dr. R. Yates.)

Medulla

The medulla consists of irregularly arranged groups of cells that have a granular cytoplasm and polygonal outlines (Figs. 20-16 and 20-17). With hematoxylin and eosin, their color is faintly purple. They react strongly to chromium salts and are therefore called chromaffin cells. Even without this specific stain, they are readily distinguished from the cortical cells by their basophilic reaction, their larger size, and their arrange-

ment. Among the cords is a network of capillaries such as is characteristic of endocrine organs.

Fine structure of the medulla. The chromaffin cells of the medulla have a relatively large nucleus, few scattered mitochondria, ribosomes, and a well-developed Golgi apparatus (Fig. 20-19). A prominent cytoplasmic feature of these cells is the presence of numerous dense granules. These granules

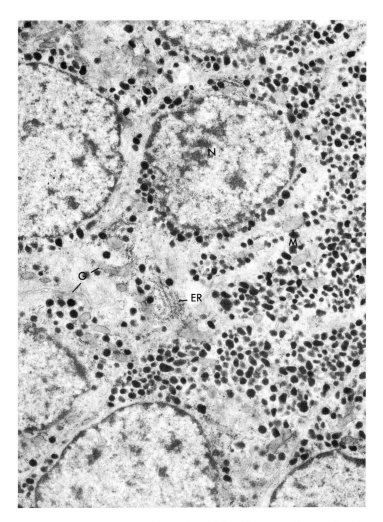

Fig. 20-19. Electron micrograph of part of adrenal medulla of hamster. These cells, known as chromaffin cells, have large nuclei, *N*, and numerous dark granules scattered throughout cytoplasm. Granules of chromaffin cells contain both norepinephrine and epinephrine. Mitochondria, *M*, endoplasmic reticulum, *ER*, and Golgi apparatus, *G*, are also shown. (×11,232.) (Courtesy Dr. R. Yates.)

apparently arise from the Golgi vesicles and are of two kinds: those containing (1) norepinephrine (dark granules) and (2) epinephrine (light granules). The Golgi vesicles containing the formed granules enlarge and migrate to the apical surface of the cell where they are eventually released. In humans the two granule types appear to be contained in the same cell. In most other species they are in separate cells.

Functions of the adrenal gland

The cortex is essential to life, and destruction or removal of the cortex results in Addison's disease, which can be fatal. It regulates electrolyte balance and maintains carbohydrate balance, affecting glycogen stores in the liver and muscles and the production of glucose from amino acid precursors in the liver (gluconeogenesis). Another important function of the cortex is the maintenance of connective tissue throughout the body. Connective tissue diseases are often dramatically arrested by the administration of glucacorticoids. Deficiency of the hormone is believed to affect adversely other functions such as blood pressure, sexual libido, and vascular permeability. The activity of the adrenal cortex is controlled in part by adrenocorticotrophic hormone (ACTH) derived from the adenohypophysis, whose effect is chiefly on the cells of the zona fasciculata and zona reticularis.

The control of the zona glomerulosa involves a number of hormonal signals, including those arising from the juxtaglomerular apparatus of the kidney. The zona glomerulosa secretes aldosterone, a hormone concerned with sodium and potassium balance. The secretion of this hormone is affected by changes in blood pressure and in the salt composition of the fluids in the afferent and efferent arterioles of the glomerulus.

The adrenal cortex also secretes sex steroids that may play a role in sexual maturation and fertility. The zona reticularis appears to be the source of these hormones.

Unlike the cortex, the medulla is not essential to life. It elaborates two substances, *epinephrine* and *norepinephrine*, which are catecholamines located in the chromaffin granules of the cells. Epinephrine increases oxygen consumption and the mobilization of glucose from glycogen that is stored in the liver. It also causes contraction of smooth muscle in some vascular beds and relaxation of others, increases cardiac output, and is active in situations of stress or emergency. Epinephrine will also stimulate the secretion of ACTH by the adenohypophysis under experimental conditions. Norepinephrine, a precursor of epinephrine, serves as a transmitting agent of adrenergic nerves regulating blood pressure of the heart and blood vessels. The human adrenal medulla secretes *both* epinephrine (E) and norepinephrine (N). The rate of conversion of norepinephrine to epinephrine depends on glucocorticoids.

PINEAL BODY

The pineal body, also known as the *epiphysis cerebri*, is a small, flattened, conical body attached to the roof of the third ventricle by a slender stalk. It is divided into lobules by connective tissue septa derived from the capsule in which it is enclosed. When stained with hematoxylin and eosin, the pineal body appears to consist of cords of epithelial cells, which are irregular in shape and have a large nucleus and pale-staining cytoplasm. These are the most numerous cells that occur in this organ and are known as *pinealocytes*. When stained with silver, they are shown to have long radiating processes that terminate in the supporting connective tissue in bulbous processes. Also present are neuroglial (interstitial) cells, which are believed to serve as supporting elements. At the sixth or seventh year in the human, the pineal body attains its maximum development, and from this time on it undergoes retrogressive changes. The human pineal body often contains concretions, *acervuli* (brain sand), which are extracellular in location and are composed of a mineralized organic matrix having a lamellate appearance.

The function of the pineal gland is not well understood. The pineal has been shown to contain *serotonin*, and *melatonin*, and several peptides. It is believed to exert a neuroendocrine function and to participate in hormonelike mediation so that it has been called "a regulator of regulating systems." The details of these processes await clarification.

21

Brain and special sense organs

BRAIN

The brain consists of many local processing circuits or centers linked together by conducting pathways. The neurons that occupy each center differ in size, form, and geometrical configuration in space. Each neuron is more than a simple unit receiving information on its dendrites and transmitting information by way of its axon. Newer concepts of the organization and function of local neuron circuits have emphasized two ideas. First, the dendritic fields of neurons are highly complicated, and a considerable amount of information processing goes on in this thicket of cellular processes called the neuropile. Second, the neuron may have different inputs confined to one region of its surface or another, and each neuron is only one small fragment in a larger functional unit made up of the interwoven processes of neurons. The idea is also beginning to emerge that local regions share some common organizational features, particularly at the synaptic level. In this chapter three familiar circuits will be considered in detail—the cerebral cortex, the cerebellar cortex, and the retina. The retina and cerebellum have clearly organized structures and are the best-understood brain circuits. The cerebral cortex is less well understood. Consideration of the retina will provide a bridge to an understanding of other sensory organs.

Neocortex

The term neocortex refers to the sheet of gray matter forming the association circuits of the most recently developed parts of the forebrain. Most brain regions can be found in one form or another throughout the vertebrate phyla but the neocortex is an exception to this rule. Fish, amphibia, and birds have little neocortex. The neocortex has greatly expanded in the human brain, and to conserve space, the surface is thrown into folds (*gyri*) separated by troughs (*sulci*). Two thirds of the cortex lies in between the fissures of these folds. Unlike the situation in the other two brain areas that will be discussed, the organization of the neocortex is difficult to understand. To start with, the fibers that carry information to (afferent) and from (efferent) the cortex enter and emerge deep in the cortex and travel together, making it difficult to trace their connections with the usual methods.

The cerebrum consists of two large, symmetrically arranged lobes or hemispheres connected by a bridge of white matter, the corpus callosum. Each hemisphere contains a central mass of white matter, the medulla, and an overlying cortex consisting of cells arranged in layers. The cells located in the cortex are arranged parallel to the surface folds. Some areas contain as few as four distinct layers, others as many as eight clearly defined zones. To illustrate the complex circuitry of the cerebral cortex, a general description of primary sensory and motor cortices will be presented (Figs. 21-1 and 21-2).

The cortex developed by outward expansion, and the fibers that carry information into and out of it penetrate through the

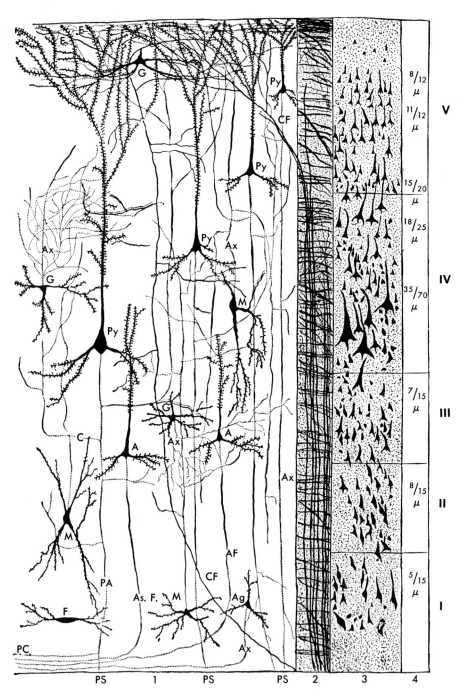

Fig. 21-1. Scheme of motor area of cerebral cortex showing effect of various staining methods. *1,* Golgi's stain; *2,* Weigert's stain; *3,* hematoxylin and eosin; *4,* relative depth of each layer. *A,* Association neurons; *Ag,* angular cells of polymorphous layer; *AF,* association fibers; *Ax,* axons; *C,* collateral; *CF,* centripetal fibers; *E,* terminal fibers; *F,* fusiform cell of polymorphous layer; *G,* Golgi cells, type II; *M,* cells of Martinotti; *PC,* collateral of pyramidal cell; *Py,* pyramidal cells; *PA,* axon of pyramidal cell; *PS,* pyramidal axons passing to cerebral medulla. Roman numerals refer to cortical layers. (After Berkley. From Jordan. Textbook of histology, D. Appleton-Century Co., Inc., Philadelphia.)

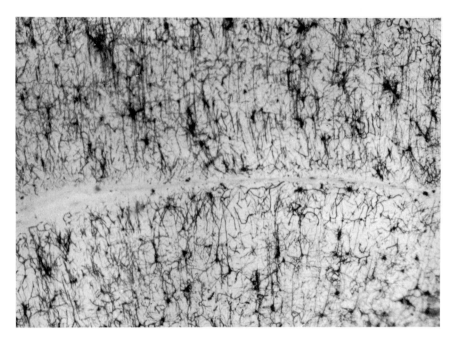

Fig. 21-2. Section of cerebral cortex showing arrangement and distribution of neurons. (Golgi method; ×140.)

depths. The input to the primary sensory cortex arrives by way of axons whose cell bodies are in the thalamus. The fibers are several micrometers in diameter and myelinated. As they enter the base of the cortex, they break into a dense arborization that extends 100 to 400 μm in both the vertical and horizontal planes about midway in the cortex (in the region referred to as area *IV*, Fig. 21-1). In addition to these connections, the cells of the cortex receive input from nonspecific thalamic nuclei, the brain stem, the basal ganglia, and the reticular activating system. In addition to all these connections, the cortical cells receive many contacts from nearby areas of cortex (short association fibers), distant cortical areas (long association fibers), and from the corresponding region in the opposite hemisphere (commissural fibers).

The outermost layer of the cortex is called the outer molecular layer (or layer I) and consists of a network of fine fibers composed chiefly of dendrites derived from cells that are located in the deep layers. These dendrites run parallel to the surface. Occasional polymorphous cells can be found in the dendritic meshes.

There are several cell layers deeper in the cortex. The output from the neocortex is relayed by way of pyramidal cells (Fig. 21-3), which form the principal neurons of the cortex. Pyramidal cells are distributed in two strata, called layers II and III and layer IV. The deepest pyramidal cells are the largest (attaining a size of 60 to 80 μm in motor cortex where they are referred to as Betz cells). The cell bodies of pyramidal cells are roughly triangular with characteristic axial and basal dendritic trunks. The smaller pyramidal cells of the superficial layers average 20 μm in width. The pyramidal cells are arranged so that their pointed apices are directed toward the surface. The cells usually have two sets of dendrites: (1) a single, long apical dendrite that ascends vertically through the cortex to branch and terminate in the outer molecular layer in a radius of 200 to 400 μm and (2) several basal dendrites that branch sparingly around the sides of the base of the cell body. These basal dendrites are distributed in the same plane as that in

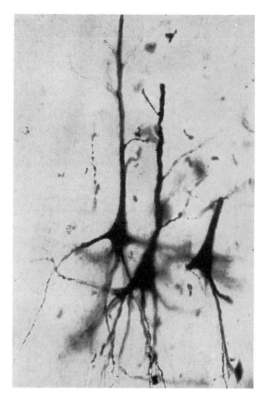

Fig. 21-3. Pyramidal cells from cerebral cortex. (Golgi method.)

cells are smaller than pyramidal cells (10 to 20 μm cell bodies) and are often called *granule cells*. They are not found in motor cortex. The granule cells are multipolar neurons that send a number of thick trunks in various directions to reach a radius of as much as 400 μm. The single thin axon is oriented vertically and rises to ramify in layer II around the pyramidal and stellate cells of that layer. Another stellate-type neuron is scattered throughout the middle and upper layers. These cells produce axon tufts that form a network around the pyramidal cell bodies, particularly in motor cortex. A third type of stellate cell is bipolar and links the most superficial and deep layers of the cortex. Other stellate cell layers can also be found with their processes oriented to link horizontal and vertical planes of the cortex.

Many maps of neocortex have been constructed on the basis of the distinctness of the cell and fiber layers and the details of cellular arrangements. The layers that make up the neocortex vary in different regions. The visual cortex is among the thinnest of the cortical areas, whereas the primary motor cortex is among the thickest due to the presence of deep pyramidal cells in layer V, the giant pyramidal cells of Betz (Fig. 21-4). The cell bodies of these neurons can be as large as 120 μm in diameter. The analyses of the structural differences between cortical areas is called cytoarchitectonics.

One brain circuit diagram that has been developed to describe the way that cortical cells are linked together is shown in Fig. 21-5. There is a basic triad of synaptic arrangements involving input fibers, principal neurons (which generate outflowing impulses to other cortical areas or to noncortical regions), and intrinsic neurons (which bind the inputs and outputs together). The relative proportions of these elements is different in sensory and motor areas. In the sensory cortex the inputs terminate mainly on the intrinsic neurons, which therefore act as an additional relay in the input pathways. This represents a final processing network within the cortex itself. Another channel for input is the nonspecific fibers that probably modulate

which the cell bodies are located. The axon of the pyramidal cells leaves the base of the cell body or large dendrite and, after giving off several short horizontal collateral branches and other long recurrent collaterals that turn back up into the cortex, plunges into white matter. The axons of the pyramidal cells have two main destinations. Some remain in the cortex and connect different parts of the cortex together. These are called *association fibers*. The other group of axons connect with regions outside the cortex and are called *projection fibers*.

In addition to the pyramidal cells there are many cells whose processes are confined to a local cortical region *(intrinsic regions)*. These cells take many forms but as a group are referred to as *stellate cells* (Golgi type II). In primary sensory cortex, intrinsic neurons are especially abundant in layer IV where they occur in a distribution corresponding roughly to the networks formed by the terminals of the afferent fibers. These

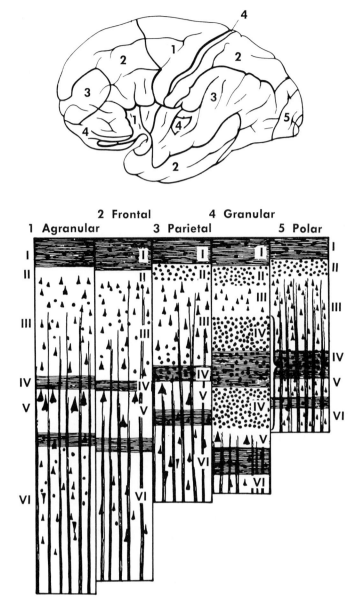

Fig. 21-4. Distribution of major types of cerebral cortex. (From Warwick, R., and P. L. Williams [eds.] 1973. Gray's anatomy, 35th [British] ed. W. B. Saunders Co., Philadelphia; Longman's Group, Ltd., Harlow, England.)

the activity of cortex through excitatory and inhibitory synapses that end on either principal or intrinsic neurons. These contacts predominate in motor and associative cortical areas. Although the basic structure of the cortex is organized in vertical columns, many cells span more than one stratum. These columns are linked together to varying degrees by axon collaterals and dendritic trees in the horizontal plane.

Cerebellum

The cerebellum is made up of two main lobes or hemispheres that are connected by a third lobe known as the vermis. Each lobe consists of several subdivisions, the lobules,

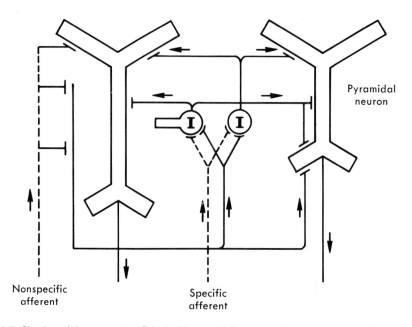

Fig. 21-5. Circuitry of the neocortex. Principal (pyramidal) neurons, intrinsic neurons, *I* (granule cells, basket cells, and bipolar cells), and inputs (specific and nonspecific afferents) make up a triad of synaptic elements. (After Shepard, G. M. 1974. The synaptic organization of the brain. University Press, New York.)

which are thrown into several transverse convolutions or folia. Like the cerebrum, the cerebellum consists of a central core of white matter, the medulla, and a thick external covering of gray matter, the cortex.

The cerebellum is a laminated region in which the brain internal structure is similar throughout and does not change appreciably in different vertebrate groups. The surface of the cerebellar cortex is thrown into folds that increase the total surface area, presumably in response to increasing demands for associative tissue involved in the maintenance of positive balance, the maintenance of muscle tone, and the coordination of rate, range, and direction of voluntary movements. Within these convolutions is a rigid geometry that is not found in other central brain regions.

The cerebellar cortex is comprised of an outer molecular layer and an inner granular layer. Between these two zones is a single layer of large conspicuous cells known as Purkinje cells (Figs. 21-6 and 21-7).

The molecular layer contains for the most part a dendritic arbor consisting of densely packed thin axons running parallel to the long axis of the folia and two types of neurons: (1) the large cortical or basket cells and (2) the small stellate cells.

1. The basket cells are relatively large multipolar cells with short, thick, branching dendrites and a long axon, which passes horizontally in the same plane as that occupied by the dendrites of the Purkinje cells. In its course it gives off five or six collaterals, which pass centrally to end in basketlike arborizations around the Purkinje cells. The basket cells are confined for the most part to the middle and outer part of the molecular layer. They are believed to be association neurons.

2. The small stellate cells are also multipolar neurons but are smaller than those just described; in addition they are more variable in size. They send out from two to five dendrites that are distributed mainly in the same plane as the Purkinje cells. A single, short, slender axon, which is horizontally placed, is

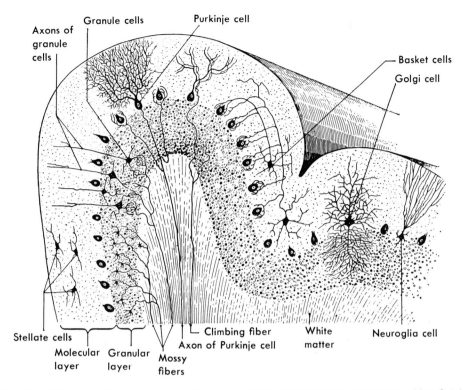

Fig. 21-6. Diagrammatic drawing of cell forms and fiber arrangement of cerebellum. (After Cajal. From Globus, R. Practical neuroanatomy. The Williams & Wilkins Co., Baltimore.)

characteristically looped and usually sends out several collaterals. These cells are distributed throughout the molecular layer; they are, however, most numerous in the outer half of this part of the cortex.

The Purkinje cells form a single layer of conspicuous neurons, which is interposed between the molecular and granular layers. These cells are histologically the most distinctive neurons that occur in the cerebellar cortex (Fig. 21-6). They are large, flask-shaped, multipolar cells that possess a thick dendrite directed toward the surface of the convolution (Fig. 21-7). Immediately on leaving the cell body, the dendrite divides into two thick branches each of which undergoes many successive dichotomous branchings. They appear at the surface as a dense profusion of fine fibrils. When viewed in its entirety, the dendrite appears fan shaped, and its characteristic expansions are placed at right angles to the long axis of the convolu-

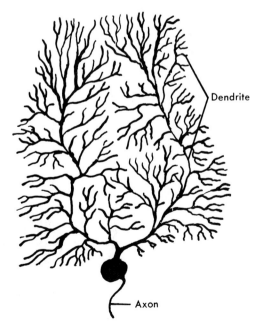

Fig. 21-7. Purkinje cell. (Redrawn from Bremer and Weatherford.)

tion. When these dendrites are examined in sections of the convolutions cut lengthwise, they are relatively much less extensive. The single axon arises from the deep surface of the cell and passes through the granular layer to the medulla. Before reaching the medulla, the axons send out several collaterals that turn back into the molecular layer and end in association with adjacent Purkinje cells.

The granular or nuclear layer contains three types of cells: (1) granule cells, (2) large stellate cells, and (3) solitary cells that are extremely small and fusiform in shape.

With routine stains the granular layer presents itself as a field of closely packed nuclei looking much like lymphocytes, with occasional clear spaces or "cerebellar islands" in which resides a complex synaptic tangle called a glomerulus. This structure involves the terminals and dendrites of granule cells and Golgi cells that make contact with incoming (mossy) fibers.

1. Granule cells are small multipolar nerve cells, which are distributed throughout the granular layer in great numbers. These cells have from two to four short dendrites, which pass toward the surface and terminate in peculiar clawlike processes that are in intimate association with small granular spheroidal masses known as eosin bodies. On reaching the surface, the axon divides into a T-shaped process, the fibers of which pass parallel to the long axis of the convolutions.

2. The large stellate cells are also multipolar neurons, with profuse dendritic processes that contribute to the molecular layer. The axons and collaterals of these cells are also profuse and contribute to the granular layer, where they end in association with the granule cells.

3. Solitary cells are scattered here and there in the cortex.

The cerebellar medulla contains three main types of fibers: (1) the axons of the Purkinje cells, which are the main efferent fibers from the cortex; (2) the climbing fibers, which are afferent and end in association with the Purkinje cells; and (3) mossy fibers, which are afferent fibers ending in mossy terminations with the granular layer.

Meninges

The brain and spinal cord are enclosed by connective tissue coverings known as the meninges. The meninges (Fig. 21-8) consist of three membranes: (1) the dura mater, (2) the arachnoid, and (3) the pia mater. In the spinal cord the dura is separated from the periosteum of the vertebrae by a space occupied by a loose fibrous and adipose tissue. This region is known as the epidural space.

1. The dura of the spinal cord is a single-layered structure made up of fibrous tissue containing a few elastic fibers. The fibers in this part of the dura are longitudinally disposed. The cranial dura consists of two layers: an outer vascular portion, serving as the periosteum, and an inner layer, the dura proper. The cranial dura forms reduplications, which extend between the cerebral hemispheres and between the hemispheres and the cerebellum. The two layers of the dura separate along the lines of attachment to form the venous dural sinuses, which receive blood from veins of the brain.

In the cord where the outer surface of the dura is not attached to the adjacent bone, the covering consists of a layer of thin mesenchymal epithelium, which serves as the lining of the epidural space. The inner surface is also lined with a layer of mesenchymal epithelium. This forms the outer wall of the subdural space.

2. The arachnoid is a loose netlike membrane that intervenes between the dura and the pia. The outer surface consists of a thin fibrous sheath, covered by a layer of epithelium. Numerous delicate strands of the membrane pass to the outer surface of the pia.

In the cranial part of the arachnoid, numerous fingerlike structures that project into the venous sinuses are to be found. They are known as the arachnoid villi.

3. The pia mater is a delicate, vascular, fibrous layer that is closely adherent to the brain and spinal cord. In the region of the roof of the third and fourth ventricles the vascular membranes that cover them are in some areas invaginated to form the choroid plexuses. Similar invaginations also occur in the lateral ventricles. The vessels of the

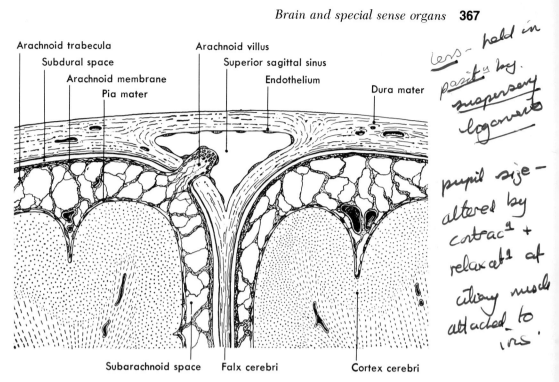

Fig. 21-8. Diagram of arachnoid and subdural spaces. (After Weed. From Bremer, F., and H. Weatherford. 1948. A text-book of histology. The Blakiston Co., New York.)

plexuses are enclosed in connective tissue, which, in turn, is covered by a granular cuboidal epithelium. The entire complex is known as the tela choroidea. The choroid plexuses are one of the main sources of cerebrospinal fluid.

EYE

On cutting the eye in a meridional horizontal plane, one may readily see the following features.

The eye is a hollow globular structure with a thick, fairly elastic wall, the inner lining of which appears darker than the remainder. It is divided into two unequal parts by a transversely placed structure, the iris. The portion between the iris and the cornea is the anterior chamber; the remainder is divided by the lens and its capsule into the small posterior chamber and the large vitreal space. (Fig. 21-9).

The curvature of the outer coat as it passes over the anterior chamber is sharper than that around the posterior part of the eye, so that the eyeball is not a perfect sphere. The coat is modified in structure also in its anterior portion, forming the transparent cornea. The anterior chamber contains a fluid, the aqueous humor.

The iris does not lie flat in the transverse plane. Its center is slightly anterior to its periphery so that it has the form of a low truncated cone. It is pierced at the center by the pupil, which is a round aperture whose dimension is variable due to a ring of muscle surrounding the opening. The posterior part of the eye contains the lens and the vitreous body or humor. The former is a smaller and more solid body lying just posterior to the iris; the latter is a jelly-like mass. The lens is suspended in this position by a group of fine fibers, the suspensory ligament. The fibers of the ligament are attached at one end to the lens capsule and at the other to the ciliary body. This is macroscopically visible as a thickening of tissue posterior to the periphery of the iris.

The optic nerve is seen as a stalk leaving the eye at a point slightly medial to the posterior pole. The thick covering of the eye ex-

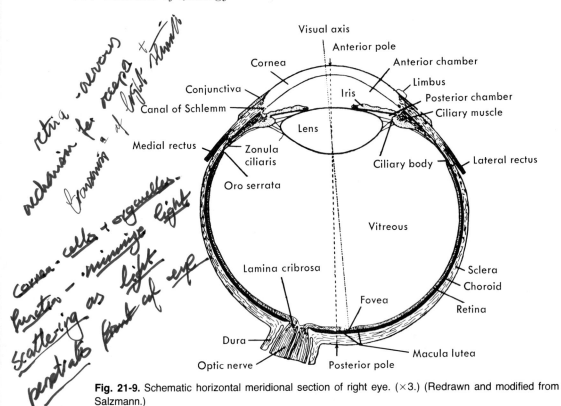

Fig. 21-9. Schematic horizontal meridional section of right eye. (×3.) (Redrawn and modified from Salzmann.)

[Handwritten margin notes: retina - nervous mechanism for receive + transmission of light stimuli; Cornea - cells + organelles - function - minimize light scattering as light penetrates front of eye; protective; nutritious; sensitive]

tends over this stalk, and in a complete dissection of the eye, the optic nerve, and the brain, one would find that the sheath of the eye extends to and is continuous with the dura mater of the brain.

Coats of the eye

On microscopic examination it is apparent that the coating of the eye has three parts as follows.

1. The fibrous coat includes the sclera covering the vitreal cavity and and the transparent cornea of the anterior chamber.

2. The vascular layer or choroid extends around the posterior chamber inside the sclera and turns inward to form the iris. The choroid in turn forms the ciliary body.

3. The retina lines the vitreal cavity. A part of the retina extends over the ciliary body and the posterior surface of the iris.

Fibrous coat. The fibrous coat consists of the sclera and the cornea.

Sclera. The sclera surrounds the vitreal cavity and extends a short distance anterior to the margin of the iris. It consists mainly of closely packed fibers and fibroblasts. At its inner margin is a layer of looser connective tissue containing pigment cells (*lamina fusca*). Elastic fibers are abundant in the sclera, especially at the points of insertion of the muscles that move the eye. At the exit of the optic nerve the sclera forms a fenestrated membrane, the *lamina cribrosa*.

Cornea. The corneal portion also consists mainly of fibers arranged in flat lamellae parallel to the surface. It has, in addition, two epithelial layers. The outer one is a thin stratified squamous epithelium (from four to six layers of cells), which rests on a relatively thick basement membrane called the anterior basal membrane (of Bowman) (Fig. 21-10). The cells and their organelles are modified to minimize light scattering as light penetrates the front of the eye. The posterior sur-

Choroid – outer – elb – jes verine
– inter – largest arteries +veins
– inner – plenu of capillaries.

Ins – cortex
amount of light →
retina

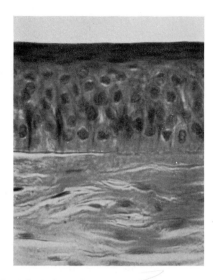

Fig. 21-10. Cornea showing stratified epithelium.

face of the cornea is covered with a mesenchymal epithelium, which consists of one layer of flattened cells and rests on an exceptionally transparent membrane called the posterior basal or Descemet's membrane.

Vascular layer. The vascular layer corresponds to the pia mater of the brain and is fundamentally a layer of loose connective tissue containing blood vessels. The part surrounding the posterior chamber is called the choroid. The anterior part forms two structures, the ciliary body and the iris.

Choroid coat. Blood vessels and connective tissue are not evenly distributed throughout the choroid. Nearest to the sclera is a layer of connective tissue with few, if any, blood vessels. The next layer contains the largest arteries and veins; the innermost layer, a plexus of capillaries. The choroid is bounded on the inside (next to the retina) by the hyaline membrane of Bruch, part of which is said to be a cuticular formation of the cells of the retina.

Ciliary body. The ciliary body is a thickening of the vascular layer to which the suspensory ligament of the lens is attached. It contains all the elements of the choroid coat except the capillary layer. In addition, it contains smooth muscle fibers, the contraction of which alters the shape of the lens. The

muscles form three groups: meridional, radial, and circular. The ciliary body is covered by a forward extension of the retina, and fibers extend from it to the capsule of the lens. These two elements will be discussed with the retina and the lens, respectively.

Iris. Anterior to the ciliary body the vascular layer forms the iris, which acts as a diaphragm to control the amount of light falling on the retina. The anterior surface of the iris is covered by flattened mesenchymal epithelium similar to the innermost layer of the cornea. The epithelium is interrupted by irregular crypts, which extend into the underlying stroma. The connective tissue of the anterior part of the stroma is a loose network of stellate cells and fine fibers. Some of the stellate cells are pigmented. Fibers are more numerous in the posterior layers of the stroma, and the cells may or may not contain pigment. In this part there are a few elastic fibers, radially arranged, and two groups of muscle fibers. One group of muscle forms the dilator, the other the sphincter, by which the size of the pupil is altered. A part of the retinal layer extends over the posterior surface of the iris.

Retina. The structures described thus far are concerned with the protection of the retina or with focusing light on it. The retina is the nervous mechanism for the reception and transmission of light stimuli.

→ telencephalon

The retina arises embryologically as a vesicular outgrowth from the forebrain. As development proceeds, the distal surface of the optic vesicle is invaginated, resulting in a two-layered, cup-shaped structure. The outer layer forms the pigmented epithelium; the invaginated portion gives rise to the remaining layers of the retina, which are, in most of its extent, ten in number.

Three main regions of the retina may be distinguished histologically and topographically: (1) the *pars optica*, lining most of the vitreal space; (2) the *pars cilaris*, covering the ciliary body; and (3) the *pars iridica*, covering the posterior surface of the iris.

Pars optica (Figs. 21-11 and 21-12). In the pars otpica, the largest part of the retina, ten

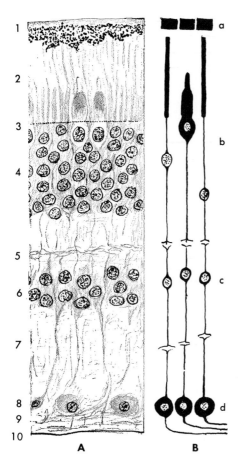

Fig. 21-11. Human retina: **A,** section of retina; **B,** isolated cells, diagrammatically presented. Numbers to left of illustration and letters to right correspond to numbers and letters in outline below.

layers have been distinguished and named as follows:

1. Pigmented epithelium   a
2. Rods and cones
3. External limiting membrane
4. Outer nuclear (granular) layer   b
5. Outer plexiform (molecular) layer
6. Inner nuclear (granular) layer
7. Inner plexiform (molecular) layer   c
8. Ganglion cell layer
9. Nerve fiber layer   d
10. Internal limiting membrane

(handwritten annotations: "receptor terminals →5." "output from retina →8." "bipolar")

The retina is, however, more easily understood when considered to be composed of a layer of pigmented epithelium and three layers of neurons with intervening strata occupied by cell processes and intrinsic cells

(Fig. 21-13). The retina is a thin sheet of nervous tissue at the posterior part of the eye, which serves as the receptor site for visual stimuli and the initial stages of processing information in the visual pathway. The entire structure of the eye is designed to collect and focus light on the retina with a minimum of light scattering.

The retina spans a depth of less than 300 μm. The nerve cells are small and are connected primarily in a vertical dimension. The main elements that form the receptive and conductive apparatus are shown in Fig. 21-11, *B*.

There are two types of receptor cells, the rods and cones, which form a sheet called the outer nuclear layer. These cells face away from the incoming light, which must pass through the outer layers of the retina to reach the receptors. The base of the retina is formed by a pigmented epithelium consisting of a single layer of cuboidal cells containing melanin in the form of rod-shaped granules. The cells send processes among the underlying rods and cones and are involved in the continual regeneration and repair of the receptor cells. In some lower vertebrates, variations in the extent of these processes and in the position of the enclosed pigment can be observed and correlated with differences in the amount of light falling on the retina, but such morphologic variations have not been established as occurring in the mammalian eye.

The rods and cones consist of a light-sensitive outer segment separated from an inner segment and containing the nucleus and the metabolic machinery of the cell. The outer segment (Fig. 21-13) is composed of a stack of flattened disks of membrane in which are inbedded the photoreceptive pigments in an orderly arrangement. The inner segment is composed of two parts. The portion nearest the outer segment is filled with mitochondria and protein synthetic machinery (polyribosomes, a Golgi apparatus, and some reticular membranes both rough and smooth). The other portion contains the nucleus and flattens into a large presynaptic region that terminates on the bipolar neurons (Fig. 21-13).

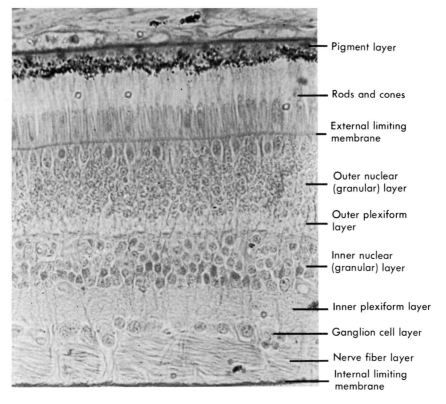

Pigment layer

Rods and cones

External limiting membrane

Outer nuclear (granular) layer

Outer plexiform layer

Inner nuclear (granular) layer

Inner plexiform layer

Ganglion cell layer

Nerve fiber layer

Internal limiting membrane

Fig. 21-12. Photomicrograph of section of human retina. (×400.)

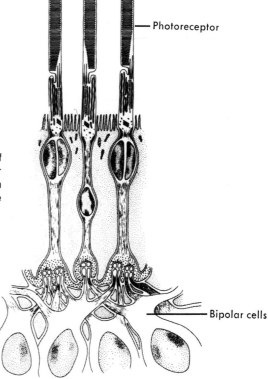

Photoreceptor

Bipolar cells

Fig. 21-13. Schematic representation of ultrastructure of retinal photoreceptors and of their connections with bipolar nerve cells. Note stacked disks in outer segments. (From Sjostrand, F. S. *In* G. K. Smelser [ed.] 1961. The structure of the eye. Academic Press, Inc., New York.)

The plates of light-sensitive pigment are replaced or repaired throughout the life of the rods and cones. In rods whole membrane disks are sloughed off at the apex of the cell and renewed from beneath. The fragments of discarded disks, are absorbed by the epithelial cells and the pigmented epithelium whose cytoplasmic processes reach down around the rods and cones. Cone disks are not replaced but are repaired by a turnover of the important components of the disks. It has been estimated that a new disk is made about once each hour from protein synthesized in the region of the inner segment just below the outer segment.

The receptors generate the input to the neuronal systems of the retina. The input is sent through a cellular process that connects the receptor site in the outer segment of the cell body to the synaptic terminals. In rods this process is short and vertically oriented (Fig. 21-13), but in the fovea the neuronal elements are displaced to one side and the connecting processes of the cones must run up to 0.5 mm to reach them. Although the process is called an axon, its fine structure is not characteristic of either axons or dendrites.

The receptor terminals are located in the outer plexiform layer. Cone endings are layers of flattened elements called *pedicles*, whereas rods form smaller round *spherules*.

The output of the retina to the brain is generated by ganglion cells. These principal neurons lie in a sheet at the inner margins of the retina. They vary in size from minute ganglion cells (12 to 15 μm in diameter) found near the fovea in the human eye to large ganglion cells whose cell bodies measure up to 3 μm. The axons of the ganglion cells pass along the inner surface of the retina and emerge to form the optic nerve. As they do so, they fail to give off recurrent collaterals, unlike most principal cells in other brain areas.

Interposed between the receptor cells and the ganglion cells are bipolar cells. The cells that connect to cone pedicles are small (8 to 10 μm in diameter) and give rise to a single trunk process that terminates in an enlargement some 5 μm across, a size that matches the cone pedicles. The other single deep process ends in several knoblike terminals in the inner plexiform layer. Bipolar cells that relay information from rods have a small cell body and a number of terminals in the outer plexiform layer. The single deep process arborizes only sparingly in the inner plexiform layer. As a rule, cone bipolar cells contact only a few cones and produce an almost 5:1 transmission to ganglion cells. There are estimated to be about 5 million cone receptors tunneling into 1 milllion ganglion cells. This arrangement is presumably responsible for the high sensitivity associated with cone systems. In the fovea where vision is most acute, the ratio of cones to ganglion cells may be less than 1:1. In contrast, rods converge in large numbers onto the bipolar cells and ganglion cells in a ratio averaging 100:1.

There are two other types of intrinsic neurons in the mammalian retina. One type is the horizontal cell, which provides a horizontal linkage between the bipolar neurons at the outer plexiform layer. The horizontal cells are related to the processing of the receptor input to the bipolar cells. These cells have cell bodies 10 to 15 μm in diameter from which ten to fifteen trunks emerge. In the central regions of the retina the horizontal cells cover a restricted field (25 μm diameter), but in the periphery the field is larger (over 100 μm). A horizontal cell may synapse with bipolar cells, other horizontal cells, and the rod and cone receptor terminals.

Another group of horizontally arranged cells influence transmission between the bipolar cells and the ganglion cells in the inner plexiform layer. These are the *amacrine* cells whose cell bodies lie in the inner nuclear layer. Some of these cells have narrow dendritic fields (less than 75 μm); others have wider fields covering 100 μm or more. The synaptic connections of the retina thus consist of a vertical flow of information from the receptors through the bipolar neurons to the ganglion cells and two tiers of horizontally arranged cells that can influence transmission in the vertical cells.

The foregoing account of retinal connections is based on electron microscopy and special preparations. Ordinary sections show a differentiation into the ten layers mentioned earlier (Fig. 21-12), but the forms and connections of many of the cells are difficult to see at the level of the light microscope.

The structure of the retina is modified in two regions, the *optic disk* and the *macula lutea* (Fig. 21-9). The optic disk is the site where the axons of ganglion cells meet and turn at right angles to their previous course to leave the eye and form the optic nerve. In the optic disk the outer layers of the retina are interrupted, and the area does not contain receptors (*blind spot*).

The macula lutea is an area near the posterior pole of the eye that appears yellow in the fresh specimen and has the shape of a shallow funnel or depression. The cells and fibers of the inner layers diverge from the outer part of this region so that the photoreceptors in the center of the shallow depression, called the fovea centralis, are not covered by as thick a sheet of neurons and cell processes. Furthermore, there are no blood vessels in the fovea. At the fovea the retina consists of a layer of small, closely packed cone cells and a few small scattered ganglion cells. This region is therefore specialized for high visual acuity. Nerve fibers leaving this area are arranged in a more orderly fashion than are the retinal fibers emerging from the peripheral retina and are less likely to be affected if the optic disk area becomes swollen.

Pars ciliaris. The pars optica of the retina ends at a point slightly posterior to the ciliary body in a thick irregular margin called the ora serrata. As it approaches this point, the retina undergoes a gradual loss of visual elements, and beyond the margin these disappear entirely. The pars ciliaris of the retina consists of two layers: the pigmented epithelium continues unchanged, and beneath it lies a layer of sustentacular cells arranged in the form of a columnar epithelium. The sustentacular cells produce fibers, some of which are gathered in a hyaline membrane bordering the cavity of the posterior cham-

ber. Other fibers enter into the formation of the ligament of the lens.

Pars iridica. The pigmented epithelium is the only part of the retina that continues beyond the ciliary body to cover the posterior surface of the iris (pars iridica). It becomes somewhat thicker in this region, and the amount of pigment contained in the cells is so great that nuclei and cell boundaries are obscured.

Contents of the eye

The fluids of the eye are extremely important, since they represent the medium through which light must pass to reach the retina. This fluid is continuously formed and circulated through the eye. Disorders of this process can cause a buildup of pressure in the eye (*glaucoma*).

The inner fluid of the eye consists of the *aqueous humor* in the anterior portion and the *vitreous body* in the posterior part of the globe. The lens is suspended within the aqueous humor by the ciliary zonules.

Aqueous humor. The region of the aqueous humor in the anterior part of the eye in front of the iris is the *anterior chamber* and the region behind the iris is the *posterior chamber*. These two areas are in communication through the pupil (Fig. 21-14). Aqueous humor is similar in chemical composition and physical properties to a protein-free plasma. The exact mechanisms by which it is formed are unknown, but secretion, dialysis, and ultrafiltration seem to be involved. In part, at least, components of the aqueous humor are secreted into the posterior chambers by the pigmented epithelium of the ciliary processes. After the aqueous humor is formed in the posterior chamber, it flows through the pupil into the anterior chamber, then diffuses through the trabecular meshwork and the angle of the iris and through the wall of Schlemm's canal (a collecting channel located in the sclera at the junction of the sclera and cornea). From Schlemm's canal the aqueous drains chiefly into the veins deep in the sclera. Usually the production of aqueous humor is balanced by outflow to maintain a pressure in the eye of 12

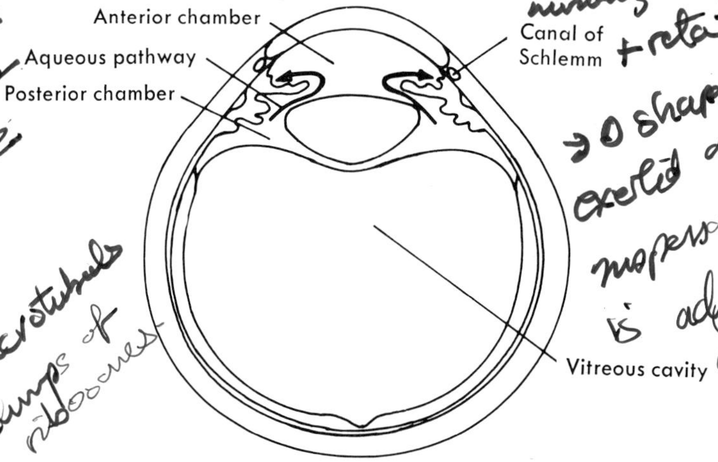

[Handwritten margin notes:]

lens - specialised to minimize light scattering + retain elasticity

→ Δ shape as tension on it by exerted on it by suspensory ligaments is adjusted by contraction of ciliary body

Δ shape needed by lens to focus light → retina at different focal lengths → "accommod."

mature lens - few microtubules + few clumps of ribosomes

Anterior chamber
Aqueous pathway
Posterior chamber
Canal of Schlemm
Vitreous cavity

Fig. 21-14. Anterior and posterior chambers of eye. (Courtesy Dr. M. D. Mann.)

to 21 mm Hg. Pressure build up usually results from blockage to outflow rather than disorders in the rate of production. Normally, aqueous humor is produced slowly at a rate of about 2 ml/min.

Vitreous body or vitreous humor. The vitreous body is a mass of jellylike transparent connective tissue consisting of a specialized collagen called *vitrosin* and glycosoaminoglycans that resembles the mucous connective tissue of the umbilical cord. The cells responsible for its production appear to be hyalocytes (vitreous cells) within the vitreous cavity. During expansion of the eye in early development the vitreous components may be made by the fetal retina and the anterior corneal epithelium. Its mass serves to hold the lens in place in front and prevent separation of the retina from its outer pigmented coat behind. The vitreous consists of fine fibers and fibroblasts in a semisolid matrix. At the edges it is denser and adheres to the internal limiting membrane of the retina, especially at the exit of the optic nerve.

Lens. The lens (Fig. 21-15) is an ectodermal structure that was originally cut off as a hollow vesicle from the epithelium. The space within the lens vesicle fills, as development proceeds, by the proliferation of epithelial cells on its posterior surface. The lens is specialized to minimize light scattering

and to retain elasticity so that it can change shape as the tension exerted on it by the suspensory ligaments is adjusted by contraction of the ciliary body. These changes in shape are necessary to focus light on the retina for objects at various distances from the eye; the process itself is called *accommodation.* The transparency of the lens is provided for by the fact that the epithelial cells which form it undergo elongation to a fibrous shape (lens fibers) and in this process lose most of their organelles and nucleus. All that is retained in a mature lens fiber are a few microtubules and clumps of free ribosomes. The remainder of the cell is filled with specific lens protein, the crystallins. The cells are not entirely inert and may persist for a lifetime. The anterior surface of the lens is covered by a cuboidal epithelium, which at the equator of the lens continues to proliferate and provides for the addition of new cells to the outside of the lens. The lens is enclosed in a capsule, which is a specialized basement membrane elaborated by the epithelial cells covering the lens. The lens capsule is always under tension, and the cells that form it are highly interdigitated. The fibers of the suspensory ligament attach at this site.

As the lens ages, the cells gradually become dehydrated, and it loses elasticity and becomes denser. As a result of aging, a loss

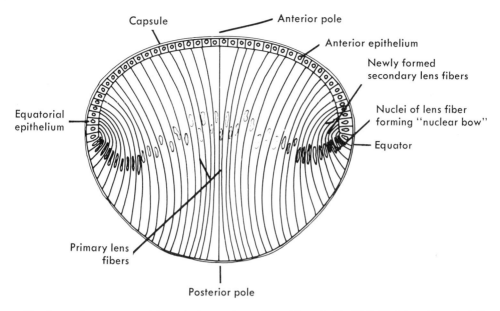

Fig. 21-15. Arrangement of fibers in human lens. (From Ham, A. W. 1974. Histology. 7th ed. J. B. Lippincott Co., Philadelphia.)

of accommodation occurs, resulting in a condition known as *presbyopia.*

Optic nerve or stalk. The optic nerve is enclosed in extensions of the pia mater and dura mater of the brain, which join the fibrous coat of the eye. The optic nerve consists of the axons of the cells of the ganglionic layer of the retina. These fibers have neither myelin nor neurilemma as long as they remain in the retina. At the optic disk they turn and leave the eyeball and at this point they acquire a myelin sheath but not a neurilemma. The optic nerve is, in fact, an extention of the substance of the central nervous system rather than a true sensory nerve, and it is more proper to call it the optic stalk.

Circulation and innervation of the eye

The retina and the optic nerve are supplied by the central artery, which passes in the optic stalk. The remainder of the eye receives blood from the opthalamic artery, which forms three ciliary vessels, supplying the choroid, sclera, iris, and ciliary bodies. Motor nerves form a plexus in the region of the ciliary body, from which are innervated the smooth muscles of the ciliary body and the iris.

EAR

The ear develops embryologically from three sources and retains throughout life a division into three parts: external ear, middle ear, and inner ear. The last-named part develops early in the course of embryonic life as a vesicle that is detached from the ectodermal covering of the head region and lies in the mesenchyme between the surface and the wall of the developing hindbrain. In this situation it becomes surrounded by bony tissue as the latter develops from the mesenchyme of the region. The middle ear develops from a diverticulum of the pharynx (first pharyngeal pouch), its ossicles being formed in the surrounding mesenchyme. The external ear is a secondary ingrowth of ectoderm from the surface, plus a projection on the surface that forms the pinna.

External ear

The pinna is an irregularly shaped flap of elastic cartilage covered by skin (Fig. 21-16), which is set on the side of the head around the opening of the external auditory meatus. The latter is a tubular channel leading to the eardrum or tympanic membrane. Its outer part is surrounded by elastic cartilage con-

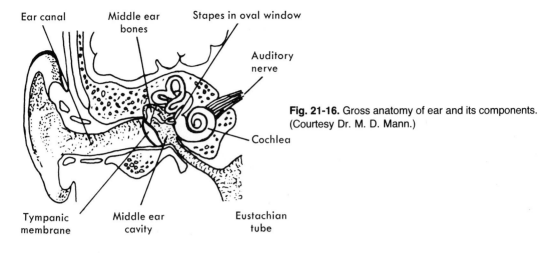

Ear canal · Middle ear bones · Stapes in oval window · Auditory nerve · Cochlea · Tympanic membrane · Middle ear cavity · Eustachian tube

Fig. 21-16. Gross anatomy of ear and its components. (Courtesy Dr. M. D. Mann.)

tinuous with that of the pinna. Its inner portion penetrates the outer layers of the temporal bone. The meatus is lined with skin that contains sebaceous and ceruminous (wax-forming) glands. Stiff hairs are present at the junction of the cartilaginous and bony parts.

Middle ear

The middle ear is a cavity in the substance of the temporal bone completely separated from the external ear by the tympanic membrane. It is in communication with the pharynx by way of the eustachian tube and separated from the inner ear by a plate of bone containing two apertures, the oval window and the round window. The former is closed by the end of one of the ossicles, the latter by a membrane, so that there is no communication between middle and inner ear. The cavity of the middle ear is crossed by a chain of three small bones, the ossicles.

The tympanic membrane is a fibrous membrane held in a groove of the temporal bone by a ring of fibrocartilage. It is covered on the outside by skin like that lining the meatus and on the inside by a layer of flattened epithelium.

The ossicles are called the malleus (hammer), the incus (anvil), and the stapes (stirrup), the names being descriptive of their respective forms. The handle of the hammer is firmly attached to the inner surface of the tympanic membrane, and its head rests on the anvil. The anvil is articulated also with

the upper end of the stirrup, and the foot of the latter is inserted into the oval window. It is by means of this chain of bones that the vibrations of the tympanic membrane are transmitted across the cavity of the middle ear to the vestibule of the inner ear.

The cavity of the middle ear is lined with flattened epithelium, which rests on the periosteum of the surrounding bone. Epithelium also covers the periosteum of the ossicles.

Inner ear

Osseous labyrinth. The cavity of the inner ear forms a series of irregular spaces in the temporal bone, the whole system being known as the osseous labyrinth. The labyrinth is bordered by a layer of compact bone, which may be separated by careful dissection from the spongy bone with which it blends. The bone is covered by periosteum, and the cavity is lined throughout by flattened epithelial tissue. It contains, besides the membranous labyrinth, a fluid called the perilymph. The labyrinth consists of a vestibular portion, semicircular canals, and a cone-shaped cochlear part. It has, in addition, a narrow outlet to the subarachnoid space, the vestibular aqueduct.

Vestibule and semicircular canals. The osseous vestibule is an irregularly rounded cavity from which the semicircular canals, the cavity of the cochlea, and the vestibular aqueduct diverge.

The semicircular canals are three in number. Two of these (the superior and posterior) are set vertically and at right angles to each other. The third canal (lateral) lies in a horizontal plane. Each is a horseshoe-shaped channel in the temporal bone, connecting at both ends with the cavity of the vestibule. One limb of each is enlarged near its connection with the vestibule to form the ampulla. The opposite ends of the superior and posterior canals join and re-enter the vestibule through a common opening; the lateral canal returns to it separately so that there are five openings from the vestibule to the system of semicircular canals.

Cochlea. The canal of the cochlea pursues a spiral course from the vestibule to the apex of a flattened cone. It surrounds a central mass of spongy bone, the modiolus, which contains the spiral ganglion. A shelf of bone projects into the canal from the modiolus, following the course of the former to its apex. This is called the osseous spiral lamina.

Membranous labyrinth. The membranous labyrinth, which lies within the osseous labyrinth, is separated from it by the perilymph and is divided functionally into two parts: the portion lying in the vestibule and the semicircular canals mediates the sense of equilibrium, and that in the cochlea is the organ of hearing. Fundamentally the structure of the membranous labyrinth is that of a closed system consisting of a sheath of connective tissue lined with flattened epithelium and containing a fluid, the endolymph. The epithelium is modified in various parts of the system to form receptors for the stimuli involved.

Utricle and saccule. The utricle and saccule are rounded sacs that lie in the perilymph of the vestibule and are held in place by trabeculae of connective tissue extending from the periosteum of the surrounding bone. They are united by a narrow duct, which has the form of an inverted V. From the apex of this duct the endolymphatic duct leads away through the vestibular sac. Another fine duct joins the saccule with the cochlear duct.

Semicircular canals. The semicircular ducts arise from the utricle. They lie within

the osseous semicircular canals, and each is attached along part of its periphery to the periosteum of the bone and is further anchored by connective tissue trabeculae.

The epithelial lining of the vestibular portion of the labyrinth contains patches of neuroepithelium. One of these is in the utricle, another in the saccule, and one in each ampulla of the semicircular ducts. The neuroepithelium contains hair cells (Fig. 21-17) and tall sustentacular cells.

Cochlear duct. One border of the membranous part of the cochlea is attached to the bony shelf of the modiolus, the lamina spiralis. The opposite border forms a wider attachment to the outer edge of the canal, thus dividing the latter into two parts, which are in communication at the apex of the spiral but not elsewhere. The upper part of the osseous canal leads from the vestibule and is known as the scala vestibuli. The lower part ends at the membrane close to the round window (secondary tympanic membrane) and is called the scala tympani. The intervening space, enclosed by the cochlear duct, is the scala media (Figs. 21-18 and 21-19). The scala vestibuli and the scala tympani are lined, as are other parts of the osseous labyrinth, by flattened epithelium resting on the periosteum of the surrounding bone. The epithelium extends, also, over the outer surfaces of the cochlear duct, where the latter is not in contact with the modiolus on the one hand or the outer wall of the osseous labyrinth on the other.

The scala media is separated from the scala vestibuli by a thin membrane, the vestibular membrane, which extends from the modiolus to the outer wall of the cochlear canal. Along this part of the wall the periosteum is thickened, forming a ligament, the lower edge of which projects toward the bony spiral lamina of the modiolus. The gap between the ligament (spiral ligament) and the lamina is closed by the basal membrane. The scala media is therefore separated from the scala tympani by three structures: the spiral ligament, the basal membrane, and the osseous spiral lamina. Between the latter and the vestibular membrane a thickening of connec-

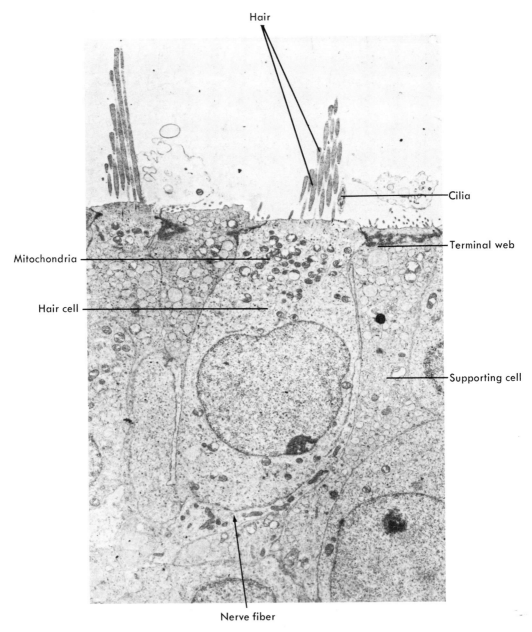

Hair

Cilia

Terminal web

Mitochondria

Hair cell

Supporting cell

Nerve fiber

Fig. 21-17. Electron micrograph of portion of sensory epithelium occurring in the macula of the saccule of mouse. (×5,000.) (Courtesy Dr. H. Nakahara.)

tive tissue called the limbus spiralis projects outward from the modiolus into the space of the scala media. The vestibular membrane is attached to the upper surface of the limbus. Its lower surface is concave, forming, with the spiral lamina, a groove known as the spiral sulcus. The space enclosed by the structures just enumerated has, in section, the form of a right-angled triangle of which the vestibular membrane forms the hypotenuse.

Histologically the different portions of the cochlear duct present striking variations from the structure of the remainder of the mem-

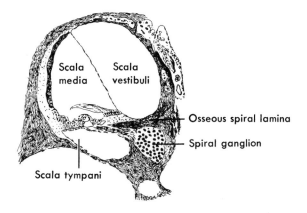

Fig. 21-18. Radial section through basal turn of cochlea.

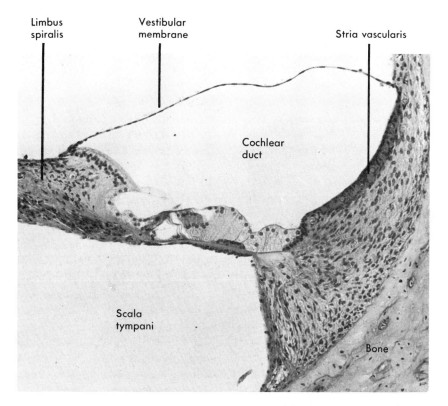

Fig. 21-19. Photomicrograph of organ of Corti. (×100.)

branous labyrinth (Figs. 21-19 and 21-20). The vestibular membrane consists of a very thin layer of connective tissue. It is covered on the outside by an extension of the mesothelium lining the remainder of the vestibule; its inner surface is also lined with flattened epithelium of ectodermal origin.

The epithelial lining of the scala media continues unchanged around the outer edge of the triangle where the duct is in contact with the border of the osseous canal. The connective tissue of this portion is much thickened, forming a relatively wide band between the epithelium and the bone. A

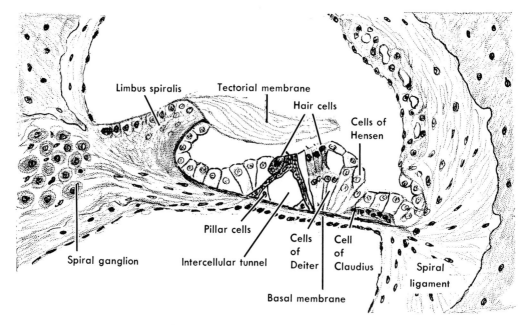

Fig. 21-20. Organ of Corti of guinea pig.

part of this layer is extremely vascular, and its lower portion is extended toward the modiolus as the spiral ligament. At the angle between the base and the outer side of the scala media, the lining epithelium changes from flattened to cuboidal or low columnar cells.

The basal membrane running from the tip of the spiral ligament to the tip of the osseous lamina is a connective tissue membrane considerably thicker than that forming the vestibular membrane. Like the latter, it has an outer covering of mesothelium that is, in this case, part of the lining of the scala tympani. The epithelium on the side toward the scala media, which is the ectodermal lining of the cochlear duct, is modified for the reception of sound waves and forms the organ of Corti. Starting at the outer edge and tracing the organ toward the modiolus, we may distinguish the following parts:

1. The cells of Claudius, which are small cuboidal cells with dark, granular cytoplasm, lie along the membrana basilaris between the latter and the cells of Hensen in that region.

2. The cells of Hensen lie next to those of Claudius, are columnar, and increase in height as they continue toward the modiolus.

3. Outer hair cells and sustentacular cells (of Deiter), as their name implies, are provided with hairlike projections from their surfaces and are the actual receptors of the organ (Fig. 21-21). They form a band three or four cells wide at the surface of the epithelium but do not reach to the basement membrane. Deiter's cells rest on the basement membrane and have narrow distal ends extending to the surface between the hair cells. They have stiff cuticular borders that give a firm support to the hair cells.

4. Two rows of pillar cells run through the length of the organ of Corti. They are tall columnar cells in which the cuticular substance forms a stiff rod. One row of these rods is inclined toward the modiolus, the other away from it so that although their distal ends meet, there is a considerable space between their bases. They thus enclose two sides of a tunnel, which is triangular in cross section, the base of the triangle being formed by the membrana basilaris of the scala media. The enclosed space is called the inner tunnel. It is crossed by naked dendrites of the cells of the spiral ganglion.

5. One row of inner hair cells lies next to

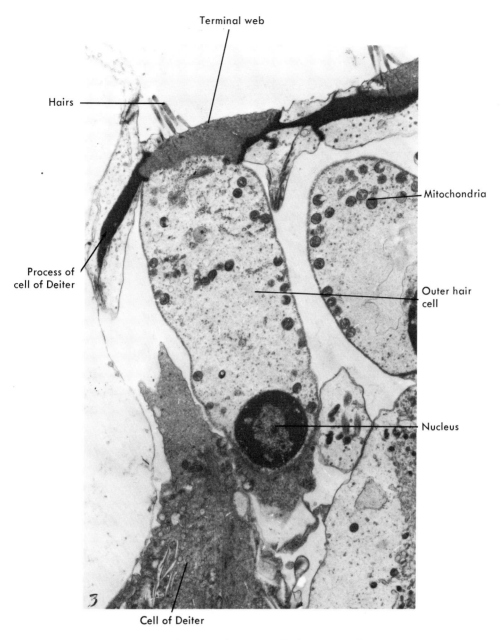

Terminal web

Hairs

Mitochondria

Process of
cell of Deiter

Outer hair
cell

Nucleus

Cell of Deiter

Fig. 21-21. Electron micrograph of portion of sensory cells from organ of Corti. (×6,000.) (Courtesy Dr. H. Nakahara.)

the inner pillar cells. These cells are usually of the low columnar type and do not reach the basement membrane. They are supported by tall columnar cells much like the cells of Hensen in appearance.

6. The spiral sulcus is lined with cuboidal epithelium. There is, however, no sharp line of demarcation between the border cells and those lining the spiral sulcus.

At the inner angle of the scala media are the osseous spiral lamina and the spiral limbus, which partially enclose the internal spiral sulcus. The periosteum of the osseous lamina extends outward from the bony shelf to meet the basal membrane. The spiral limbus is composed of connective tissue and projects into the space enclosed by the scala media. Its apical convex surface is covered by columnar cells that have a thick cuticular border. Its lower surface is covered by cuboidal cells. From the border between these two surfaces projects the tectorial membrane, which extends into the scala media and rests on the portion of the organ of Corti that contains the hair cells (Fig. 21-21). The tectorial membrane is a noncellular structure composed of fine fibers in an adhesive matrix. It is believed to be attached, in life, to the organ of Corti, although the two are almost always separated in fixed preparations.

The spiral ganglion, situated in the osseous lamina, is composed of bipolar nerve cells. The dendrites of these cells pass toward the organ of Corti, forming a conspicuous band of myelinated fibers in the lamina. As they leave the latter, they lose their myelin sheaths. Some of them cross the inner tunnel, others pass below it, and both groups end in arborizations among the hair cells. The axons of the cells of the spiral ganglion carry impulses to the appropriate region of the brain (Fig. 21-20).

Sound waves are transmitted to the organ of Corti as a result of movements of the tympanic membrane. Such vibrations are transmitted to the perilymph of the vestibule by the movement of the ossicles of the middle ear. The movement of the perilymph causes movement of the basal membrane of the organ of Corti, and the consequent alteration of position of the hair cells in relation to the tectorial membrane generates the

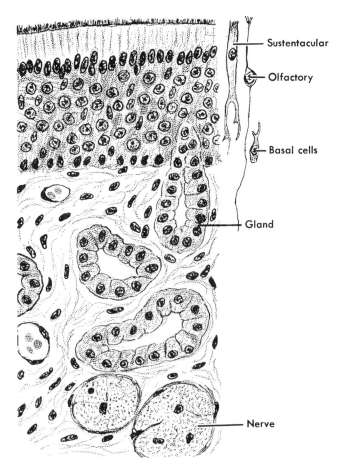

Sustentacular

Olfactory

Basal cells

Gland

Nerve

Fig. 21-22. Olfactory mucosa of rabbit. (After Jordan.)

stimulus that is transmitted to the brain as sound.

OLFACTORY ORGAN

The receptors for olfactory stimuli or sensations of smell are located in the nose. This organ also functions as a part of the respiratory system, since air passes through it into the trachea by way of the nasopharynx. The nose consists of two passageways separated by the nasal septum. Each passage may be divided into a vestibule lined with skin and a nasal cavity that opens into the nasopharynx through an aperture known as the choana. The outline of the nasal cavity is irregular, its lateral margin having three longitudinal elevations of the surrounding tissue. These are the conchae or the turbinate bones. The lining of the cavity is, for the most part, columnar or pseudostratified epithelium but may contain some patches of stratified squamous epithelium.

The olfactory part of the nose is an area of neuroepithelium extending from the superior concha across the roof of the nasal cavity and part way down the septum. The epithelium in this region appears as stratified columnar and contains sustentacular cells, olfactory cells, and basal cells (Figs. 21-22 and 21-23).

Sustentacular cells

Sustentacular cells are tall columnar cells that form the superficial layer. Their basal portions are extended in irregular branching processes among the olfactory and basal cells. Their apical ends contain pigment granules, are ciliated, and have a distinct cuticular bor-

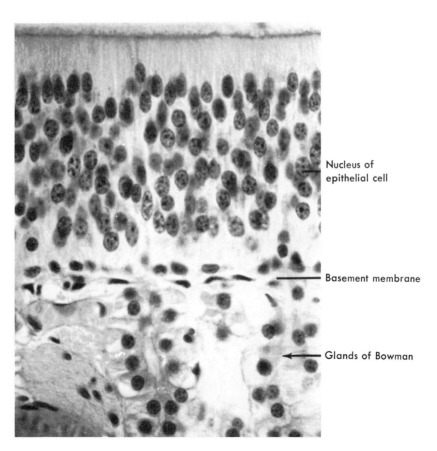

Fig. 21-23. Olfactory mucosa of fetal pig. ($\times$640.)

Nucleus of epithelial cell

Basement membrane

Glands of Bowman

der. The nuclei of the sustentacular cells are oval and lie for the most part in a zone between the surface of the epithelium and the nuclei of the olfactory cells. Some oval nuclei may be found scattered among the deeper layers.

Olfactory cells

The olfactory cells are true nerve cells, bipolar in form. Their dendrites extend to the surface of the epithelium, passing through minute openings in the cuticle and ending in a tuft of cilia. A layer of mucus secreted by Bowman's glands covers the cell surfaces and is swept along by ciliary action to permit removal of absorbed chemicals. The perikarya are small rounded elements with spherical nuclei. They form a broad band below the zone of oval nuclei called the zone of round nuclei. The cells contain abundant granular endoplasmic reticulum, many mitochondria, and an extensive Golgi apparatus. The axons of the olfactory cells pass inward through the lamina propria where they may be seen as large groups of nonmyelinated fibers. They terminate in the olfactory bulb.

Basal cells

The basal cells are thought to be reserve sustentacular cells. They are short, irregularly shaped cells, which form a layer next to the lamina propria. Like the sustentacular cells, they have oval nuclei. Their distal ends form short processes that extend among the branched ends of the sustentacular cells.

The lamina propria of the olfactory mucosa contains glands that open into the surface through wide ducts. The epithelium lining the glands (of Bowman) has the appearance of serous-secreting tissue but sometimes contains mucus.

The olfactory mucosa has a rich blood supply, the veins of which drain into the superior longitudinal sinus.

Index